Visit our website

to find out about other books from Churchill Livingstone and our sister companies in Harcourt Health Sciences

Register free at
www.harcourt-international.com

and you will get

- the latest information on new books, journals and electronic products in your chosen subject areas

- the choice of e-mail or post alerts or both, when there are any new books in your chosen areas

- news of special offers and promotions

- information about products from all Harcourt Health Sciences companies including W. B. Saunders, Churchill Livingstone, and Mosby

You will also find an easily searchable catalogue, online ordering, information on our extensive list of journals...and much more!

Visit the Harcourt Health Sciences website today!

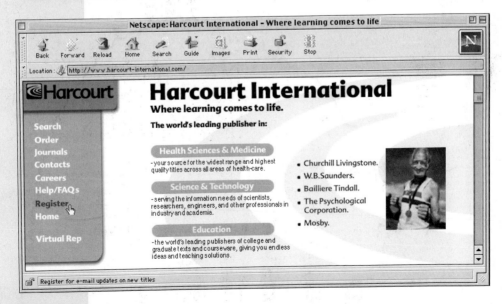

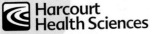

A PRACTICAL GUIDE
FOR MEDICAL TEACHERS

Commissioning Editor: Laurence Hunter
Project Development Manager: Janice Urquhart
Project Manager: Frances Affleck
Design direction: Erik Bigland
Illustrated by: MTG Design & Illustration

A PRACTICAL GUIDE FOR MEDICAL TEACHERS

Edited by

John A. Dent MMedEd MD FRCSEd

Acting Director, Clinical Skills Centre, Senior Lecturer in Orthopaedic
and Trauma Surgery, Ninewells Hospital and Medical School, University of Dundee,
Dundee, UK

Ronald M. Harden MD FRCP(Glas) FRCPC FRCSEd

Professor of Medical Education
Director, Centre for Medical Education, University of Dundee;
Teaching Dean, Faculty of Medicine, University of
Dundee, Dundee, UK;
Director, Education Development Unit,
Scottish Council for Postgraduate Medical and Dental Education

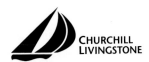
CHURCHILL
LIVINGSTONE

EDINBURGH LONDON NEW YORK PHILADELPHIA ST LOUIS SYDNEY TORONTO 2001

CHURCHILL LIVINGSTONE
An imprint of Harcourt Publishers Limited

© Harcourt Publishers Limited 2001

 is a registered trademark of Harcourt Publishers Limited

First published 2001

ISBN 0 443 06273 0

British Library Cataloguing in Publication Data
A catalogue record for this book is available from the British Library

Library of Congress Cataloging in Publication Data
A catalog record for this book is available from the Library of Congress

Note
Medical knowledge is constantly changing. As new information becomes available, changes in treatment, procedures, equipment and the use of drugs become necessary. The editors, contributors and the publishers have taken care to ensure that the information given in this text is accurate and up to date. However, readers are strongly advised to confirm that the information, especially with regard to drug usage, complies with the latest legislation and standards of practice.

The
publisher's
policy is to use
**paper manufactured
from sustainable forests**

Printed in China

PREFACE

Significant changes have recently occurred in both healthcare delivery and in the context and methods in which medicine is taught and learned. These changes have brought considerable challenges to all those involved in medical teaching. Although most clinicians in principle are enthusiastic towards clinical teaching, recent change has often required them to prioritise their clinical practice or research responsibilities and as a result time and energy for clinical teaching have been eroded. At the same time changes in the content and style of delivery of medical education have made it less possible for established clinicians to teach in the style to which they were previously accustomed. So is it possible to re-interest clinicians in medical education when they are already under pressure from other contractual obligation?

It is the purpose of this book to address this task by bridging the gap between the theoretical aspects of medical education and its attendant jargon, and the practical delivery of enthusiastic teaching. This book is an attempt to help clinicians especially, and other healthcare teachers in general, in their understanding of contemporary educational principles and to provide practical help for them in the delivery of the variety of teaching situations which characterise present day curricula.

If it is to continue to be delivered in the context of a hospital-based medical school or an expanded ambulatory care service, medical education will require the continued support of an expanded cohort of clinical teachers conversant with the ethos and techniques of modern medical education. Key concepts and appropriate tips must, therefore, be presented in a digestible form, without unnecessary jargon, in a way which indicates both their immediate relevance and practical implications. Once it has been shown that an increased knowledge about a particular educational topic can be put to practical use then clinicians' interest is engendered and further study in the field stimulated. Present observations suggest that current changes have eroded the number of clinicians willing to be involved in teaching. There is therefore no time to lose to prevent a generation of practising clinicians from missing the opportunity of making their contribution to the education of doctors for tomorrow.

Although the thrust of this book is towards undergraduate medical education, the principles described and the examples supplied are just as relevant to teaching in other healthcare professions and to postgraduate medical education. Some readers may wish to make many changes, others may wish to introduce one or two aspects, but all involved in teaching in the healthcare disciplines will benefit from this view of current developments in medical education, from practical tips and from the quotes and references which will

encourage them as practical medical teachers.

I would like to thank Gillian Dewar and Sarah Rennie for their help in the development stage of the book.

J. A. Dent
Dundee 2000

CONTENTS

CONTRIBUTORS

Raja C. Bandaranayake MBBS (Ceylon) PhD(London) MSEd(SoCal) FRACS
Chairman, Department of Anatomy, College of Medicine and Medical Sciences, Arabian Gulf University, Manama, Bahrain

Mark G. Brennan BA MA AKC DHMSA FCollP FRSH
Lecturer in Medical and Dental Education, University of Wales College of Medicine, Cardiff; Senior Lecturer in Medical Ethics, Royal College of Surgeons in Ireland, Dublin

Stuart Cable MSc BA(Hons) RGN
Researcher/Lecturer, School of Nursing and Midwifery, University of Dundee, Dundee, UK

Joy Rebecca Crosby MPhil BSc(Hons) DipMedEd DipAdEd
Lecturer in Medical Education, University of Dundee, Dundee, UK

Alan T. Davidson BSc(Hons) Ceng MICE MIStructE
Director of Quality Assurance, University of Dundee, Dundee, UK

Margery H. Davis MB ChB MRCP
Senior Lecturer in Medical Education, Centre for Medical Education, University of Dundee, Dundee, UK

John A. Dent MMedEd MD FRCSEd
Acting Director, Clinical Skills Centre, Senior Lecturer in Orthopaedic and Trauma Surgery, Ninewells Hospital and Medical School, University of Dundee, Dundee, UK

Charles D. Forbes MB ChB DSc MD FRCP
Professor of Medicine, University of Dundee, Ninewells Hospital and Medical School, Dundee, UK

Ronald M. Harden MD FRCP(Glas) FRCPC FRCS
Professor of Medical Education and Director, Centre for Medical Education, University of Dundee; Teaching Dean, Faculty of Medicine, University of Dundee, Dundee, UK

Ian R. Hart MB ChB MSc FRCPC FRCP(Glas) FACP MACP
Professor Emeritus, University of Ottowa, Canada

E. Anne Hesketh BSc(Hons) DipEd
Senior Education Development Officer, Education Development Unit (Scottish Council for Postgraduate Medical and Dental Education), University of Dundee, Dundee, UK

Jean S. Ker BSc(Hons) MB ChB DRCOG DFFP MRCGP
Lecturer in Medical Education and General Practitioner, Faculty of Medicine, Dentistry and Nursing, University of Dundee, Dundee, UK

Jennifer M. Laidlaw DipEdTech MMEd
Assistant Director, Education Development Unit (Scottish Council for Postgraduate Medical and Dental Education), University of Dundee, Dundee, UK

Iain McA Ledingham MD(Hons) FRCS(Ed) FRCP(Ed and Glas) FInstBiol FCCM FRSE
Professor of Medical Education, Faculty of Medicine, Dentistry and Nursing, University of Dundee, Dundee, UK

Grant C. Leslie BSc PhD
Senior Lecturer (Physiology), Department of Anatomy and Physiology, The University of Dundee, Dundee, UK

Sean McAleer BSc DPhil
Lecturer, Centre for Medical Education, University of Dundee, Dundee, UK

I. Chris McManus MA MD PhD FRCP
Professor of Psychology and Medical Education, University College London, London, UK

Neil K. McManus BSc(Hons)
Computer Scientist, Education Development Unit, Scottish Council for Postgraduate Medical and Dental Education, University of Dundee, Dundee, UK

Marion E. T. McMurdo MB ChB MD FRCP(Edin, Glas)
Professor of Ageing and Health, Department of Medicine, Ninewells Hospital and Medical School, Dundee, UK

David C. Old DSc PhD FIBiol FRCPath
Reader in Medical Microbiology, Infection and Immunity Group, Molecular and Cellular Pathology Department, University of Dundee Medical School, Ninewells Hospital, Dundee, UK

Sarah Rennie MB ChB BMSc(Hons)
Surgical Pre-Registration House Officer, Perth Royal Infirmary, Perth, UK

Ann Sefton AO BSc(Med) MB BS PhD DSc
Professor in Physiology, Associate Dean (Curriculum) in the Faculties of Medicine and Dentistry, University of Sydney, Australia

David Snadden MCISc MD FRCGP
Director, Postgraduate General Practice Education and Senior Lecturer, Tayside Centre for General Practice, University of Dundee, Dundee, UK

Alistair Stewart MSc PhD
Educational Consultant, Centre for Medical Education, University of Dundee, Dundee, UK

Frank Sullivan PhD FRCP FRCGP
Professor of Research and Development in Primary Care, Dundee University, Dundee, UK

Chapter 1
Teaching and learning medicine

J. A. Dent

Introduction

It is generally true that clinicians enjoy teaching students. However, the recent pace and scale of change in both medical practice and medical education have left many feeling less available or less able to enjoy teaching students than they used to. A brief reflection will quickly indicate that the context in which medicine is practised and taught today has recently changed radically and is likely to change further during the 21st century. What are the trends which have contributed to this change?

The context of change

Figure 1.1 illustrates the key areas in which fundamental changes have occurred. These interact with each other and have a direct bearing on how medicine is practised and learned. The changes include the following:

- Medical knowledge has increased exponentially.
- The role played by information technology has developed.
- The pattern of disease is different.
- The approach to health-care delivery has changed.
- Society in general has altered.
- Patients' expectations of doctors in particular have changed.
- There have been changes in professional roles and boundaries.
- The attitudes of doctors to work have changed.
- The student body in many medical schools is different from what it used to be.

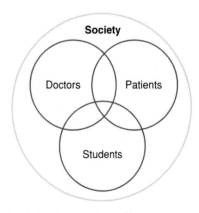

Fig. 1.1   Interaction of key areas

All these have contributed to produce a change in what is required of a doctor and therefore in the way in which medicine should be taught and learned.

Changes in medical knowledge

Traditionally the medical course was structured as a progression from the basic sciences to the medical sciences. Although this was initially acceptable, recent advances in these disciplines have greatly increased the content of the scientific aspect of the curriculum. The subsequent development of research-orientated medical schools during the last century has further contributed to the enormous increase in medical knowledge. New specialties have appeared so that the potential knowledge base of medicine has risen exponentially in the last decade. The pattern of disease seen in practice has also changed. There are fewer acute infections but an ageing population has led to an increase in problems of chronic ill health. Such changes mean that it is unreasonable to attempt to teach the entirety of medical knowledge in an undergraduate medical course. Although recent developments in medicine are usually more relevant there has been a reluctance to remove older topics from the curriculum. As a result the course becomes progressively unable to produce competent doctors.

Change in health-care delivery

The style of practice for most doctors has changed. In the community large group practices have replaced the individual, well-known family physician while in hospital shift systems have replaced the constantly available junior doctor and to some extent jeopardised the continuity of in-patient care.

An increased multiprofessional awareness has influenced the extent to which cooperation with nurses and with the other professions allied to medicine is expected so that professional isolation and stereotyping have become inappropriate in modern medical practice.

Finally there has been a shift of health-care delivery towards community settings and ambulatory care and away from the wards.

"It has been realised for many years that an undergraduate course such as this suffers from the chronic disorder 'curriculopathy'"

Guilbert 1985

Changes in patients' expectations

Recent years have seen a move away from a hierarchical to a more open society with ready media access to all aspects of medical practice and education. As a result patients are well informed about health and disease and about the choice of treatment available. They no longer wish to be the passive recipients of medical opinion but prefer to share in decision-making. They and their relatives expect courteous communication and appropriate attitudes from their medical practitioners.

Doctors can no longer, therefore, expect to practise in an authoritarian or paternalistic manner but must change the attitudes to both practice and patients which may have caricatured them in the past.

Accountability is now expected from all those perceived as being in positions of privilege or responsibility. The efficiency of a treatment must be known and its cost-effectiveness proven. Best evidence-based medicine is being adopted.

In both the undergraduate and postgraduate arenas accountability is also required by funding bodies such as the Scottish Higher Education Funding Council (SHEFC), the General Medical Council (GMC) and Specialist Advisory Committees (SACs) as well as by students and trainees.

Finally, while health promotion and disease prevention are seen as priorities in some areas of society, it is universally demanded that disease and illness are met with the most advanced methods of health care available irrespective of cost. While in many instances this is possible, society in general has become less tolerant of real or perceived deficiencies in health-care delivery and, rather than being quiescent, has become increasingly litigious.

Changes in doctors themselves

Despite endeavouring to espouse a more approachable style, individual doctors are now less likely to be readily available to patients as contemporary attitudes to work, leisure and restricted hours of duty are adopted.

When at work the pressures to deliver a clinical service and demands to provide accountable training

Both doctors and patients can experience difficulties when dealing with someone from a different ethnic group. . . . A lack of shared culture means differences in beliefs and expectations, as well as more obvious language issues. Future doctors are expected to 'be more aware and respond sensitively to the culturally determined expectations of their patients'.

Gill & Green 1996

opportunities for trainees have made it more difficult for senior staff to focus on teaching. At the same time junior doctors, now engaged in faster training programmes and with protected time for research and postgraduate education, may have fewer opportunities to prioritise undergraduate teaching and be less experienced themselves in clinical procedures.

A further change in working practice impacts on doctors today. The theoretical components of postgraduate qualifications, the Continuing Medical Education (CME) requirements of doctors in general and the possibility of periodic re-accreditation require that self-directed learning (SDL) skills be acquired early as a tool for life-long learning.

A final change in medical practice relates to professional roles and boundaries where some work traditionally done only by doctors is now taken over in certain situations by nurse practitioners, surgeon's assistants and a multiprofessional team approach to patient care.

Changes in students

It has been reported that medical courses contribute to the disillusionment and demoralisation of students by deadening their initial enthusiasm for medicine and failing to prepare them adequately for the diversity of problems with which they will be presented as professionals (Godfrey 1991). In the UK the GMC has indicated the need for a medical course which will produce doctors with appropriate attitudes to medicine and learning and will fit them for a lifetime of professional self-education (General Medical Council 1993). Courses emphasising self-directed learning, problem solving and the development of critical thought serve students better than ones which demand only spoon-feeding and factual recall.

Students' expectations of both the quality and administration of undergraduate teaching are also higher than in the past and course review and monitoring are becoming established aspects of medical schools.

"There is no denying the striking difference between the bright, interesting 18-year-olds seen at interview and the weary, disillusioned, unquestioning absorbers of information seen during the clinical years"

Fraser 1991

A further change is that students today come from a wider range of social, ethnic and financial backgrounds than previously and have attained a greater variety of personal and academic achievements. A sizeable group will be studying in a culture and language which are not their own. These students are often disadvantaged in communication and interpersonal skills and may have cultural problems with fundamental aspects of the course such as physical examination.

All these changes to the context in which medicine is being practised require corresponding changes to be made in how medicine is taught and learned.

The response to change

It is inappropriate to continue to rely on the usual time-honoured methods of teaching. A broader approach to undergraduate and postgraduate education is necessary to prepare doctors for practice in the new millennium. The innovations outlined below go some way towards meeting the challenge of change.

A new curriculum

But what should the content of a revised curriculum be? The 'core' plus 'options' approach has been formally advocated as a way of reducing curriculum overload and of introducing the possibility of choosing additional topics as self-selected special study modules (SSMs) (General Medical Council, 1993).

Innovative curricula have been described which seek to decrease the amount of factual knowledge presented and provide opportunities for choice; they also aim to include vertical and horizontal integration of the disciplines and to function in hospital and community learning environments. They seek to define learning outcomes and emphasise skills and attitudes as well as knowledge (Harden, Davis & Crosby 1997).

Medical education must respond to the context in which it operates (Towle 1998):

- Teach scientific behaviour as well as scientific facts
- Promote the use of information technology
- Adapt to the changing doctor–patient relationship
- Help future doctors to shape and adapt to change
- Promote multiprofessional teamworking and care
- Help future doctors handle broader responsibilities
- Reflect the changing pattern of disease and health-care delivery
- Involve health service employers and users.

"The first challenge, therefore, is how to create an educational system which is better able to respond to changes in the outside world than has been the case to date"

Towle 1998

New learning situations

Today fewer patients are available in hospital for clinical teaching as contemporary practice and government reforms promote day-case surgery and early discharge back to the community (Crombie 1991). A transfer of structured clinical teaching to other locations of patient care is therefore required. New learning opportunities are being developed in community contexts, ambulatory care and day surgery which illustrate that traditional professional skills can be learned in contemporary health-care situations (Murdoch Eaton & Cottrell 1998).

The emphasis on skills and attitudes in innovative curricula requires the special approach to teaching and learning to be adopted in clinical skills centres while practical courses providing on-the-job learning prepare students near the end of the medical course to become practising junior doctors.

New educational strategies

A variety of educational strategies appropriate for adult learning can be adopted in place of 'spoon-feeding'. Self-directed learning, problem-based learning (PBL), integrated learning and multiprofessional learning are examples.

Traditional methods of teaching are not necessarily suitable for dealing with an enlarging volume of material; indeed it has been shown that student learning styles deteriorate when they come into contact with the medical curriculum (Coles 1985)! Pleas for a decrease in the number of lectures are not new. Studies have shown that students place little value on lectures as a method of learning, preferring instead that teaching should become more self-directed, containing PBL and small group tutorials (Dent 1993). Some medical schools have already decided to move away from traditional teaching styles completely and adopt the PBL approach introduced by McMaster University (Spaulding 1969). Such an approach may not suit all students so some medical schools have set up PBL as an optional, parallel course which students can follow if they wish.

However, facilitating student learning may prove more difficult than traditional teaching. Questions must be asked as to what a change will entail and whether such a change will be acceptable to students and staff.

Methods of changing the style of teaching are becoming better known although not all have found general acceptance. Unfamiliarity with the techniques and mistrust of the implicit radical changes probably conspire to slow this development.

New tools and aids

Research in medical education has led to a better understanding of how students learn. Advanced approaches to education and new tools to aid learning have evolved and these will become the main themes of teaching medicine in the 21st century (CHIME 1999).

The importance of information technology as a tool for life-long learning and for accessing information has been realised (Cox, Dawson & Hobbs 1992). The role of study guides is being developed in postgraduate as well as undergraduate courses. The use of self-video in acquiring communication skills and exploring issues of attitude and behaviour is progressing.

New curriculum themes

Communication skills, attitudinal and ethical issues, preparation for practice, teamwork and the role of evidence-based practice should all find a place in a revised curriculum. All these will help new doctors in their relationships with patients and in developing a multiprofessional approach to health-care delivery in which problem-solving is the doctor's role but decision-making is a joint activity between doctor and patient (Towle 1998).

New methods of assessment

A new approach to learning requires a new approach to assessment and in this field innovative assessment instruments are appearing which can sample widely and test objectively in a diversity of competencies or outcomes. Extended matching items (EMIs) are beginning to replace shorter multiple choice questions and the objective structured clinical examination (OSCE) has found a place in a variety of qualifying examinations.

The concept of portfolio assessment has been introduced (Mathers et al 1999) and the role of formative assessment established in the development of student learning.

New Support Structures

Finally it is realised that little can be accomplished in the field of medical education without appropriate staff development and adequate support structures for students.

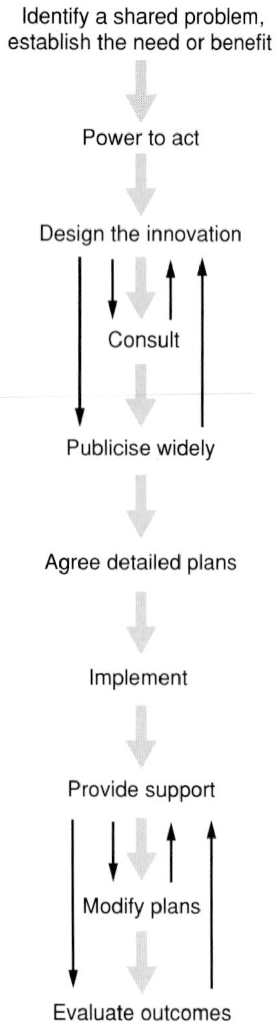

How to manage change

Medical education has responded to the change in context of medical practice with far-reaching innovations. The need for change has been largely acknowledged and potential barriers have been identified (Harden 1998). But how can these new approaches be implemented by clinicians to help them enjoy teaching students again?

Teaching is often the first casualty if there is a conflict for the lecturer's time with research or clinical work. In some cases prioritising the role of teaching may require a change in the staff structure of a medical school, but whatever is the case change is here to stay and is now an integral part of organisational life and education. 'We can look around', suggest Pritchett and Pound (1997), and see 'many would be refugees from change, people looking around from all the stress. Yet there is no place to run. No back door. No escape from reality.' 'The bottle neck to change in medical education is not lack of understanding innovative ideas, but rather a lack of understanding of the innovative process and factors which facilitate the process. A capacity to manage change is required' (Lazarus & Harden 1985).

Gale & Grant (1998) suggest that change is possible and practicable. They describe ten steps (see Fig. 1.2):

Identify a shared problem, establish the need or benefit

Power to act

Design the innovation

Consult

Publicise widely

Agree detailed plans

Implement

Provide support

Modify plans

Evaluate outcomes

Fig. 1.2   Core activity (redrawn from Gale & Grant 1998)

- Establish the need for or benefit of the change. This must be shared by all upon whom the change will have an impact.
- Look at the sources of power to act or to move the change forward and the forces which might hinder it.
- Design the innovation taking into account its feasibility, the resources needed, an appropriate timescale and those involved in the change.
- Consult widely with all those affected by the change.
- Publicise the change widely, taking feedback with a view to amending the proposal.
- Agree detailed plans to implement the change with those concerned.
- Implement the proposals using an appropriate implementation strategy.
- Provide support in dealing with difficulties and maintaining change.
- Modify the plans, redesigning the system in the light of experience.
- Evaluate the outcomes.

Any clinician involved in medical education who is about to embark on a programme of change needs an understanding of the teaching and learning process and of the range of methods and tools available. This book seeks to introduce such concepts; they might at first appear daunting but it is hoped that with increasing familiarity clinicians will become more and more at ease with them and will continue to share their experience and enthusiasm for medicine with those who will be the doctors of tomorrow.

References and further reading

CHIME 1999 21st century medicine: challenges facing medical schools and NHS trusts. http://www.chime.ucl.ac.uk/21cmed.htm

Coles C R 1985 Differences between conventional and problem-based curricula in students' approaches to studying. Medical Education 19:308–309

Cox J J, Dawson J K, Hobbs K E F 1992 The electronic information revolution and how to exploit it. British Journal of Surgery 79:1004–1010

Crombie A L 1991 The changed status of hospital and undergraduate medical education. British Journal of Hospital Medicine 45:127

Dent J A 1993 Towards the substitution of a programme of self-directed learning for a conventional lecture course. MMedEd thesis, University of Dundee

Fraser R C 1991 Undergraduate medical education: present state and future needs. British Medical Journal 303:41–43

Gale R, Grant J 1998 Manifesting change in a medical education context: guidelines for action. AMEE Medical Education Guide no. 10

General Medical Council 1993 Tomorrow's doctors. General Medical Council, London

Gill P S, Green P 1996 Learning for a multicultural society. British Journal of General Practice 46:704–705

Godfrey R 1991 All change? Lancet 338:297–299

Guilbert J J 1985 Les maladies du curriculum. Revue d'Education Médicale 4:13–16

Harden R M 1998 Change – building windmills not walls. Medical Teacher 20:189–191

Harden R M, Davis M H, Crosby J 1997 The new Dundee curriculum: a whole that is greater than the sum of the parts. Medical Education 31:264–291

Lazarus J, Harden R M 1985 The innovative process in medical education. Medical Teacher 7:333–342

Mathers N J, Challis M C, Howe A C, Field N J 1999 Portfolios in continuing medical education – effective and efficient? Medical Education 33:521–530

Murdoch Eaton D, Cottrell D 1998 Maximising the effectiveness of undergraduate teaching in the clinical setting. Archives of Diseases in Childhood 79:365–367

Okell C C 1938 Grain's and samples. Lancet i:107–108

Parsell G J, Bligh J 1995 The changing context of undergraduate medical education. Postgraduate Medical Journal 71:397–403

Pritchett and Pound 1997 The stress of organisational change. Pritchett & Associates, Tyne & Wear, UK

Spaulding W B 1969 The undergraduate medical curriculum, McMaster University. Canadian Medical Association Journal 100:639–664

Towle A 1998 Continuing medical education: changes in health care and continuing medical education for the 21st century. British Medical Journal 316:301–304

SECTION 1
CURRICULUM

Chapter 2
Planning a curriculum

R. M. Harden

Introduction

Curriculum planning and development is very much on today's agenda for undergraduate, postgraduate and continuing medical education.

The days are now past when the teacher produced a curriculum like a magician produced a rabbit out of a hat, when the lecturer taught whatever attracted his or her interest and when the students' clinical training was limited to the patients who happened to present during a clinical attachment. It is now accepted that careful planning is necessary if the programme of teaching and learning is to be successful.

What is a curriculum?

A curriculum is more than just a syllabus or a statement of content. A curriculum is about what should happen in a teaching programme – about the intention of the teachers and about the way they make this happen. This extended vision of a curriculum is illustrated in Figure 2.1.

Curriculum planning can be considered in ten steps (Harden 1986b). They have been used as headings to divide this chapter and are reviewed here in the context of the trends in medical education.

Identifying the need

The relevance or appropriateness of educational programmes has been questioned. It has been argued that there is often a mismatch between what is expected

"Curriculum is in the air. No matter what the problem in medical education, curriculum is looked to as the solution"

Davidoff 1996

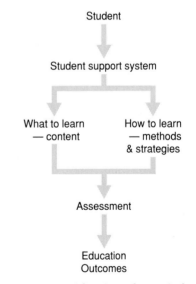

Fig. 2.1   **A wider view of a curriculum**

The ten main headings in this chapter provide a useful checklist for planning and evaluating a curriculum.

of the young doctor and the competencies gained from the training programme.

The need has been recognised to emphasise not only sickness salvaging, organic pathology and crisis care, but also health promotion and preventative medicine. Aspects of medical care which have not been adequately addressed in the past include:

- communication skills
- health promotion and disease prevention
- clinical procedures such as cardiopulmonary resuscitation
- the development of attitudes and an understanding of ethical principles.

A range of approaches can be used to identify the curriculum needs (Dunn, Hamilton & Harden 1985):

- The wisemen approach. Senior teachers and senior practitioners from different specialty backgrounds reach a consensus.
- Consultation with the stakeholders. The views of members of the public, patients, government and other professions are sought.
- A study of errors in practice. Areas are identified where the curriculum is likely to be deficient.
- Critical incident studies. Individuals are asked to describe key medical incidents in their experience which represent good or bad practice.
- Task analysis. The work undertaken by a doctor is studied.
- Study of star performers. Doctors recognised as 'star performers' are studied to identify their special qualities or competencies.

Establishing the learning outcomes

Since the work of Bloom, Mager and others in the 1960s and 1970s, the value of setting out the aims and objectives of a training programme has been accepted. In practice, lists of aims and objectives are often used only as window dressing. They are ignored in planning and

"Needs assessment is a central part of a systematic approach to developing educational projects"

Levine et al 1984

Remember that if you don't know where you are going, you can't know how to get there.

implementing the curriculum. There are a number of reasons for this:

- The list of objectives is usually extensive, time-consuming to produce and of only limited assistance in decisions about the curriculum.
- The commonly accepted classification – knowledge, skills and attitudes – does not reflect clinical practice. Most clinical competencies incorporate all three domains.

Despite these problems, the underlying principle has much to recommend it. One of the big ideas in medical education today is the move to the use of learning outcomes as a tool in curriculum planning. An outcome-based approach to education is discussed in Chapter 3.

In outcome-based education:

- The learning outcomes are defined.
- The outcomes inform decisions about the curriculum.

There is a move away from a process model of curriculum planning, where what matters is the teaching and learning experiences and methods, to a product model, where what matters is the learning outcomes and the product and where there is increasing clarity of focus for learning.

Agreeing the content

The content of a textbook is outlined in the contents pages and in the index. The content of a curriculum is found in the syllabus, in the handouts relating to the topics covered in lectures and in students' study guides. Traditionally there has been an emphasis on knowledge. Increased recognition is now being made of skills and attitudes.

The content of the curriculum can be analysed from a number of perspectives:

- subjects or disciplines (in a traditional curriculum)
- body systems, e.g. the cardiovascular system (in an integrated curriculum)
- the life cycle, e.g. childhood, adulthood, old age

If you go from this book with only one idea it should be the concept of outcome-based education.

"A move from the 'How' and 'When' to the 'What' and 'Whether'"

Spady 1994

"I've seen many schools that purport to emphasise communication skills, appropriate attitudes and health promotion In their curriculum. In looking inside these schools, however, it didn't take long to see that their business was actively teaching content in medicine, surgery and other disciplines – with the noble aims listed above receiving little direct attention"

Senior teacher

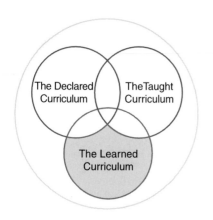

Fig. 2.2   The hidden curriculum

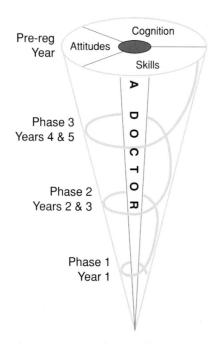

Fig. 2.3   A spiral curriculum

- problems or tasks (in a problem-based or task-based curriculum)
- learning outcomes (in an outcome-based curriculum)

Grids can be prepared which look at the content of a curriculum from two or more of these perspectives.

No account of the curriculum content would be complete without reference to the concept of the hidden curriculum. The 'declared' curriculum is the curriculum as set out in the institution's documents. The 'taught' curriculum is what happens in practice. The 'learned' curriculum is what is learned by the student. The 'hidden' curriculum is the informal learning in which students engage and which is unrelated to what is taught (see Fig. 2.2).

Organising the content

One assumption in a traditional medical curriculum is that students should first master the basic sciences of anatomy, physiology and biochemistry and then the applied sciences of pathology, microbiology and epidemiology. Once they have achieved this they move on to a study of clinical medicine. A common criticism of this approach is that students may not see the relevance of what is taught to their future career as doctors. Once they have passed the examinations in the basic sciences, students tend to forget or ignore what they have learned.

It has been advocated that the curriculum should be turned on its head, with students starting to think like a doctor from the day they enter medical school. In a vertically integrated curriculum, students are introduced to clinical medicine alongside the basic sciences in the early years of the programme. The students continue to look at the basic sciences as applied to clinical medicine in the later years.

A spiral curriculum (see Fig. 2.3) offers a useful approach to the organisation of content (Harden & Stamper 1999). In a spiral curriculum:

- There is iterative revisiting of topics throughout the course.

- Topics are revisited at numerous levels of difficulty.
- New learning is related to previous learning.
- The competence of students increases with each visit to a topic.

Deciding the educational strategy

Much discussion and controversy in medical education has related to education strategies. Should the curriculum be integrated or discipline-based? What is the role of problem-based learning? How much of the curriculum should be based in the community? The SPICES model for curriculum planning (Fig. 2.4) offers a useful tool to consider these strategies (Harden, Sowden & Dunn 1984). The model:

- represents each strategy as a continuum, thus avoiding the polarising of opinion
- acknowledges that schools vary in their approach to different strategies
- is useful in planning a new curriculum and in evaluating and changing an existing one.

Student-centred learning

In student-centred learning, what matters is what the student learns rather than what is taught. Students are given more responsibility for their own education. This is discussed further in Chapter 13.

Problem-based learning (PBL)/Task-based learning (TBL)

PBL is a seductive approach to medical education as described in chapter 14. Eleven steps can be recognised in the PBL continuum between information-orientated and task-based learning (Harden & Davis 1998).

In TBL the learning is focused round a series of tasks which the doctor may be expected to do (Harden et al 1996). Examples are the management of a patient with abdominal pain and the management of the unconscious patient. TBL is a useful approach to integration and PBL in clinical clerkships (Harden et al 2000).

Student-centred	Teacher-centred
Problem-based	Information-oriented
Integrated or inter-professional	Subject or discipline-based
Community-based	Hospital-based
Elective-driven	Uniform
Systematic	Opportunistic

Fig. 2.4   SPICES model

In planning a curriculum ask teachers to identify where they think they are at present on each continuum and where they would like to go.

"TBL offers an attractive combination of pragmatism and idealism: pragmatism in the sense that learning with an explicit sense of purpose is seen as an important source of student motivation and satisfaction; idealism in that it is consonant with current theories of education"

Harden et al 1996

"We strongly favour true integration of the course, both horizontal and vertical"

General Medical Council 1993

"The community involves a potential broadening of perspective"

Boaden & Bligh 1999

Implementing an adaptive curriculum may not be as difficult as you think.

Integration and interprofessional teaching

Integrated teaching is a feature of many curricula (General Medical Council 1993). It is discussed further in Chapter 15. Eleven steps on a continuum between discipline-based and integrated teaching have been described (Harden 2000). There is also a move to interprofessional teaching where students look at a subject from the perspective of other professions as well as their own (Harden 1998).

Community-based

There are strong educational and logistical arguments for placing less emphasis on a hospital-based programme and more emphasis on the community as a context for student learning (Boaden & Bligh 1999). Many curricula are now community-orientated with students spending 10% or more of their time in the community.

Electives

Elective programmes are now firmly established and valued by staff and students in many medical schools. They have moved from being a fringe event to an important educational activity. They can be viewed as one type of special study module (SSM) as described in Chapter 5. Electives and SSMs are designed to meet the needs of individual students.

A newer concept is the idea of the adaptive curriculum. This is an approach to curriculum planning where teaching and learning can be adjusted to the varying needs of individual students. Students spend different amounts of time studying a unit depending on their learning needs.

The features of an adaptive curriculum are:

- The learning outcomes are made explicit and the learning experiences are matched to the students' individual needs.
- Students' mastery of the core is assessed before the end of the course, and at a time when further study of the core can be arranged.

- Feedback is given to students and further studies are organised to meet the students' needs.

Systematic approach

Factors encouraging a move to a more systematic approach to medical education include:

- the increasing complexities of specialist medical practice
- the need to ensure that all students have had comparable learning experiences
- the move to outcome-based education where the learning experience and curriculum content are planned to correspond to the learning outcomes
- the concept of a core curriculum which includes the competences essential for medical practice.

A range of paper and electronic methods may be used to record encounters students have with patients. Such records are analysed to see if there are gaps or deficiencies in the students' experiences.

Deciding the teaching methods

There is no panacea, no magic answer to teaching. A good teacher is one who makes good use of a range of methods, applying each method for the use to which it is most appropriate. Later chapters of this book describe the tools available in the teacher's tool kit:

- The lecture and whole class teaching remain powerful tools if used properly. They need not be passive.
- Small group work facilitates interaction between students and makes possible cooperative learning, with students learning from each other. Small group work is usually an important part of problem-based learning.
- Independent learning can make an important contribution. Students master the area being studied, while at the same time they develop the ability to work on their own and to take responsibility for their own learning.

There is no holy grail of instructional wizardry which will provide a solution to all teaching problems. The teacher's tool kit should contain a variety of approaches, each with its strengths and weaknesses.

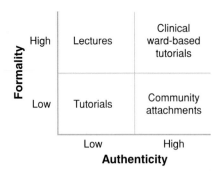

Fig. 2.5   Teaching situations

A significant development in recent years has been the application of the new learning technologies. Computers may be used as a source of information, as a medium for presentation of interactive patient simulations, and as a method of facilitating and managing learning.

Teaching and learning experiences can be rated in terms of:

- authenticity, with theoretical approaches at one end of the spectrum and real-life ones at the other
- formality, with different levels of formality and informality.

Teaching situations can be located in each quadrant of the formality/authenticity grid (see Fig. 2.5).

Preparing the assessment

Assessment is a key component of the curriculum. The significant effect that examinations have on student learning is well documented.

Issues that should be addressed in assessment include:

- What should be assessed?
  - The outcome model provides a useful framework
- How should it be assessed?
  - Which methods should be used?
  - How can one determine whether students have achieved the appropriate level of competence?
- What are the aims of the assessment process?
  - To pass or fail the student, to grade the student, to provide the student and teacher with feedback or to motivate the student?
- When should students be assessed?
  - At the beginning of the course to assess what they already know or can do, during the course or at the end of the course?
- Who should assess the student?
  - The teacher, other teachers in the same institution, teachers from other institutions, a national board or the students themselves?

These issues are addressed in more detail in later chapters.

Communication about the curriculum

Failure in communication between teacher and student is a common problem in medical education (see Fig. 2.6). Teachers have the responsibility to ensure that students have a clear understanding of:

- what they should be learning – the learning outcomes
- the range of learning experiences and opportunities available
- how and when they can access these most efficiently and effectively
- how they can match the available learning experiences to their own needs
- whether they have mastered the topic or not, and if not, what further studies and experience are required.

Communication can be improved in a number of ways:

- the provision of clear curriculum documentation with learning outcomes, timetables and annotated lists of learning resources included
- the use of study guides as a method of communication with the student
- the development of a curriculum map which identifies the areas to be studied and relates these to the courses where they are most appropriately learned.

Promoting an appropriate educational environment

The educational environment or 'climate' is a key aspect of the curriculum. It is less tangible than the content studied, the teaching methods used or the examinations. It is none the less of equal importance. There is little point in developing a curriculum whose aim is to orientate the student to medicine in the community and to health promotion, if the students perceive that what is valued by the senior teachers is hospital practice, curative medicine and research. In the same way it is difficult to develop in students a spirit of teamwork and

Failure to keep staff and students informed about the curriculum is a recipe for failure.

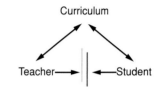

Fig. 2.6   Failure in communication

"The establishing of this climate is almost certainly the most important single task of the medical teacher"

Genn & Harden 1986

collaboration if the environment in the medical school is a competitive rather than a collaborative one.

Tools to assess this educational environment in medicine have not been readily available (Genn & Harden 1986). Recently, Roff et al (1997) have described the Dundee Ready Education Environment Measure (DREEM) which can be used for this purpose.

Managing the curriculum

Curriculum management has become more important in the context of:

- an increasing complexity of the curriculum
- integrated and interdisciplinary teaching
- increasing pressures on staff with regard to their clinical duties, teaching responsibilities and research commitments
- shortage of resources to support teaching
- rapid changes taking place in medical education and medical practice
- increasing demands for accountability.

In the context of undergraduate medical schools it is likely that:

- Responsibilities and resources for teaching will be at a faculty rather than departmental level.
- An undergraduate medical education committee will be responsible for planning and implementing the curriculum.
- A teaching dean or director of undergraduate medical education will be appointed who has a commitment to curriculum development and implementation.
- Staff will be appointed with particular expertise in curriculum planning, teaching methods and assessment to support work on the curriculum.
- Time and contributions made by staff to teaching will be recognised.
- A staff development programme will be instituted.
- An independent group will have responsibility for academic standards and quality assurance.

A number of approaches to curriculum development management can be recognised (Harden 1986a).

The style of management must be designed to suit the institution within which it has to operate.

"Medical school deans should identify and designate an interdisciplinary and interdepartmental organisation of faculty members"

American Association of Medical Colleges 1984

- The architect approach. The emphasis is on the plans with a clear statement of expected learning outcomes.
- The mechanic approach. The emphasis is on the teaching methods and educational strategies. There is more concern about how the curriculum is working rather than where it is going. The educational strategy may itself become the goal of the curriculum rather than a means to an end.
- The cookbook approach. Consideration is given to the details of the content and how much of each component or ingredient is included. The emphasis is on the individual components rather than on the overall curriculum where the whole should be greater than the sum of the parts.
- The railway timetable approach. The emphasis is on the timetable, what courses are held and when, and the duration of each course. This simplistic view of curriculum planning ignores many of the real challenges facing medical education.

A final word: don't expect to get the curriculum right first time. The curriculum will continue to evolve and will need to change in response to changes in medicine (see Chapter 1).

Summary

The development of a teaching programme can no longer be left to chance. A curriculum must be carefully planned. Ten questions have been identified which need to be addressed:

1. the need the training programme is intended to fulfil
2. the expected student learning outcomes
3. the content to be included
4. the organisation of the content including the sequence in which it is to be covered
5. the educational strategies to be adopted – integrated teaching is an example
6. the teaching methods to be used including large group teaching, small group teaching and the use of new learning technologies

For the curriculum to be successful a mixture of approaches is required, with the emphasis varying at different times in the development of the curriculum.

"A little known fact is that the Apollo moon missions were on course less than 1% of the time. The mission was composed of almost constant mid-course corrections"

Belasco 1996

7. assessment of the students' progress and of the teaching programme
8. communication about the curriculum to all the stakeholders including the students
9. the educational environment
10. management of the curriculum.

References and further reading

Association of American Medical Colleges 1984 Physicians for the 21st century: Report of the Project Panel on the General Professional Education of the Physicians and College Preparation for Medicine. Journal of Medical Education 59 Part 2:1–208

Belasco J A 1996. In Simon J, Parker R A dictionary of business quotations. Hutchinson, London

Boaden N, Bligh J 1999 Community-based medical education: towards a shared agenda for learning. Oxford University Press, New York

Davidoff F 1996 Who has seen a blood sugar? Reflections on medical education. American College of Physicians, Philadelphia, Pennsylvania, p 46

Dunn W R, Hamilton D D, Harden R M 1985 Techniques of identifying competencies needed by doctors. Medical Teacher 7(1):15–25

General Medical Council 1993 Tomorrow's doctors: recommendations on undergraduate medical education. General Medical Council, London

Genn J, Harden R M 1986 What is medical education here really like? Suggestions for action research studies of climates of medical education environments. Medical Teacher 8(2):111–124

Harden R M 1986a Approaches to curriculum planning. ASME Medical Education Booklet no. 21. Medical Education 20:458–466

Harden R M 1986b Ten questions to ask when planning a course or curriculum. Medical Education 20:356–365

Harden R M 1998 Effective multi-professional education: a three dimensional perspective. Medical Teacher 20(5):402–408

Harden R M 2000 The integration ladder: a tool for curriculum planning and evaluation. Medical Education 34:551–557

Harden R M, Crosby J R, Davis M H, Howie P W, Struthers A D 2000 Task-based learning: the answer to integration and problem-based learning in the clinical years 34:391–397

Harden R M, Davis M H 1998 The continuum of problem-based learning. Medical Teacher 20(4):301–306

Harden R M, Laidlaw J M, Ker J S, Mitchell H E 1996 AMEE Medical Education Guide no. 7 Task-based learning: an educational strategy for undergraduate, postgraduate and continuing medical education, part 1 & 2. Medical Teacher 18(1):7–13 and 18(2): 91–98

Harden R M, Sowden S, Dunn W R 1984 Some educational strategies in curriculum development: the SPICES model. Medical Education 18:284–297

Harden R M, Stamper N 1999 What is a spiral curriculum? Medical Teacher 21(2):141–143

Levine H G, Cordes D L, Moore Jr D E, Rennington F C 1984 In: Green J S, Grosswald S J, Suter E, Walthall D B (eds) Continuing education for the health professions. Jossey Bass, San Francisco

Roff S, McAleer S, Warden R M, Al Qahtani M et al 1997 Development and validation of the Dundee Ready Education Environment Measure (DREEM). Medical Teacher 19(4):295–299

Spady W. G 1994 Outcome-based education: critical issues and answers. American Association of Schools Administrators, Arlington, Virginia

Chapter 3
Curriculum goals

J. R. Crosby

Introduction

Although the goals of a medical school curriculum may be complex they will probably seek to:

- produce future doctors
- utilise modern educational methods
- comply with governing body regulations: for example, in the UK the General Medical Council (GMC)
- ensure that a number of students pass the course
- meet consumer expectations.

Whilst all goals are important this chapter will focus on the curriculum goal of producing future doctors. All curricula, whether by design or not, produce doctors, although the nature of the (doctor) product may be unspecified (Harden et al 1999). The type of doctor a school wishes to produce may vary. This variety may be due to differences in health-care provision, resources available or other expectations (goals) of the schools. The type of training required for a doctor practising in the African heartland might be different from that of a doctor working in a westernised inner-city laboratory.

A medical school should be explicit in stating its goals. Does the school wish to produce students able to progress into hospital practice, general practice, laboratory-based work or research-based activities, or a combination of all four? In stating these goals other parameters should also be considered. What competencies will the doctor possess? What basic skills, including personal transferable and

"A goal is 'the end towards which effort is directed' "

Webster's Dictionary

communication skills, are required? Do students need to be competent in research? Do they need to be orientated to health care in the community as well as the hospital?

A curriculum may define its product specifically by adopting outcome-based education.

What is outcome-based education?

Outcome-based education has developed from a fundamental rethinking of the structure and function of education (McNeir 1993). Although a simple agreed definition of outcome-based education does not exist, Cohen (1994) stated simply that in outcome-based education 'product defines the process'. In traditional medical education students are exposed to a specific segment of the curriculum. The student is then assessed regarding the specific segment of the curriculum learnt. Students then progress to the next segment of the curriculum. In contrast to this input–output model of education, outcome-based education specifies the outcomes students should be able to demonstrate upon leaving the system (McNeir 1993). Outcomes relate to the question 'what is a graduate?' and emphasise what a learner knows and can do as a result of learning. They are concerned with what a student achieves as opposed to what the teacher intends to teach. In this way outcome-based education is linked to mastery learning. However, the goal of outcome-based education is not only mastery of specific tasks but also the application of information and the attainment of greater independence in learning (Fitzpatrick 1991).

There are four main characteristics of outcome-based education (Terry 1996):

- Outcomes are clearly identified.
- Achievement determines progress.
- Multiple instructional strategies and authentic assessment tools are used.
- Students are given time and assistance to reach their potential.

"An outcome is 'something that follows as a result or consequence' "

Webster's Dictionary

Outcomes do not preclude or minimise the importance of knowledge but rather determine the relevance of the information. This relevance can be seen as the major difference between outcomes and objectives. Objectives are frequently statements with no reference to their ultimate end-point. For example, Mager stated that objectives have four key components.

- the act: e.g. to list
- the content: the anatomical pathway of the respiratory system
- the condition: from the palate to the alveoli
- the criteria: as stated in *Gray's Anatomy*.

The degree of specification of objectives has frequently prompted surface learning with students having little understanding of why they have to learn the material, other than to pass the examination.

Outcomes allow both a broad perspective of what is to be achieved by the students as well as the specifics. For example:

- Exit outcome: To diagnose and manage patients with asthma.
- Intermediate outcome: Take a respiratory history of a patient. Perform a general inspection of chest and respiratory system.
- Introductory outcome: Describe airway physiology, in a written form, including reference to relevant anatomy of the respiratory system.

The introductory level outcomes may involve the statement of traditional-type objectives.

The advantages of outcome-based education
Harden et al (1999) stated 12 reasons for adopting outcome-based education:

1. relevance
2. controversy
3. acceptability
4. clarity
5. provision of framework
6. accountability

"The knowledge which a man can use is the only real knowledge, the only knowledge which has life and growth in it and converts itself into practical power. The rest hangs like dust about the brain or dries like rain off stones"

Froude 1818–94

Consider what kind of doctor you would like to treat you.

7. self-directed learning
8. flexibility
9. assessment
10. participation
11. evaluation
12. continuity of education.

Specifying outcomes

Developing outcomes

Who should be responsible for specifying outcomes? University staff may take a lead role in specifying the outcomes. However, the opinion of a variety of different groups should be sought and these should include patients, community health groups, recent graduates, current students, doctors in the hospital and community, representatives of employers and other health-care professionals. Support from all of these is required to ensure that the outcomes generated are appropriate. Consultation will also maximise the adoption of outcome-based education and will ensure that it is agreed and understood by the organisers and teachers who will deliver it.

The methods these groups use to generate the outcomes can be based on the techniques used to determine educational need. A variety of methods can be adopted. Diversity of approach is recommended rather than one single form.

Different groups may be used in different ways. Some groups may be asked to generate outcomes whereas other groups may be asked to critique and refine work already conducted.

Stating outcomes

Several stages have been identified in specifying outcomes. The first step is to determine the outcomes expected at graduation, exit outcomes (Spady 1994). Outcomes should be stated in broad terms then developed into more specific terms. This is known as the design down process.

The exit outcome can be considered as the first level of outcome specification:

"An ongoing system . . . that includes staff accountability, effective leadership and staff collaboration"

Spady 1988

Design down:

- Exit outcomes
- Phase outcomes
- Course/attachment outcomes
- Lesson outcomes

- *Level 1*
  - — A graduate should demonstrate appropriate attitudes, ethics and understanding of legal responsibilities.

This may be further specified:
- *Level 2*
  - — Demonstrate an ethical and moral approach.
  - — Display appropriate attitudes and behaviour.
  - — Recognise and respond to legal responsibilities.
  - — Be aware of human rights issues.

Each of these may then be further specified e.g. under 'Display appropriate attitudes and behaviour':
- *Level 3*
  - — Behave in ways that demonstrate confidentiality, integrity, truthfulness and respect towards patients and colleagues.
  - — Deal compassionately and sensitively with dying patients and their relatives.
  - — Listen dispassionately to complaints made about performance, seek expert independent advice, and respond constructively and promptly (Preece 1999).

This activity may determine that the teaching programme and assessment currently designed and implemented is allowing the student to meet and be assessed in the outcome. However, the process may highlight areas of neglect. Ethics, personal development, transferable skills and so on may not feature as prominently as expected or may not be adequately assessed. If a series of outcomes are felt to be of importance there is then an obligation to ensure changes in the curriculum to facilitate learning of these outcomes.

Specifying stage of attainment

Although exit outcomes are the first key step in outcome-based education it is impractical to think that students could learn or be assessed on all aspects of a 5-year course at the end of that period. Although exit outcomes are emphasised they may be sequenced over time. A design down process is adopted whereby the outcomes are mapped to different areas of a programme.

"A tightly articulated framework of program, course unit outcomes that derive from the exit outcomes"

Spady 1994

- *"Identify exit outcomes*
- *Allocate exit outcomes to programs*
- *Identify program outcomes*
- *Identify course outcomes*
- *Identify unit outcomes*
- *Identify lesson outcomes"*

Glatthorn 1993

For example, young doctors after several years of postgraduate training may be expected to carry out a lumbar puncture for therapeutic purposes unsupervised. On qualification at the end of a 5-year undergraduate programme they may be expected to take a lumbar puncture for diagnostic purposes unsupervised. After 3 years they may be expected to have an understanding of the technique and indications for its use. After the first year they should have an awareness of the technique and of the relevant anatomy and physiology.

In order to specify to staff and students the level of each outcome a scale of achievement is required. Fitzpatrick (1991) developed a three-point scale for school attainment:

- developing a knowledge base
- demonstrating practical application
- transferring learning to new situations.

These stages reflect not only how the programme develops but also the level of student achievement and the change in the teacher's role. This simple scale of attainment may be applicable in the medical environment, especially in the later clinical phases when students may be presented with clinical dilemmas and decisions not previously encountered.

In the medical arena potential scales have already been developed. Many medical schools will have determined the practical procedures they expect students to be able to undertake and the level of competence expected. The Core Clinical Competencies Medicine Project (1999) documented how medical schools in the UK graded the stage of achievement for practical skills:

1. The students have been **exposed** to the skill and understand the basic sciences associated with the skill but may not have attempted it for themselves. *They may have read about the skill or seen it performed.*
2. The students have been **involved** and may have **assisted** with the skill. *They have been taught through active demonstration, interactive, video, computer-assisted learning programme and so on.*

 Try not to reinvent the wheel.

3. The students have **attempted** the skill for themselves. *They have performed the skill on a model (supervised or unsupervised) or on a patient with supervision.*
4. The students are **competent** to perform the skill. *They are able to perform the skill without supervision.*
5. The students are **proficient**. *They can perform the skill routinely without supervision and may be able to teach the skill or explain it to other learners.*

Once the outcomes have been specified and an explicit statement made of the level of competence required at different stages of the course, the coverage in the curriculum can be programmed.

Implementing outcomes

Moving from idealism to realism
Seldom does a medical school have the luxury of designing a new curriculum on a blank canvas. The introduction of outcome-based education has to be sensitive to curriculum design and resources already in place. The implementation of outcome-based education can be considered in two different settings:

- a totally new curriculum with no historical background
- adaptation of established curriculum.

Most undergraduate courses are not new. The palette to which outcome-based education is added has already had many colourful predecessors. In adopting outcome-based education it is important to recognise the form to be adopted. Spady and Marshall (1991) suggest that there are three forms of outcome-based education: traditional, transitional and transformational.

Traditional model
The basic tenet of the traditional form is that curriculum design has come before development of the outcomes. This may occur for the majority of curricula for which outcome-based restructuring is being considered. Programme constraints will dictate the degree of adoption of the outcome-based philosophy (Terry 1996).

Spady and Marshall (1991) considered that the danger of the traditional approach is that the demonstration of outcomes is often limited because instruction is restricted to a particular unit that is an end in itself. There is also a danger that the original curriculum is still present with only selective elements being taught with more clarity.

Although Shanks (1992) suggests that there are weaknesses in adopting this approach, Spady and Marshall still consider that a traditional model may be effective in improving student achievement.

Transitional model

A transitional approach is a pragmatic model for established curricula that wish to move towards outcome-based education. This is an intermediate stage between the traditional and transformational models. Only a partial shift to outcome-based education is observed.

Transformational model

A transformational model where the curriculum is totally based on the attainment of outcomes can seldom be achieved in an established curriculum model. The transformational model is usually observed after a lengthy period of time or in schools where the curriculum has not been previously established.

The degree of adoption of outcome-based education may be dependent on the size of curriculum development and commitment of personnel. The exit, phase, year and course outcomes have to be matched to learning opportunities in the curriculum for the outcome to be achieved. This may result in a little change in the learning programme; alternatively it may require a larger change.

Displaying the outcomes

Spady (1988) suggested that one of the key elements of outcome-based education is the public nature of the outcomes. The statement of outcomes must be obvious not only to staff and students but also to managers,

"Clearly defined, publicly derived exit outcomes that students must demonstrate when leaving the school"

Spady 1994

administrators, governing bodies, consumer groups and associated professionals.

The statement of outcomes should not be restricted to a simple list of the expected exit outcomes but should also show how these are to be achieved (see Fig. 3.1).

One of the best ways of displaying the elements of the outcome-based model is through a curriculum map. A curriculum map may be analogous to a road map with a statement of destinations (exit outcomes), possible means of transport (learning opportunities, i.e lectures, ward work and so on), the company offering the transport (course organiser and teachers), schedule of times of transport (educational timetable), means of knowing arrival at destination, e.g landmarks (feedback on attainment of outcomes). Medical schools may decide on similar exit outcomes (destinations) but the method and means of arriving at that outcome may vary depending on local resources and educational philosophy.

The curriculum map should encompass all the elements identified by Spady (1994):

- exit outcomes
  — clear statement of exit outcomes
  — progression of learning towards exit outcomes
- curriculum content and structure
  — courses/modules
  — timetable
  — contribution by departments
- instructional delivery
  — types of learning opportunity
  — teachers who may deliver teaching
- student assessment
  — stages of assessment and how they relate to the outcomes
- student placement and advancement
  — feedback on progression to exit outcomes.

The development of an outcome-based curriculum has the advantage of:

- making explicit the outcome expected (Ross & Davies 1999) and thus increasing transparency and accountability

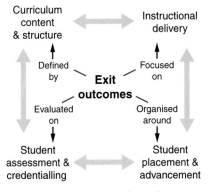

Fig. 3.1   The outcome based education model (after Spady 1988)

Consider computer packages as a method for displaying outcomes.

- transparency, allowing the identification and potential resolution of the differences between the curriculum planned, implemented and experienced (Lowry 1993)
- facilitating integration of previous discipline-based departments; exit outcomes by their inclusive nature encourage horizontal and vertical integration of courses
- facilitating greater student autonomy; the statement of exit outcomes and progression to the exit outcome may increase an awareness of the rationale for learning
- encouraging curriculum development and refinement to reflect the evolving nature of health care.

Due to the potential complexity of the curriculum map the use of an electronic system is advised (Ross & Davies 1999).

Performance assessment and outcome based-education are closely related paradigms (Friedman Ben-David 1999). In order that outcomes are adequately assessed the methods used should match the learning method. For some practical outcomes, objective observational scales may be used: for example, assessing communication skills and practical procedures using the Objective Structured Clinical Examination. Knowledge outcomes may be more appropriately measured by paper-based examinations. Some broad-based outcomes may be best assessed through continuous monitoring of performance and may utilise portfolio-based assessment methods. Outcome-based educational programmes that require both learning and performance to be considered may require the development of new assessment methods (Friedman Ben-David 1999).

A key component of outcome-based education requires giving students more time, if required, to master material (Spady 1994). Careful planning of both course and assessment is needed in order to fulfil this requirement.

Current examples of health care learning outcomes

Governing bodies, consumer groups and medical schools are beginning to endorse the importance of stating expected outcomes of students. The following are some examples of broad exit outcomes which have already been generated.

World Health Organization (WHO)

WHO made a simple resolution (WHA48.8) regarding the key outcomes expected of a doctor:

- care-provider
- decision-maker
- communicator
- community leader
- manager.

Dundee Medical School (Scotland, UK)

Twelve outcomes have been generated and categorised under three headings (Harden et al 1999):

- Outcomes related to the performance of tasks expected of a doctor
    — application of the clinical skills of history-taking and physical examination
    — undertaking practical procedures
    — investigation of patient
    — management of patient
    — health promotion and disease prevention
    — communication with patients, relatives and other health-care team members
    — application of appropriate information retrieval and handling skills
- outcomes related to the approach adopted by the doctor in performance of the tasks
    — application of an understanding of basic and clinical science as a basis of medical practice
    — incorporation of attitudes, ethical stance and an understanding of legal responsibilities
    — use of critical thinking, problem-solving and decision-making skills, clinical reasoning and judgement
- outcomes related to professionalism
    — an acceptable level of professionalism and understanding of the role of the doctor
    — an aptitude for personal development.

Brown University (USA)

Brown University has developed nine outcomes that encapsulate the desirable qualities of a medical school graduate:

- effective communication
- basic clinical skills
- using basic science in the practice of medicine
- diagnosis, management and prevention
- life-long learning
- self-awareness, self-care and personal growth
- social and community contexts of health care
- moral reasoning and clinical ethics
- problem-solving.

American Association of Medical Colleges (AAMC)

The AAMC stated the following outcomes. Physicians must be:

- altruistic
- knowledgeable
- skillful
- dutiful.

Training of doctors in the Netherlands

A blueprint detailing the objectives of undergraduate medical education in the Netherlands was devised (Metz et al 1994). Although the term outcomes was not used the general objectives stated covered four broad outcome areas:

- medical aspects
  — humans in somatic, mental and social respects
  — problem recognition and description
  — history
  — physical examination
  — process of medical problem-solving
  — additional investigations
  — management
  — attending
  — reporting and making records
  — prevention

- scientific aspects
  - principles
  - meaning of scientific approach
  - advancement and maintenance of professional competence
- personal aspects
  - doctor–patient relationship
  - functioning as a doctor
  - balance between work and private life
- aspects related to society and the health-care system
  - functioning of health care
  - medical ethics
  - legal regulations
  - financial aspects.

Summary

The setting of explicit outcomes for students is a current trend observed in medical schools. In recent years British medical schools have concentrated on the educational delivery of undergraduate programmes: for example, whether to adopt problem-based learning or more traditional methods of teaching.

Outcome-based education aims to consider what skills, knowledge and attitudes are desired of a student or junior doctor. The statement of explicit outcomes not only has the advantage of making the curriculum clear to students but also provides an opportunity of ensuring greater continuity.

When outcome-based education is adopted, the outcomes require to be formulated and specified. Differing levels of outcome specification will be found, from a broad to a specific perspective. The use of a curriculum which is analogous to a road map is recommended as a method for displaying outcomes.

References and further reading

Association of American Medical Colleges 1998 Report 1 Learning objectives for medical student education guidelines for medical school. Association of American Colleges, Washington

Brown University 1997 An educational blue-print for the Brown University School of Medicine: competency-based curriculum, 3rd edn. Brown University School of Medicine

Cohen A M 1994 Relating curriculum and transfer. New directions for community colleges, no. 86 22(2)

Core Clinical Competencies Medicine Project 1999 Department of Education and Employment. ISBN 0853161887

Dunn W R, Hamilton D D, Harden R M 1985 Techniques for identifying competencies needed of doctors. Medical Teacher 7:15–25

Fitzpatrick K A 1991 Restructuring to achieve outcomes of significance for all students. Educational Leadership 48(8):18–22

Friedman Ben-David M 1999 Assessment in outcome-based education. Part 3, AMEE no. 14 Outcome-based Education, pp 26–30

Glatthorn A A 1993 Perspectives and imperatives Outcome based education: reform and curriculum process. Journal of Curriculum and Supervision 8(4):354–363

Harden R M, Crosby J R, Davis M H 1999 An introduction to outcome-based education. Part 1, AMEE no. 14 Outcome-based Education, pp 7–16

Lowry S 1993 Medical education. BMJ Publishing Group, London

McNeir G 1993 Outcome-based education, tool for restructuring. Oregon School Study Council Bulletin, Eugene, 36(8)

Mager R 1962 Preparing instructional objectives, 2nd edn. David Lake, Belmont, CA

Metz J C M, Stoelinga G B A, Pels Rijcken E H, van der Brand B W M 1994 Blueprint 1994: training of doctors in the Netherlands. University of Nijmegen, ISBN 90 373 0261 0

Preece P 1999 Outcome-based education. Unpublished material. University of Dundee

Ross N, Davies D 1999 Outcome-based learning and the electronic curriculum at Birmingham Medical School. Part 4, AMEE no. 14 Outcome-based Education, pp 30–36

Shanks J 1992 Unintended outcomes: curriculum and outcome based education. Paper presented at the annual meeting of the American Research Association

Spady W G 1988 Organising for results: the basis of authentic restructuring and reform. Educational Leadership 46(2):4–8

Spady W G 1994 Outcome-based education: critical issues and answers. American Association of School Administrators. ISBN 0 87652 183 9

Spady W G, Marshall K J 1991 Transformational outcome-based educational curriculum restructuring. Educational Researcher 6:9–15

Terry P M 1996 Outcome-based education: is it mastery learning all over again, or is it revolution to the reform movement? Paper presented at the 7th Annual Midwest Education Society (CIES) Conference, Indiana

Chapter 4
The core curriculum

R. M. Harden

Introduction

A powerful new idea in medical education is the concept of a core curriculum with special study modules. This is a key recommendation of the General Medical Council in their 1993 report to UK medical schools, 'Tomorrow's doctors'. The aim is to tackle the most important challenge facing medical educators today – the problem of information overload.

The amount of information available to the health-care professions is expanding at an alarming rate. In addition to an average of four new journals published every day, we have the rapid development of the Internet and other electronic sources. It has been estimated that information in the biosciences is doubling every 20 months. If this is true, by the end of a doctor's career there will be a million times more information available than when he or she qualified – a sobering thought.

Even if this is a gross overestimate the implications are still significant:

- Teachers and trainers must recognise that students cannot learn everything. More has to be covered in the time available and no longer will it be possible to cover all of the curriculum content in the same depth. Teachers need to spell out more clearly than they have in the past what is expected of the student – the learning outcomes (see Chapter 3).
- The emphasis in the core curriculum will be on clearly defined breadth rather than on depth. Learning outcomes should reflect the core competencies expected of the student or trainee and should be

"The most striking feature of the new proposals is the introduction of the concept of 'core and options'"

Lowry 1992

"Until an attempt is made to circumscribe the requirements of the course in respect of factual quantum, the unconfined overload of the curriculum will prevail and will continue to deny students the educational opportunities to which they are entitled"

General Medical Council 1993

"We move towards a curriculum that is no longer all embracing, but containing a core which is more rigorously defined than has been customary"

General Medical Council 1993

Combining a core programme with options or electives is useful in planning a curriculum.

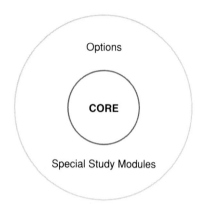

Fig. 4.1   Areas of study

These ideas can help you to liberate your curriculum from its present factual overload.

agreed by all stakeholders. Students should also have the opportunity to study some areas in more depth through electives, options or special study modules (see Chapter 5 and Fig. 4.1).

- Teachers should help students to improve the efficiency of their learning through:
  — study skills courses (see Chapter 37)
  — the use of study guides (see Chapter 18)
  — clearly stated and presented learning outcomes (see Chapter 3)
  — a more systematic structured curriculum (see Chapter 2)
  — appropriate training in information technology (see Chapter 25).
- Students and trainees need to continue their learning after they have completed their basic training. They should acquire the skills and motivation to do so.
- Teachers should remain vigilant that the curriculum does not become overloaded, and that there is enough space and time for students to meet higher-level objectives, and to reflect on and think about what they are studying. There is a tendency for overload to occur insidiously; every 3 years or so the load factor in the curriculum needs to be reassessed.

In this chapter we explore how a core curriculum is the answer to the problem of information overload, and discuss:

- what a core curriculum is
- the concepts behind a core curriculum
- the development of a core curriculum
- special study modules (SSMs) or options and the relation between them and the core
- myths of the core curriculum
- assessment and the core.

What is a core curriculum?

The core curriculum is that part of the total field of areas covered in the curriculum which all students should study and master. The core has been defined in terms of:

- Essential or key aspects of a subject or discipline. For some subjects such as internal medicine or general surgery the core may be fairly extensive.
- Key or essential disciplines. All disciplines, however, are likely to be included in the core.

For some specialties, the core learning outcomes will be more limited but still important.

- The curriculum necessary to achieve the learning outcomes required for competence for practice. For example, core clinical skills can be identified which all doctors should have, e.g. measurement of blood pressure, cardiopulmonary resuscitation, management of a patient with abdominal pain.

  The features of a core curriculum are that:

- It is common to all students, as distinct from topics in the self-selected part of the curriculum which students may or may not choose to study.
- It covers competencies essential for the practice of medicine which, if lacking in a doctor, result in him or her being incompetent.
- It requires a high standard of mastery before satisfactory completion of training.
- It covers skills and attitudes as well as knowledge.
- It provides a foundation for study in subsequent stages of the curriculum or phases of education.

The concepts behind a core curriculum

A number of concepts underpin the idea of the core curriculum – the 'seven Cs' (Harden & Davis 1995):

- certification/credibility
- capability/competence
- comprehensiveness/communication
- consistency
- constructivism/continuum
- choice/career
- compacted curriculum.

"Mastery of the core curriculum should allow the student to prescribe current drugs in a way that maximises the chances of efficacy while minimising the chances of causing harm"

Nierenberg 1990

The core can be thought of as the breadth of the curriculum.

"... core curriculum as a prerequisite for excellence and fairness in education"

Hirsch 1993

Certification/credibility

The core curriculum is a public statement of what is expected of students if they are to complete their training satisfactorily. This is consistent with the idea of mastery learning. The concept of a core curriculum reflects the trend towards greater accountability for educational institutions. The curriculum has to be credible in the eyes of the stakeholders including the consumers.

Capability/competence

Higher education has been criticised as being too theoretical, with graduates on qualification lacking the skills necessary to practise in their profession. The 'education for capability' movement focuses on the need to include in the curriculum those studies relevant to the competencies required by graduates when they take up a post in their profession. These competencies are addressed in a core curriculum.

Comprehensiveness/communication

Implicit in the concept of a core curriculum is that all essential aspects of the subject will be mastered. This notion of comprehensiveness has been the driving force for the specification of a core curriculum in a range of areas such as cancer medicine, neurology and clinical skills.

The core curriculum communicates those aspects of the subject that should be mastered by the student. All students work to achieve the same curriculum objectives but they take different amounts of time to do so.

Consistency

Another dimension of certification and standards reflected in the core curriculum is the concept of consistency or uniformity.

A concern in medical education is that students, particularly in the later years of their undergraduate programme and in their postgraduate training, have widely varying experiences. It has been demonstrated that in hospital practice and in the community, this cannot be left to chance.

Appropriate experiences may not just happen – they have to be planned. The core curriculum includes the experiences which should be common to all students.

Consistency is important at the level of the individual school or training institution. It may also be relevant at a national or international level – the concept of a global core curriculum.

Constructivism/continuum of education

The core curriculum is the important starting-off point for the wider exploration of a topic in the later phases of the curriculum. In the constructivist psychology of learning, the student builds new knowledge on existing knowledge (Hirsch 1993). New knowledge is acquired just as a tree acquires new leaves. A weak and poorly growing tree will not easily continue to generate new leaves.

This constructivist approach is key to the continuum of learning. The core learned as an undergraduate student constitutes the building blocks for postgraduate education and for later life-long learning.

Choice/career

A concern sometimes expressed about a core curriculum is that it removes the element of student choice. This would be true if the curriculum comprised only the core. As the term implies, there are areas to be studied beyond this core. These options were referred to by the General Medical Council as 'special study modules'. The GMC recommended that the curriculum should spell out the core unambiguously and restrict study of it to two-thirds of the total curriculum time available. This makes it possible for students to study areas of particular interest to them in the remaining third. Experience has shown that this is a very real advantage to the core and SSM model. All students master the same core but choose for SSMs those fields of medical practice where they wish to gain

"The strategy which elicited the widest discussion at the August 1993 World Summit on Medical Education was the development of a global core curriculum, flexible and adaptable to change and allowing a large and open menu of options"

Warren 1993

"Core knowledge increased the students' ability to question"

Hirsch 1993

"Curriculum compacting is a flexible, research-supported instructional technique that enables high-ability students to skip work they already know and substitute more challenging content"

Reis & Renzulli 1992

The core in an area should not be defined exclusively by the department concerned.

further experience, perhaps with a view to a career choice.

Compacted curriculum

Another concept relevant to the core curriculum is that of the compacted curriculum. The identification of the core competencies to be mastered makes it possible to look seriously at whether some students can complete their studies in a shorter period of time if the elements are compacted. Students with appropriate previous experience may be able to master the core in less time or may need to complete fewer SSMs to reach the same level of competence.

The development of a core curriculum

The reasons for defining a core curriculum and the underlying educational philosophy underpinning it are clear. The actual task of specifying the core, however, is not an easy one. Teachers need sufficient motivation and the necessary time and effort to commit to the task. A range of approaches are available and these have been summarised in Chapter 2.

Here are some hints which may help:

- Don't reinvent the wheel. Look at what other teachers have done and build on or adopt this. Many examples of core curricula are now available.
- Work as a team. Involve staff with a particular interest in the subject or topic and individuals from a different background but with an interest in curriculum development. Staff with an interest in primary care should be included as well as staff with a hospital base.
- Use a variety of approaches or techniques when setting about the task. Different approaches bring their own perspective.
- Involve students in the process. Students can play an important role in curriculum planning.

- Identify or recruit staff who have experience of curriculum planning, who will give the necessary educational support and will facilitate the completion of the work.
- Use an outcome-based model. This will make the identification of the core curriculum easier. It should be relatively easy to get agreement on learning outcomes at a general level. Further details can then be added.

Factors to be considered when you determine the core include:

- the importance of the topic to the tasks undertaken by a doctor
- the commonness of the problem
- the extent to which one can generalise from the subject to other topics in medicine.

Special study modules (SSMs) or options

SSMs or options provide students with the opportunity to study an area in depth. They allow teachers to indulge themselves in interacting with students in their area of research, knowing that the students are covering the breadth of medicine elsewhere in the curriculum.

The content area studied in an SSM is optional. It should be noted, however, that an SSM or elective can contribute to the achievement of the core learning outcomes (see Fig. 4.2).

Examples of core learning outcomes addressed in SSMs or electives are:

- use of information technology (in a search for data)
- development of communication skills (in the presentation and report of work completed)
- teamworking (in collaborative working on a project).

A balance should be achieved in determining the core. Emphasise priority areas, but do not ignore other areas which may currently be neglected.

"The greatest educational opportunities will be afforded by that part of the course which goes beyond the limits of the core, that allows students to study in depth the areas of particular interest to them, that provides them with insights into scientific method and the discipline of research and that engenders an approach to medicine that is constantly questioning and self-critical. This part of the course we refer to in terms of 'special study modules'"

General Medical Council 1993

Aspect of Curriculum	Component of curriculum	
	Core curriculum	SSM or elective
Content	Core	Optional
Learning Outcomes	Core	Core and optional

Fig. 4.2 Contribution of SSM to learning outcomes

Take care to protect time allocated in the curriculum for special study modules.

Relationship between core and SSM

SSMs can be related to the core curriculum in four ways (Harden & Davis 1995).

Integrated
The SSMs are integrated into core course modules. Each module has elements which are core and others which are optional. In the options, students choose to look at the core from different perspectives.

Concurrent
SSMs run concurrently with the core, e.g. one day or afternoon per week. These are independent and are not related to the core.

Intermittent
Blocks of time, usually of several weeks' or months' duration, are scheduled for SSMs. This work is unrelated to students' study of the core.

Sequential
Each block of core is followed by an SSM. Students choose to study the core in more depth or to study subjects unrelated to the core. They may be directed to further study of the core if they have not yet reached the required mastery of the core.

Myths of the core curriculum with SSMs

The concept of a core curriculum with SSMs is often misunderstood. There may be unnecessary concern about this approach to curriculum planning. Some of the common myths are described below.

Myth 1 A core curriculum will trivialise medical education.
NO Mastery of the core across the breadth of medicine is a significant task. At the same time, students develop an in-depth understanding in selected areas.

It is important that all concerned with the planning and implementation of a core curriculum and SSMs are fully informed about the concept and its advantages. Allow time to confront any misunderstandings and objections.

Myth 2   The core curriculum is about amassing factual knowledge.

NO   Essential knowledge is part of the core curriculum. Students must develop an understanding and be able to apply this knowledge in practice. Mastery of the core also entails a wider vision of competence which includes key skills and attitudes.

Myth 3   The options or SSMs are relatively unimportant components of the curriculum and need not be taken seriously by the student.

NO   Students through their in-depth studies in SSMs acquire essential core competencies. Some of these are listed above. SSMs can be rigorous and demanding and this can be reflected in their assessment.

Myth 4   The core curriculum is about the major specialties in medicine and ignores the minor specialties. It is restrictive and represents an unacceptable narrowing of the curriculum.

NO   All specialties can be included in a core curriculum. The question is to what depth study is appropriate at a particular stage of students' training. Students may learn, for example, about the role of plastic surgery and when patients should be referred but not the operative details. Disciplines can contribute to the core curriculum in many ways. Plastic surgeons may contribute, for example, to the theme of wound management, and urologists to the theme of impotence.

Myth 5   Standards will fall with less expected of the students.

NO   High standards in the core areas of the course will be required of all students. No student will be able to move on to the next phase of the course without mastery of the core. Appropriate standards should also be set for the SSM part of the course.

"Attitudes of mind and of behaviour that befit a doctor should be inculcated and should imbue the new graduate with attributes appropriate to his/her future responsibilities to patients, colleagues and society in general"

General Medical Council 1993

"Those who think of core knowledge as 'rote learning of isolated facts' are simply misinformed or have too little faith in teachers"

Frazee 1993

"The core must be tested rigorously, in the interests of the public and of the integrity of professional standards"

General Medical Council 1993

"To hold that disagreements are so fundamental that any core selected is bound to be arbitrary is a recipe for inertia or anarchy."

Kirk 1986

Myth 6   The concept of core curriculum and options is applicable only to the undergraduate curriculum.
NO   Most of what has been written about core and options has been about undergraduate education but the concept is equally applicable in postgraduate or continuing medical education.

Myth 7   It is not possible to get agreement on what contributes to the core.
NO   Significant progress has been made in the definition of core in a wide range of topics in medicine. If, after due discussion, there is no agreement about an area, it is likely that it is not core.

Myth 8   The core curriculum is drab and uniform and threatens the richness and diversity of a curriculum in medicine.
NO   The core need not be dull or boring. The only limit to excitement and stimulation is the imagination of the course developer and presenter. The SSMs add an additional sparkle and challenge.

Myth 9   One cannot define the core curriculum because of the rapid changes taking place in medicine. What is true today may be proved false tomorrow.
NO   The core curriculum should be part of a living evolving curriculum. It should not be static but should change as required.

Myth 10   A core curriculum takes away the autonomy of the teacher and ignores the fact that the individual teacher knows best what should be included in the curriculum.
YES/NO   This is only partly true. There is an element of uniformity achieved in the core curriculum but this is desirable. There is, however, ample scope for the individual teacher with regard to content and how this is presented.

Assessment and the core

There are important implications of a core curriculum for student assessment:

- What is assessed must reflect the core curriculum.
- Students should be expected to reach a high standard in the core components of the curriculum. In practice this means a pass mark of 80–90% for the essential or 'inner core'. For less important aspects – 'the outer core' – a standard of 60–80% may be acceptable.
- Students should be required to demonstrate mastery of the core in one phase of the curriculum before moving on to the next part of the course – 'assessment to a standard'.

Summary

The core curriculum is an important strategy in the battle against information overload. The core curriculum is about the competencies required of all students. It is not only about facts, but also includes core skills and attitudes.

Ideas underpinning the concept are certification and credibility, capability and competence, comprehensiveness and communication, consistency, constructiveness and the continuum of education, choice and career, and a compacted curriculum.

The core curriculum, which is concerned with breadth, is closely linked in curriculum planning with special study modules. These allow students to study an area in depth. SSMs at the same time help students to develop core competencies of independent learning.

References and further reading

General Medical Council 1993 Tomorrow's doctors: recommendations on undergraduate medical education. General Medical Council, London

Harden R M, Davis M H 1995. The core curriculum with options or special study modules. AMEE Education Guide no. 5. Medical Teacher 17:125–148

Hirsch E D 1993. The core knowledge curriculum – what's behind its success? Educational Leadership, May: 23–25

Kirk G 1996 The core curriculum. Hodder and Stoughton, London

Lowry S 1992 Strategies for implementing curriculum change. British Medical Journal 305:1482–1485

Nierenberg D W 1990 A core curriculum for medical students in clinical pharmacology and therapeutics. The Council for Medical Student Education in Clinical Pharmacology and Therapeutics. Clinical Pharmacology, 48, 6:606–610

Reis S M, Renzulli J S 1992 Using curriculum compacting to challenge the above-average. Educational Leadership October: 51–57

Warren K S 1993 Change and the curriculum. Lancet 342: 488

Think of the curriculum and assessment as the wheels of the bicycle. They only work if pointing in the same direction.

"The aim of correcting the curriculum overload by the introduction of the core and special study module concept would be wholly frustrated if the present examination system were to continue"

General Medical Council 1993

Chapter 5
Electives, options and special study modules

C. D. Forbes

Introduction

Self-selected studies form the part of the curriculum which can be classified as non-core. It is very likely that medical schools will develop them in different ways, which may include special study modules, assignments or electives. Self-selected studies should occupy about a third of the curriculum time and provide a unique opportunity for students to personalise their self-learning in areas of specific interest in which they will have the opportunity to:

- study in greater depth topics of their choice
- take responsibility for their own learning
- develop a questioning and critical approach to learning
- gain experience in information retrieval and analysis
- acquire or improve on various personal, clinical and laboratory skills of their choice.

Self-selected studies should be integrated throughout the course with the opportunity for students in any year to apply for any of the modules offered in prior years.

Special Study Modules

Organisation

Special study modules (SSMs) should be offered in a range of topics including:

"The kids we bring into medical schools are wonderful with the highest possible qualities. We then submerge them in facts and beat the imagination out of them"

K Calman 1997

"Learning without thinking is useless. Thinking without learning is dangerous"

Confucius 551–478 BC

- basic medical scientific topics
- clinical science topics
- community/primary care and psychiatry subjects
- clinical practice across all specialties
- non-medical topics, e.g. language, legal and ethical studies and information technology.

Self-proposed SSMs should also be an option.

SSMs may last from 1 week up to 8 weeks in a single block of full-time study or they may be designed to take place in a longitudinal fashion in protected time each week during the course of a year.

Organiser

The key to the success of this aspect of the curriculum is to excite staff about the concepts of SSM teaching. An instructional booklet must be prepared and examples given of potential SSMs so potential supervisors understand that:

- SSMs should be set up with teams of colleagues.
- Teaching SSMs takes place in time that was once allocated to other standard teaching and not in addition to it.
- They must produce a booklet containing course material and a programme for the student.
- They are responsible for the final assessment of the students' performance.
- The SSM is not an opportunity to add more 'core' material in their own subject.

Budget

SSMs are usually set up by supervisors using their own departmental resources. Inevitably there are minor additional expenses which can be met by the medical school. In general terms these modules replace existing teaching commitments for most teachers, so additional payment to supervisors is not required.

When looking for staff to set up SSMs, start by identifying those who currently do little teaching and have time to organise others.

Produce an explanatory leaflet to inform and stimulate potential SSM organisers.

Allocation and choice

With a long list of choices and a range of SSMs of varying popularity a computer program is required to match an equitable mix of topics to a list of transferable choices made by the students.

Phase 1

In the first year of the medical course, subjects are usually offered in the basic sciences. All the modules are 'beyond the core' and cover areas that would not normally be taught. In addition, students may be stimulated by offering some modules which give an introduction to clinical practice such as professional nursing and midwifery, lifting and handling, and dealing with aggression in patients. Modules may also be offered in languages, ethics and law. In addition a major effort must be made to ensure that all new students are offered training in information technology to develop competence in word processing skills, statistics, graphics and powerpoint presentations.

Phase 2

In the second and third years of the course a large menu of SSMs is offered. Topics should include some appropriate for large group work: for example, surgery beyond the core, travel medicine, practical medical French, smoking and the role of health promotion or sports medicine.

Others are highly specialised small group modules and might include: care of people with learning disabilities, hand surgery or forensic psychiatry for beginners.

In addition, self-proposed modules may be offered.

Students are expected to undertake a range of modules to include some in hospital and some in general practice. It is important that they choose a range of modules to include basic sciences, specialist clinical practice and community. Students must be dissuaded from choosing 'easy options' in subjects in which they are already competent.

Phase 3

At this stage of the curriculum a larger portion of time is devoted to SSMs. These should be divided between:

- Hospital. Clinical attachments in hospital are designed to give experience beyond the core. At this stage senior students should be encouraged to play a role in teaching juniors.
- General practice. As most of medicine is covered within general practice and the majority of patients are to be found here, this experience is of major value.
- Theme-based. These show how developments in science impact on knowledge in the medical curriculum. A range of career options can be demonstrated, including science, pharmaceutical industry or medical publishing.

Examples of theme-based SSMs include:

- New drugs. This topic gives the student an insight into how new drugs are developed and which ones are selected for further evaluation.
- Surgical management. This takes an in-depth look at imaging, endoscopy and minimal invasive surgery.
- New advances in the management of cancer. This focuses on treatment with new anti-cancer drugs and drug regimens with an assessment of the risks and benefits. There is an emphasis on terminal care management when drug and other therapies have failed.
- Laboratory investigations. This topic examines the optimal way to investigate patients using appropriate laboratory tests and looks at how to interpret results. Attention is paid to the overuse and abuse of these services.
- Acute care. This module re-emphasises community and hospital-based acute medicine and surgery and ensures that students recognise the seriously ill or traumatised. Part of the course covers advanced trauma life support (ATLS) and advanced cardiac life support (ACLS).

Produce a special leaflet to tell the student how to apply and where to get the information, and give examples of topics.

Agree with all staff involved on the basic standard format of assessment. Encourage them to give realistic marks.

- Neurosciences, drug dependence and addiction. This examines drug dependency and drugs misuse in clinical practice; shows the neurobiological basis of addictive behaviour and demonstrates how such patients can be looked after both in the hospital and in the community.
- Assessment of medical evidence. Students are encouraged to read new publications in a variety of areas and to understand how meta-analysis works. The importance of evidence and guidelines to improve clinical practice is also stressed.

Self-proposed SSMs

These topics range widely depending on the initiative of the student but will usually fall within the following categories:

- Clinical practice topics
- Community medicine, primary care and psychiatric topics
- Medical sciences topics
- Ethical and legal topics
- Skills topics
- Medical education topics.

For self-proposed SSMs the student is required to find a supervisor and produce a summary of what is to be achieved. A brochure containing details of what is required and what the assessment of the module will entail is necessary for the supervisors. All these modules require a major educational content which may include acquisition of hand skills.

The module should be full-time and occupy the student for approximately 4 1/2 days per week. There should be a minimum contact time with the module supervisor of 3 hours per week. The module must have an end product, e.g. a report, a presentation or a demonstration of the techniques or skills acquired.

Multiprofessional SSMs

Some SSMs, such as ethics, law, languages, IT skills, counselling, addictive behaviours, violence in the home and eating disorders, lend themselves to being made available to students from other health-care groups. Tentative attempts to run these courses are encouraging but they do require more thought, planning and finance.

Assessment

As there is a wide and diverse range of SSMs it is not possible to define a rigid set of assessment criteria. However, assessment should include key aspects and can be weighted appropriately:

- Quality of material submitted or presented ... 60%
- Interest and motivation of the student ... 10%
- Critical thinking ... 10%
- Information retrieval ... 10%
- Reliability ... 10%

These, of course, are flexible assessments and will not fit conveniently into every type of module. A grading system is used for the final mark which students must realise is relevant to their final assessment in the medical course. The marking of the module is the responsibility of the internal assessor but external examiners are appointed to look at overall quality. A credit system of grades must be devised to encourage all students to take as many modules as possible. As in the 'core' parts of the course, poor performance or failure to attend in modules must result in the student repeating the year.

Assignments

The aims and objectives of the assignment are:

- to develop personal interest and ownership of learning
- to develop self-regulated learning skills
- to encourage self-management to facilitate deep learning in a topic of personal future work
- to enhance research skills.

Develop a computer program to help students choose their SSMs rationally.

Organisation

An assignment is organised as a longitudinal SSM and occupies the fourth year of the course. A protected half-day per week is assigned and spread over the whole year, equivalent to a full-time 4-week block. This provides students with a lot of thinking time to develop ideas on a particular theme, and also with the opportunity to discuss ideas with colleagues and staff. It is important to learn the constraints of working to a time schedule, to do the research and prepare the report.

Assignments involve not only supervisors and medical staff but may also include nursing and therapy staff, biochemists and scientists in other disciplines. Staff should not see supervision as a major chore as contact time with the student is quite small and spread over the whole year. Students require instruction on what is required of them and this is given in a comprehensive booklet. The list of staff who volunteer is posted and students then approach the individual of their own choice to discuss the project. These projects can range from an extensive in-depth review of the literature of a particular pertinent problem or undertaking a project under supervision which might involve the searching of case notes and analysis of data. Some more ambitious projects involve students collecting blood or other samples from patients, usually at specialist clinics which are held on one day per week. There are therefore a wide range and variety of projects which might include:

- antibiotic treatment of sore throats
- informed consent for gastrointestinal endoscopy
- intravenous cannula insertion and aftercare by junior house officers
- methicillin-resistant *Staphylococcus aureus* (MRSA) eradication regimens.

The assignment gives the individual student the opportunity to have a sustained one-to-one relationship with a member of staff who is responsible for marking the assignment and ensuring its completion.

Assignments have proved popular with both staff and students. Some reports may go on to be published in peer-reviewed journals but topics need to be varied each year as such material may be plagiarised by succeeding students.

It is of course important to ensure that the supervisor sees candidates intermittently as the project runs continuously throughout the year. Candidates must also remember that they have to submit by the agreed date and achieve a pass mark to proceed into the next year. The size of the project will vary greatly depending on the amount of data generated but about 10 000 words (30 × A4 pages), including diagrams and references as appropriate, are reasonable. The student is encouraged to use the style of paper adopted in the *British Medical Journal*, starting if possible with a structured abstract stating objective, design, setting subjects, results and conclusion. The main report should be broken down into an introduction, method, results and conclusions with references and appendices.

It is also important that the student's report is a high-quality presentation, and for those who are not computer-literate at the start of the fourth year, this is an excellent opportunity to work on the word processing skills which are critical for every medical graduate.

Assessment

The project is marked on a grading system from A to G; each letter is equivalent to the words excellent, very good, satisfactory, just adequate, marginal fail, definite fail and bad fail. The grade is entered on the central progress report card of each student.

Electives

An elective is a period which enables students in the later years of the medical course to follow prolonged studies of their own choosing.

Travel arrangements

Part of the discipline of the elective is that students are expected to make their own arrangements, including contacting a home or overseas institute, identifying a local supervisor and making arrangements to travel. Often this takes some time and arrangements for

Ensure you have a preliminary report at about the half-way mark to know that individuals have started the work.

"So it is in travelling; a man must carry knowledge with him, if he would bring home knowledge"

Samuel Johnson 1709–84

Make sure students start planning early as travel documentation may take a year to prepare.

electives need to start a year in advance of the date of travel. Students will often get ideas and examples from each other. The reports of satisfactorily completed electives are made available in the library and from these students in subsequent years can gain an idea of what is on offer, a contact name, and also hints about the financing of travel and accommodation. Faculty approval must always be obtained before the student leaves, to ensure that the place chosen is reasonably safe and that there is the potential for learning.

Funding

For the majority of students, no central financial support is available and raising money themselves is part of the learning process. Funds can be obtained from commercial and charitable sources who can be quite generous, especially if the candidate is going to the Third World. A variety of travel grants may be made available from charities and also from the Royal Colleges and some large companies. It is important for students to have a current passport, apply for a visa and work permit in reasonable time, and arrange medical insurance.

Immunisation

Students should also be encouraged to check up on the immunisation required and to initiate their vaccination programme. Some countries still require a current chest X-ray and physical examination.

Students are, responsible for organising this usually through their family doctor, the local travel clinic or the university health service. It is important to re-emphasise that because a number of immunisations may be necessary, they must be done logically and appropriate time allowed. In particular immunisation against hepatitis B and A is required and several months may be needed to prove that it has been effective.

Medical indemnity

Medical defence unions will usually provide cover to destinations other than the USA and Canada. If North

American destinations are planned, then it is usual for the host institute to provide cover.

Civil or military unrest

Many countries of the Third World are inherently unstable and it is important to check in the news whether they are currently experiencing any unrest. If this is so, the elective should be cancelled. It is worthwhile thinking in advance of who might help if things go wrong; this would usually be the consular mission in the country and contact should be made with them in advance. The addresses of British missions can be obtained from the Diplomatic Service List which is available in public libraries and local telephone directories in the countries concerned. It is also available from the Foreign and Commonwealth Office (telephone number 0207 270 3000).

Risk of exposure to HIV

An official letter should be sent to every student going overseas to indicate the risk of exposure to human immunodeficiency virus (HIV) and related infections. Students should also be encouraged to take clean needles and syringes should they require any medication to be given by injection. They should also be warned about the problems of blood transfusion and blood or body fluids in contact with skin. In the event of exposure to HIV-infected body fluids a starter pack of the appropriate antiviral drugs should be available.

Student's report

Students should be aware that they will need to submit a written report within 4 weeks of completing the elective. The report should contain detailed information about the attachment, what was seen, what was done and other information of educational value, including details of how the elective was planned and the name of the contact person, with addresses, telephone numbers, fax and e-mail. It is very helpful if a camera is taken abroad to record the professional and social aspects of the elective.

"To be trained is to have arrived; to be educated is to continue to travel . . . a challenge to get better all the time"

K Calman 1997

Supervisor's report

Students are given an assessment form to complete by the local supervisor and this must be returned to the medical school.

Students must understand that they are ambassadors for their medical school and country and appropriate standards of behaviour and diligence are expected. We have found that this part of the course is one of the most interesting, exciting and educational of the whole medical course. It is still remarkable to see how far students travel and the experience they gain.

Summary

Curriculum changes represent a huge challenge for all medical teachers, especially as improvements are usually to be made within existing budgets. Self-selected studies give staff and students a new dimension for teaching and learning. The possibilities are limitless and significantly empower students who enhance their own profile of knowledge and skills. Staff believe that they will significantly improve the quality of the new graduates and hence their competitiveness in the future.

References and further reading

Anon 1993 The overseas elective: purpose or picnic? Lancet 342:753–754

Bissonette R P, Alvarez C A 1991 American medical students broaden their horizons in the Third World. World Health Forum 12:49–54

Calman K 1997 Utopia and other destinations

Downie R, Macnaughton J 1999 Should medical students read Plato? Medical Journal of Australia 170:125–127

Fletcher G, Agius R M 1995 The special study module: a novel approach to undergraduate teaching in occupational medicine. Occupational Medicine (Oxford) 45:326–328

Harden R M, Davis M H, Crosby J R 1997 The new Dundee medical curriculum: a whole that is greater than the sum of the parts. Med Educ 31:264–271

Heck J E, Wedemeyer D 1991 A survey of American medical schools to assess their preparation of students for overseas practice. Academic Medicine 66:78–81

Northrup R S 1991 Preparing students for overseas electives. Academic Medicine 66:92

Taylor C E 1994 International experience and idealism in medical education. Academic Medicine 69:631–634

Wilkinson D, Symon B 1999 Medical students, their electives, and HIV. British Medical Journal 318:139–140

SECTION 2
LEARNING SITUATIONS

Chapter 6
Lectures

J. A. Dent

Introduction

The lecture has been the classical mechanism of tertiary education for centuries and, together with bedside teaching, formed the traditional picture of medical school. Recent developments have seen the introduction of alternative learning situations into the modern medical curriculum but a place remains for lectures although their role and style can be changed. A lengthy monologue promoting the memorisation of factual information with little emphasis on understanding or application is unlikely to be appropriate in the contemporary learning environment.

The role of lectures

Although a lecture may usually be thought of as a mechanism of imparting factual knowledge it probably has a more important role in stimulating students' interest and so enabling additional self-directed learning in the topic.

Context

An effective way of stimulating interest and promoting learning is by using a study guide. In this way the role of a particular lecture can be set in the context of the whole of the course and its content related to other lectures or to additional material which is being presented in alternative learning situations.

"Lecture: process by which the notes of a teacher become the notes of a student without passing through the minds of either"

Michael O'Donnell

Content

What to include

Not all course material designated as being 'core' needs to be presented as a lecture and indeed much may be more appropriately presented in other ways. Questions of ethics or patient management, for instance, lend themselves to learning in small group discussion sessions while factual information relating to the pathological or pharmacological aspects of a condition may be more efficiently presented as self-directed learning or interactive computer-assisted learning (CAL) programs.

Relevance and application

The material presented should be shown to be relevant to the course and related to material presented elsewhere. The relevance of the content should be made obvious to the students and any key points should be emphasised.

Variety

When they are integrated into a course lectures should not spoon-feed students with pre-digested facts (Fig. 6.1). Instead even the classic didactic lecture can be used in a variety of more interesting roles:

- Overview. An 'overview' of the entire body system in health and disease can be given in an introductory lecture as an advance organiser to the whole course. A 'flavour' of the system is given and key features can be highlighted which will be expanded later as the course progresses.
- Core. A series of lectures can be used to present the core content of the course.
- Non-core. An occasional lecture may be used to introduce material 'beyond the core'. This may illustrate wider aspects of the topic being studied and include recent research developments.
- Assessment material. The style of assessment material to be used in forthcoming examinations can be introduced and examples worked through with the whole class.
- Patient presentations. These can be used to illustrate general aspects of a case history to the whole class or

"Some experience of popular lecturing had convinced me that the necessity of making things plain to uninstructed people was one of the very best means of clearing up the obscure corners in one's own mind"

Huxley T. H. 1825–95

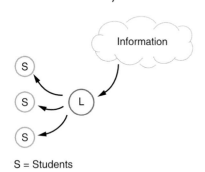

S = Students

L = Lecturer

Fig. 6.1 Didactic lecture information

to discuss the impact of an illness and its management on an individual. The lecture then assumes an interactive role as the students engage with the patient and lecturer by questions, answers and discussion (see Fig. 6.2).

- Shared lecture. Two or more lecturers may share the session to present different or multiprofessional approaches or opinions on a topic, e.g. a general practitioner and an orthopaedic surgeon on the management of osteoarthritis.
- Mini-symposium. Several participants can take part to demonstrate various approaches to the management of a clinical problem.

Format

Duration
Studies have shown that students' attention deteriorates after 45 minutes. Lectures should be timed to last no longer than this and should include time for answering any questions. Lectures with more than one participant can last longer but it should be remembered that students will be better prepared if they have a break before their next session starts.

Structure
The lecture should be structured so that its role in directing students to the aims of the course and the realisation of objectives is clear.

Advance organiser
An outline of the proposed content of the lecture should be given at the beginning so students know what is to come and are able to pace themselves for the session.

Sections
The lecture should be divided into separate sections to break up the total time available. A classic method is described as 'set, body, close'. Initially the form of the lecture is described. This is followed by the main content of the lecture. Any questions can next be answered

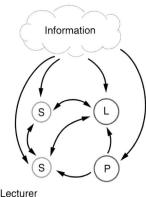

L = Lecturer

S = Students

P = Patient

Fig. 6.2 Interactive lecture

"Say what you are going to say, say it and then say what you have said"

Advice to a young preacher

Always end your lecture with a summary of the content rather than on a discussion of some free-for-all-point raised as a question.

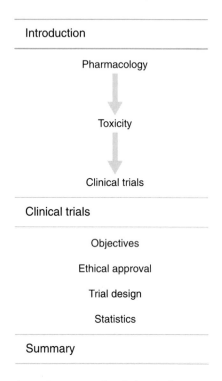

Fig. 6.3   Example of classical method of lecturing (redrawn from Brown & Tomlinson 1979)

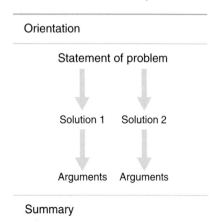

Fig. 6.4   Example of problem centred method of lecturing (redrawn from Brown & Tomlinson 1979)

before the session closes with a reiteration of the main points.

The construction of the central portion of the lecture may vary. Brown and Tomlinson (1979) described:

- The classical method. This divides the lecture into sections and subsections. It is easy to plan and take notes from but also easily becomes boring (see Fig. 6.3, which takes the example of drug development and trial).
- The problem-centred method. This first states a problem and then argues for and against various solutions, promoting enquiry, cross-referencing and formation of a conclusion (see Fig. 6.4).
- The sequential method. This consists of a series of linked statements which lead to a conclusion (see Fig. 6.5).

Lesson plan

A lesson plan should be available to students either as a handout or a website which indicates:

- Aims and objectives. These terms are often confused and used synonymously. However, 'aims' indicate the general direction in which a students' studies are leading (e.g. to understand how to manage a patient in pain), whereas 'objectives' relate to goals which should be attainable either after the lecture or in the near future (e.g., to be able to list four drugs which help to control pain and describe their method of action).
- Summary. The main points of the lecture can be listed.
- Self-assessment questions. These can be presented during the lecture or in the lesson plan for students to use in their own time to assess their understanding of the topic presented.
- Directions to background reading and other material.

Presentation

Presentation skills

It is not an exaggeration to think of the lecturer as a performer who has to entertain the audience.

Attention to several key points will make this easier to accomplish.

Where to stand

- Choose where you are going to position yourself in the lecture theatre and whether you are going to stand, sit or be able to walk around. Do you wish to be behind a podium or bench or nearer to and more in contact with the audience?
- Are you near the microphone and is it at the correct height for you?
- Are you obstructing the audience's view of the screen for slides or the overhead projector?

How to speak

- It should be clearly stated at the beginning whether the lecturer intends students to take notes or not. Taking down every word verbatim should be discouraged but if it is expected that notes are to be taken then an appropriate pace of lecturing should be adopted and new words clearly indicated. If the role of the lecture is to paint a general overview then only the occasional word need be written down and the pace and style of lecture can be quicker and more colloquial.
- It is fatal to read a lecture if student concentration is to be maintained but some notes will help you to keep the main points in view and are invaluable to fall back on if interrupted or diverted.
- Variations in pitch and speed make a lecture more engaging.
- Be sure you are audible at the back of the auditorium.
- The occasional appropriate joke or reference to a current social event are other strategies which may help you break up the style of your lecture and recapture students' attention.
- Do not be afraid to pause to allow students to catch up if they are being expected to take detailed notes.
- If visual aids are being used these should be cued into your notes so that they are not forgotten or brought in at the wrong time.

 "Don't:
- **A**nnoy
- **B**ore
- **C**onfuse
- **D**istract
- **E**xhaust"

Robert D. Acland

Ensure that you have arrived at the correct lecture theatre to avoid beginning your lecture with the wrong audience!

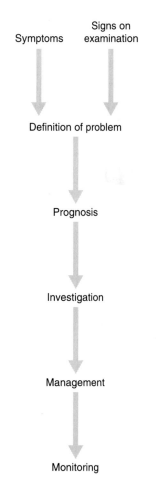

Fig. 6.5   The sequential method (redrawn from Brown & Tomlinson 1979)

"No sleep is so deeply refreshing as that which, during lectures, Morpheus invites us so insistently to enjoy. From the standpoint of physiology it is amazing how quickly the ravages of a short night or a long operating session can be repaired by nodding off for a few seconds at a time"

P. B. Medawar 1979

Keeping in contact with the audience

- Maintain eye contact with the audience but not with any particular student as this can be disturbing.
- Look around various sections of the audience in turn.
- Do not speak to the walls or the projector.
- If circumstances are favourable it is possible to walk around the lecture theatre and speak from different points at the back or towards the middle instead of always from the front. This may be especially helpful if using slides so that you can check that the features illustrated can be seen from the back.
- Appropriate use of gestures may enliven your presentation and maintain attention.
- If using a projector do not stand at the back next to it to talk but use a remote control so you can be positioned within sight of the audience as they look at the slides.
- Beware of dimming the house lights completely as you will lose eye contact with the audience and encourage sleep!

Questions

- At certain points in the lecture it should be possible to stop and ask questions in order to clarify any points which may have been confusing or to check on students' understanding of the material so far.
- At times particular questions can be asked to individual students but this may appear threatening and it may be best to ask questions to different areas of the auditorium in turn to help maintain interest.

Some final points

- **Don't** fidget or fiddle with loose change and car keys in your pockets!
- **Do** avoid repetitive mannerisms or hesitations such as 'er', 'um"'and 'OK?'

Aids

Any additional material presented in a lecture must be of good quality or else it will be a distraction.

Slides

Slides can be used to illustrate clinical features, radiographs, results of investigations or aspects of surgical or other lines of management. They must be the correct way round and the right way up! Photomicrographs and diagrams or pictures of prosections may be helpful in illustrating basic sciences but line slides and tables should be used cautiously as they are often overcrowded and may be impossible to read. Attention should be paid to the size of the words, the type of font and the colours used on the slides (Laidlaw 1987). Slides are often illegible from the back of the theatre if you use colours which are too pale or too similar. Pale print on a dark ground tends to dazzle and be difficult to read, as are words written entirely in capital letters. Double projection is probably less popular now than it used to be. It requires considerable skill if a meaningful flow of slides is to be constructed. One useful technique is to have line slides on one side and illustrative material on the other. It is important that both frames are advanced together as the chance of getting the two projectors out of synchrony with each other will quickly destroy the most carefully prepared lecture.

Flip charts, blackboards and wipe-clean boards

These will be of little use in a lecture theatre as anything written on them must be big enough to be visible at the back.

Handouts

A lesson plan may be given at the beginning of a lecture to give an outline of the content:

- Comprehensive handouts avoid students having to take extensive notes but encourage lack of concentration.
- Skeletal handouts which require to be filled in encourage the audience to pay more attention to the material being presented.

Other interactive material to promote audience participation may be distributed to use in question and answer sessions during the lecture.

It is best to stand or sit to one side of the overhead projector otherwise you will probably be obstructing the view of part of the audience.

Overhead projector

Care must be paid to the amount, size and clarity of writing presented by the overhead projector (OHP) (Laidlaw 1987). It should not be:

- too small
- too crowded
- too scribbled.

The OHP can also be used to present previously drawn diagrams or tables which can be built up by removing successive layers of masking or adding successive layers of pre-drawn or coloured acetate sheets. Points gathered from interaction with the audience can be written down on the OHP as they are raised.

Computerised presentation

Computer programs such as 'Microsoft PowerPoint' can remove the expense of producing slides and presentations can be quicker to prepare than OHP acetate sheets. Material can even be added during the course of the lecture as new points are raised by interaction with the audience. It is important, however, that technical assistance is available and that breakdowns can be dealt with promptly. The lecturer must have practised to become familiar with the computer program used. Again attention must be paid to colour, crowding and the type and size of fonts used. The use of additional visuals such as 'Clip Art' or scanned-in photographs and video clips help to enliven the presentation (Crosby 1994).

Headsets

Radio headsets have been used to receive sounds from a patient or manikin which would normally be heard by only one person. Heart or intrauterine sounds can be transmitted to the whole audience and subsequently discussed.

Video, closed circuit TV and teleconferencing

The lecture can be used to view short sections of previously recorded video or closed circuit TV presentations from another site such as an operating theatre. Interactive teleconferencing from several locations may form part of the event.

Website

Copies of handouts, illustrations, PowerPoint slides and references to other resource material can subsequently be made available at a website for students to access after the lecture. Directions to additional learning resources can also be given.

Challenges

If you have forgotten your presentation notes or slides it may be necessary, if you cannot restructure the style of your lecture immediately, to apologise and reschedule your lecture for another day. For the majority of challenges, however, it is simply a matter of keeping calm and not being afraid to stop until the disturbance is over or you have refound your place in your presentation notes. Interruptions and technical faults provide a test of the lecturer's skill in holding the floor and it may be wise to work out a personal strategy for dealing with some of these before being faced with them:

- interruptions
  — late arrivals
  — unexpected questions
  — paging system
  — talking on the back row
  — students falling asleep
- technical failures
  — OHP bulb blows
  — projector remote control failing to function
  — computer crash
  — house lights failing to dim
  — blackouts being inadequate for the use of slides.

By always making a point of arriving early to familiarise yourself with the equipment many of these disasters can be averted.

Staff development

Everybody thinks they can lecture adequately and consequently interest in staff development sessions on

If you are unsure of the answer to a question raised ask the student to meet you later rather than stalling.

lecturing is low. However, while it is probably true that anyone can lecture many can be helped to lecture better by rehearsing the use of the techniques mentioned earlier in this chapter and by paying attention to the use of visual aids. Other strategies include:

- peer review and constructive feedback of a lecture including its content and presentation
- opportunities to watch yourself lecturing on video and for self-critique
- induction session for new lecturers including video of a lecture
- examples of good and bad lecturing, interactive session.

Summary

In a modern curriculum a lecture is only one of several ways of imparting factual information. As such its role in the context of the entire course must be made clear. As well as presenting core material, lectures can also be used to give an overview of the course, present assessment material and make patient presentations which may involve a shared presentation with multiprofessional participation. However it is used, the lecture should be clearly structured, have defined aims and objectives and be accompanied by an explicit lesson plan. To lecture effectively requires that attention be paid to presentation skills and the use of any visual or technical aids. Even when all is prepared the lecturer must be able to deal with any unforeseen challenges which indicate that attendance at staff development sessions in lecturing may be more valuable than originally perceived.

References and further reading

Amoto D, Quirt I 1990 Lecture handouts of projected slides in a medical course. Medical Teacher 12:291–296

Brown G, Tomlinson D 1979. How to improve lecturing. Medical Teacher 1:128–135

Butler J A 1992 Use of teaching methods within the lecture format. Medical Teacher 14:11–25

Crosby J 1994 Twelve tips for effective electronic presentation. Medical Teacher 16:3–8

Laidlaw J M 1987 Twelve tips for users of the overhead projector. Medical Teacher 9:247–251

"educationalists must change their use of the lecture time in order to improve student learning, [and] achieve the higher-order educational objectives"

J. A. Butler 1992

Laidlaw J 1987 Twelve tips on preparing 35 mm slides. Medical Teacher
    9:389–393
MacLean I 1991 Twelve tips on providing handouts. Medical Teacher 13:7–12
Medawar P B 1979 Advice to a young Scientist. Harper & Row
O'Donnell M 1997 A sceptic's medical dictionary. BMJ Publishing Group,
    London

Chapter 7
Small group sessions

I. McA. Ledingham   J. R. Crosby

Introduction

Small group work is one of a variety of educational methods for promoting student learning. The reason for adopting the small group approach has to be carefully considered. Other learning situations are detailed in this section of the book. Problem-based learning and self-directed learning are covered in Section 3.

The recent trend to small group work is indicative of the movement from a teacher-centred approach to education to a more student-centred approach (see Chapter 3). However, the reasons for choosing small groups should be dictated by the educational objectives of the session. The organiser of a course or programme has to be clear about the rationale for using small group work and the outcomes expected of this method. The use of small groups will also be influenced by resource availability e.g. rooms, facilitators, resource material etc.

Students tend to learn in different ways and a range of learning situations may ensure appropriate learning for all (University of Toronto website). A mixed approach to the learning situation is often appropriate and may be positively encouraged. The use of both lectures and small groups may be complementary to the learning process.

Why would you use a lecture and why a small group?

What is a small group?

Small group work is characterised by student participation and interaction (Crosby 1996). It is possible to have a small number of students and a tutor and yet participation by the students remains minimal. This may be better called a lecture (albeit for a small number of students). In addition to participation, small group work is also characterised by group work on a task and reflection on the work completed.

Ideally effective small group work occurs when there is a small number of students. It is impossible or very difficult to ensure the participation of a large number of students in a group. If the number increases too much the group may be split into two groups. The number of students in a group does not conform to any hard and fast rule. Some experienced tutors may be able to facilitate many students whereas an inexperienced tutor may feel more comfortable with fewer students. Numbers in small groups are, however, frequently fixed by curriculum demands and the generation of grouping based on a yearly intake. A tutor may not be able to dictate the preferred size of a group.

Why small groups?

There are advantages to using small group teaching over larger class activities or independent learning. The following are a few examples:

- It familiarises students with an adult approach to learning, a generic skill they will need for the rest of their professional lives.
- It encourages students to take responsibility for their own learning. Teacher-centred models of learning tend not to encourage students to take responsibility for their own learning.
- It promotes deeper understanding of material. Small group work allows students to bring to the group their own prior learning and perceptions (or misconceptions) of material previously learnt. Learning can then develop from this point.
- It encourages problem-solving skills.
- It encourages participation. The nature of social interactions means that they are usually more enjoyable than solitary pursuits. The element of

The size of a small group is less important than the characteristics of the group.

"When adults teach and learn in one another's company, they find themselves engaging in a challenging passion and creative activity"

Brookfield 1986

"With undergraduate medical education currently carrying a health warning because of the stress and anxiety exhibited by students and young graduates, any educational process that promotes enjoyment of learning without loss of basic knowledge must be a good thing"

Bligh 1995

Think – how do you learn?

enjoyment and its influence on motivation may encourage students to learn.

- It develops
  — interpersonal skills
  — communication skills
  — social teamworking skills
  — presentation skills.
- It encourages an awareness of different views on issues and has the potential to encourage an attitude of tolerance.

Personal understanding of an educational issue can be attained in a number of ways but small groups make it possible to turn such understanding into a 'coherent, rational and professionally defensible position that can be clearly articulated' (Walker 1998).

Notwithstanding these advantages, small group work should only be adopted when it is the most efficient approach to achieve these benefits/objectives. It should not be considered as a panacea for learning. There are disadvantages of small group work. Invariably the emphasis on understanding rather than rote regurgitation results in more time being spent to master the topic area. This can sometimes be problematic, time constraints being a feature of modern life.

The expertise of the tutor may also be considered as a potential problem. The role of the tutor can be crucial to the success of any small group work. Staff may be more familiar with traditional modes of teaching and may need training in the specific role of a small group tutor. The logistics of running small groups may be difficult, as more teachers, more rooms and more resource material may be required. The preparation of resource material to support small groups is also an important part of the process and requires considerable time and expertise.

What kind of small group session?

In the context of a medical undergraduate curriculum a variety of small group sessions may be relevant. At one end of the spectrum is the structured, teacher-centred, tutorial group usually focusing on an identified task

(Entwistle & Thompson 1992) and often pursuing a series of conclusions (a differential diagnosis perhaps or a patient management plan). At the other end is the unstructured, student-centred, discussion/dialogue group (Christensen 1991), the principal purpose of which is to exchange views on a topic and promote reflection (attitudes to patient care perhaps or interpersonal communication). Between these two extremes all manner of group structures and functions exist, limited only by the imagination and creativity of the course organisers and individual tutors. Examples include:

- seminars
- workshops
- clinical skills sessions
- communication skills sessions
- problem-based learning tutorials
- clinical teaching sessions
  — ward-based
  — ambulatory care/ outpatient-based
  — community-based
- support groups
  — students
  — tutors.

The majority of these small group sessions are dealt with in detail elsewhere in this book. The main focus of the present chapter is those elements that are common to all small group, student-centred activities. The text can, of course, only serve as an introduction to actual practice in a variety of settings.

All such activities must complement the institution's overall curricular strategy, address specific course objectives and enhance the educational programme. The sessions should be seen to be an integral component of the course content and relate appropriately to the other learning opportunities on offer. For example, the week's work may be framed around a patient problem. The lectures and small group work, both theoretical and practical, contribute to an understanding of the patient's problem. Key to the success of small group work is the tutor, working either alone or in collaboration with a co-tutor.

What is the role of the tutor?

Traditional tutorial role

In the case of the traditional tutorial group the tutor normally states the objectives of the session (usually known to the participants beforehand), initiates the process, invites learner input (often prepared), promotes discussion and brings the session to an appropriate close. Throughout the session the tutor 'leads from the front' (often literally) and is clearly in control. This format is familiar to most medical teachers and is one in which the tutor's effectiveness is derived from a combination of innate ability, content expertise, teaching experience and personal enthusiasm. Such learning groups are of undoubted value in selected circumstances. The range of discussion, however, may be relatively narrow, the contribution to self-learning limited and interaction between learners at best patchy.

Facilitated tutorial role

Increasingly, small group learning signifies a process in which the learners together provide much of the initiative, explore options, test hypotheses, develop solutions, elaborate on-going actions (including clinical investigations and treatment) and review outcomes. Role-playing and the performance of practical procedures may be an integral part of such sessions. The role of the tutor in these circumstances varies according to the stage of academic development of the learners, their familiarity with the process, their maturity as a group, and the frequency and duration of the tutorials. If the small group session is one of a linked series, say within an 'organ/system/problem-based' course, continuity of contact with a single tutor or pair of tutors has much to recommend it. This is often seen to be a problem for busy clinical teachers but experience shows that where teaching responsibilities are taken seriously at institutional and individual level, appropriate solutions can usually be found which do not adversely affect the teacher's other functions.

"Leaders can model... manual, intellectual and communication skills, and learners can safely rehearse and refine these capabilities"

Westberg & Jason 1996

"I will hand on precepts, lectures and all other learning ... to those pupils duly apprenticed and sworn"

Hippocratic Oath c.460–377 BC

Requirements of a tutor

Preparation

Tutors will wish to confirm the details of their role as perceived by the course organisers and ensure that they are properly briefed on the specific objectives of the small group session. Tutor guides containing this kind of information are a feature of modern educational programmes. They will then obviously rehearse the content and context of the session and in this connection will have regard to the 'learner factors' previously cited, particularly their stage of development and degree of comfort with the small group process.

If tutors are not seasoned campaigners in small group learning activities (and there are only a few answering this description in any medical school) then they would be wise to acquire some basic expertise. Appropriate staff development programmes should be on offer in all medical schools to meet the needs of aspiring teachers. These may take the form of specific courses or 'on the job' training and may include the opportunity to join experienced tutors at work (Hekelman et al 1994). Evidence suggests that the basic skills of small group facilitation may be acquired in 12 to 24 hours of experiential training. Studies have also shown that while content expertise may be useful in small group teaching facilitation skills are essential. This is particularly so in the early years when learners stand to derive the greatest benefit from acquiring the skills and habit of independent self-learning.

A few practical points remain. Tutors should be the first to appear at the appointed hour not the last (regrettably all too common). Preferably, they should make a point of turning up at least 15 minutes before the session starts in order to check the venue, the seating and the resources, to trouble-shoot and last but by no means least, to set an example.

Conduct of the session

The success of small group learning may be judged by the extent to which trust is created and collaboration

"over two-thirds of academic and clinical staff had received no formal training in teaching skills"

Preston-Whyte et al 1999

The clinician as role model exerts a potent influence – for good or bad.

"A fundamental feature of effective facilitation is to make participants feel that they are valued as separate, unique individuals deserving of respect"

Brookfield 1986

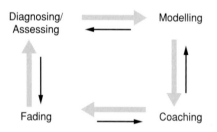

Fig. 7.1 Cyclical leadership roles in small groups (redrawn from Collins, Brown & Newman 1989)

fostered. This is critical in the case of a linked series of tutorials but should be aspired to in all instances.

As with all such events the opening few minutes can make or mar the entire session. In 'one-off' situations or early in a series the tutor will wish to set the scene, state the objectives and suggest some basic ground rules. At this and subsequent stages of the session the tutor should endeavour to visualise the students' learning needs specifically from their point of view. Recollection of the tutor's own learning experiences may assist in this regard. It may also be useful for the group to discuss the tutor's role and the fact that this will change as the learners become increasingly competent at handling their own affairs. Ultimately the tutor may merge with the group such that an observer might have difficulty distinguishing tutor from learner (see Fig. 7.1 cyclical leadership roles). This is the greatest challenge for the traditional teacher, who is likely to be initially uncomfortable with the thought of losing control and allowing the session to become untidy or 'even worse'.

Issues of importance during the discussion itself include:

- participation of all group members (may require control of dominant students and encouragement of quieter ones; a co-tutor may be particularly helpful in this regard)
- critical thinking (assimilation, interpretation and synthesis of information)
- articulation of thoughts/views (an essential generic skill)
- learner interaction (enhancement of understanding, growth of mutual respect and promotion of teamworking)
- review of objectives ('keeping on track')
- intermittent summary of achievements (encouragement of reflection)
- observation of agreed time constraints (development of time management skills).

The emphasis on these and other individual issues will vary with circumstances and some goals may only realistically be achieved in the context of serial sessions.

Conclusion

Whatever small group model is envisaged the importance of according sufficient time to bring the session to an appropriate ending cannot be exaggerated. In a 'stand alone' traditional tutorial this may require only a few minutes but in the kind of session which forms the main focus of this chapter considerably more time may have to be allocated. Feedback to learners is critically important and is widely regarded as one of the strengths of the small group process. Reference may be made not only to general points and particular details of the learning content of the session but also to the conduct of the session. The latter may on occasion prompt later counselling of individual students where specific difficulties have been identified that are best dealt with away from the group. In the case of a series of interconnected sessions (e.g. a problem-based model) there will also be a need to agree the topics for discussion at the next session.

What is the role of the student?

The student is, of course, the key figure in any learning event but the positive commitment of the individual learner is absolutely critical to the success of small group learning. As in the case of the tutor the learners must accept the principle of this form of learning and realise that what they get out of the process directly reflects what they put into it. This will include undertaking prior reading, actively and constructively contributing to the conduct of the session and effectively reflecting on the issues raised. The student also has an increasingly important role in assessment and evaluation.

It should be remembered that student groups may function entirely satisfactorily in the absence of a tutor.

Assessment

Assessment of learners engaged in small group activities can be tricky and requires careful consideration. The learners will certainly want to be informed of the nature of the assessment and whether it will be formative or

"Group methods succeed or fail to the extent that work is accomplished"

Walton 1997

Feedback needs to be linked to actual observation of learners' performance, timely, descriptive of specific behaviours, potential in supportive, non-judgemental ways, and when possible tied to the learner's self-assessments.

summative or both. They will also want to know who is responsible for the assessment. If the tutor is involved, particularly in summative assessment, this may act as a barrier to the creation of trust within the group and tend to inhibit the spontaneity of discussion. Some learners may be less inclined to 'take the risk' of revealing ignorance if they believe their every utterance is being carefully monitored and scrutinised. Tutors need to be aware of these sensitivities and be prepared to confront the problem – for example, by openly discussing their role in assessment as part of the group process. (It may help to indicate that the tutor's performance will also be assessed and therefore, since they are all 'in the same boat', they may as well 'pull on the oars' together.)

The details of assessment will be discussed in Section 6. In general, it is relatively straightforward to construct an instrument for assessing the performance of the group as a whole, particularly if the assessment is formative. The first step is to identify the performance to be assessed. Performance may relate to:

- the attainment of the objectives or task – the product
- the working of the small group – the process (team working, collaboration etc.)

Attainment of the objectives can be assessed in traditional ways, while assessing the group process may be more challenging. This can be achieved in a variety of ways:

- Student self-reporting. Given key guidelines students may report on the success of teamworking and individual contributions.
- Tutor observations. Most small group assessments occur spontaneously and informally. The dominant or quiet members are easily spotted. These observations, whilst necessary to ensure appropriate facilitation of the group, may also be used to assess the development of the student.
- External or co-tutor observations. A third party may be asked to observe and assess the group process. These observations may involve more in-depth analysis of interaction and frequency of contributions by both students and staff.

The difficulty arises in assessing the abilities of individual learners especially if the small group sessions are part of a series involving and specifically encouraging teamwork. A recent study (Heathfield 1999) has shown that the learners themselves may assist in this process and, in effect, decide the relative merit of individual performance on the basis of :

- attendance
- contribution of ideas
- research, analysis and preparation of material
- contribution to cooperative process
- support and encouragement of team members
- practical contributions to end-product.

The individual items can be graded and, if accepted as an ongoing part of the small group continuum, can assist individual learners develop and enhance their abilities, become aware and reflective of attitudes (both their own and their peers), and improve their competence as team players.

Evaluation and development

Course monitoring

It goes without saying that small group sessions need to be evaluated as much as any other part of the educational programme. The points to be taken into consideration can be considered under the following headings:

- Evaluation of the product: the achievement of the tasks. This may be best achieved by assessment results related to the objectives of the session. A variety of methods may be used – for example, an objective structured clinical examination (OSCE) to evaluate the success of small group work in developing communication skills.
- Evaluation of the process: the method used to achieve the objectives (small group work). This point may be best elicited in either a free text response or Likert-type questionnaire. Questions to ask may include:
  — Did all the group participate?

"We need to continue to develop ways of assessing what we truly value rather than only valuing what we can more easily assess"

Heathfield 1999

Likert type: the grading of questions/statements using a numerical scale, e.g. between 1 and 5, where 1 = strongly disagree and 5 = strongly agree

— Did you take responsibility for your own learning?
— Did the group work effectively?
— Did anyone dominate?

Support groups

Much has been written recently about the need for undergraduate medical students and young graduates to be supported as they face the increasing pressures of professional life, particularly when responsibilities in their private lives may also weigh heavily upon them. In Section 7 the topic of learner support is addressed in detail. It is also worth reflecting on the need for support amongst teachers, particularly when taking on new and unfamiliar tasks.

To quote Alcoholics Anonymous, the important first step is to realise that help is required and then to take steps to seek help (Walton 1997). There is little merit in soldiering on alone when other more experienced colleagues are around and are willing to assist (Hekelman et al 1994). Both you and those dependent upon you for their learning will benefit from support which is appropriately offered. Most medical schools do in fact offer such assistance but there is still a tendency for teachers to be unwilling or ostensibly too busy to avail themselves of it. Both medical schools and teachers might with advantage review their approach to this aspect of staff development.

Summary

Small group work is a powerful educational tool. As with all teaching instruments its benefits are maximised when used skilfully in carefully considered situations. The reasons for its deployment have to be clear to both tutor and learner. Advantages include the encouragement of independent self-learning, critical thinking and awareness of the views of others. Successful small groups are based on the creation of trust, fostering of collaboration and achievement of work.

In the context of a medical undergraduate curriculum the range of small group sessions is limited only by the imagination of the course organisers and tutors. Clinical teaching is invariably small group in character but educational strategies and teaching methods need to be geared to the overall objectives of the curriculum. Staff development is an important part of this process. One of the greatest opportunities of small group work is that of constructive feedback.

As always assessment and evaluation are critical components of this form of education and should be directed at both the group and its individual members. Increasingly effective methods are being developed to meet this challenge.

References and further reading

Bligh J 1995 Problem-based, small group learning. British Medical Journal 311:342–343

Brookfield S 1986 Understanding and facilitating adult learning. Jossey Bass, San Francisco

Christensen C R 1991 Promises and practices of discussion teaching. In: Christensen C R, Garvin D A, Sweet A (eds) Education for judgement: the artistry of discussion leadership. Harvard Business School, Boston, pp. 15–34

Collins A, Brown J S, Newman S E 1989 Cognitive apprenticeship: teaching the craft of reading, writing and mathematics. In: Reswick L B (ed.) Knowing, learning and instruction: essays in honor of Robert Glaser. Lawrence Erlbaum, Hillsdale, N J, pp. 453–494

Crosby J 1996 AMEE Medical Education Guide no. 8 Learning in Small Groups. Medical Teacher 18:189–202

Entwistle N, Thompson S, 1992 Guidelines for promoting effective learning in higher education. Centre for Research on Learning and Instruction, Edinburgh

Heathfield M 1999 How to assess group work. The Times Higher Educational Supplement, March 26: 40–41

Hekelman F P, Flynn S P, Glover P B, Galazka S S 1994 Peer coaching in clinical teaching: formative assessment of a case. Evaluation of Health Professions 17:366–381

Preston-Whyte M E, Clark R, Peterson S, Fraser R C 1999 The views of academic and clinical teachers in Leicester Medical School on criteria to assess teaching competence in the small-group setting. Medical Teacher 21(5): 500–505

University of Toronto Website: http://snow.utoronto.ca/learn2/intoll.html

Walker M 1998 Small group teaching in the medical context. In: Peyton J W R (ed.) Teaching and Learning in Medical Practice. Manticore, Herts, pp. 139–154

Walton H J 1997 ASME Medical Education Booklet no. 1 Small group methods in medical teaching. Medical Education 31:457–464

Westberg J, Jason H 1996 Generic concepts and issues. In: Westberg J, Jason H (eds) Fostering learning in small groups. Springer, New York, pp. 9–10

Chapter 8
Clinical skills centres

I. McA. Ledingham   J. A. Dent

Introduction

Competency in clinical skills is part and parcel of being a doctor. Acquiring the necessary competency takes time, patience and practice in a range of suitable settings. Mastery of the process requires that students:

- understand how the body functions in health and disease
- appreciate that patients are individual, sensitive human beings whose response to disease is as varied as their fingerprints.

It also requires that tutors:

- deliver effective instruction
- act as appropriate role models.

Clinical skills are slowly acquired. Most are vulnerable to disuse atrophy. In the absence of practice the useful half-life of resuscitation skills is measured in months. Until recently medical students acquired skill in both communication and clinical examination largely at the bedside of patients in hospital. Their level of achievement was dependent on individual motivation, access to patients and quality of teaching; competency in clinical skills, as such, was rarely assessed. As a result, the ability of newly qualified doctors to perform even routine clinical procedures efficiently and effectively was very variable. First aid and resuscitation skills were notoriously limited. Such deficiencies undoubtedly contributed to stress amongst young medical practitioners and probably less than optimal care of

'Practice makes perfect' is as relevant in the context of clinical skills as with any other group of skills.

"Medical schools cannot rely on clerkship experiences alone to provide adequate basic skills training"

Ledingham & Harden 1998

"The resuscitation skills of MRCP candidates in 1994 and 1996 were objectively assessed as unsatisfactory. More should be done to raise standards"

Chin et al 1997

patients. The opportunity to correct these deficiencies after graduation was often limited.

The dawn of a new era

All this is changing. Recognition of inadequate or incomplete competence in clinical skills amongst medical graduates has led to a radical review of the approach to clinical teaching (Bligh 1995). The need for medical students and young graduates to receive structured and systematic teaching and to be assessed in a comprehensive range of clinical skills is now widely accepted. In the undergraduate curriculum appropriate learning opportunities are offered at an early stage and become progressively more sophisticated as the student's experience and knowledge base increase. A student's ability to demonstrate proficiency in clinical skills is now considered to be as important a determinant of progress as any other component of the curriculum. At postgraduate level the Royal Colleges and other educational bodies in the UK, and equivalent institutions overseas, are modifying their clinical examinations to make them more valid, reliable and fair. Clinical skills are generally assessed by one or other of the many variants of the objective structured clinical examination (OSCE) (see Chapter 33).

What do we mean by clinical skills?

Knowledge, skills and attitudes have each been defined as being of equal importance in the training of a doctor (GMC). Aspects of each of these are combined in the term 'clinical skills', which includes the following abilities:

* communication and history-taking
* professional attitudes and awareness of the ethical basis of health care
* physical examination, procedural and clinical laboratory skills
* diagnostic and therapeutic skills
* resuscitation

"Psychological distress is linked to confidence amongst SHOs in performing clinical tasks"

Williams et al 1997

"Being a successful doctor extends far beyond mere academic ability. Care, compassion and competence are equally important attributes"

GMC 1993

"Essential dimensions of competent clinical skills performance:
- *application of underpinning knowledge and understanding*
- *self-regulation and monitoring*
- *safe practice*
- *effective communication*
- *effective use of time"*

Core clinical competencies in medicine, Project report, October 1998

"A clinical skills centre reduces the difficulties encountered in medical and nursing colleges in ensuring adequate exposure to clinical problems"

Dacre et al 1996

- critical thinking, reasoning and problem-solving
- teamworking, organisation and management
- information technology.

Although the principal focus of this chapter will be the teaching of medical students and doctors, one of the major strengths of clinical skill centres is the opportunity they afford for multi- and interprofessional learning. The extent to which individual institutions offer these learning opportunities in a clinical skills centre depends on the available physical facilities and human resources (both in the centre and elsewhere) and, indeed, on the degree of commitment to this particular component of the overall teaching programme.

The development of clinical skills centres

The new approach to clinical teaching has had a variety of consequences. The most obvious has been the proliferation of clinical skills centres in which students receive training in a systematic, safe and protected fashion using effective educational strategies appropriate to their specific needs and level of experience. Experience has shown that improved acquisition of knowledge accompanies the development of clinical skills competency so that clinical skills centres are now seen to be complementary to real patient encounters in conventional clinical settings (Ledingham & Harden 1998).

Many health-care institutions have set up clinical skills learning facilities either by adapting existing space or constructing new, purpose-built areas. Physiotherapy gymnasia, former wards and even dusty garrets have been converted to this end (Bradley & Bligh 1999, Dacre et al 1996). An example of a purpose-built unit is illustrated in Figure 8.1. In this centre (Dundee) there is a mixture of demonstration rooms, resuscitation suites, a simulated ward, consultation rooms and specialised treatment areas. The variation in size, design and use of clinical skills facilities reflects differences in teaching strategy, availability of space and funding priorities.

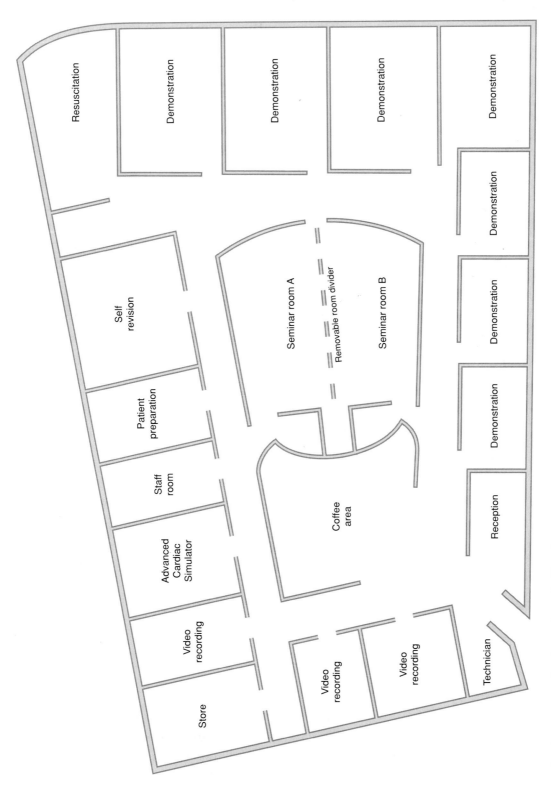

Fig. 8.1 Example of a purpose built unit

A clinical skills centre benefits from being:

- readily accessible to major users
- of adequate size
- designed, furnished and equipped to meet a range of perceived needs
- attractive to students, staff and patients
- provided with appropriate telecommunication links, and audiovisual and computer facilities.

Staff

Staffing of clinical skills centres is very variable. Some centres operate as 'drop-in' facilities to be used by clinicians according to their individual inclination. In this situation technical staff are required principally to prepare the teaching rooms and equipment and to maintain and restock as needed (Bullimore 1998). By contrast, other centres offer a comprehensive teaching programme and are responsible for providing tutors whose principal professional commitment is to teaching. This has the advantage of ensuring the educational construction and content of the clinical skills session and that students receive adequate exposure to 'core' clinical skills teaching under the supervision of a group of enthusiastic trained tutors (Scherpbier et al 1997).

A common compromise involves a small, multidisciplinary team of skills centre tutors and clinicians who together develop and coordinate delivery of the learning programmes in collaboration with convenors of the various systems. The advantage of this model is that of wider ownership of the teaching programme although the clinicians will require to undertake relevant staff development, often supplemented by appropriate 'on the job' training.

Equipment

Educational aids for clinical skills teaching have advanced beyond all recognition in recent years. Perhaps the most impressive technological advances have been in relation to manikins, telecommunications and computer facilities.

Clinical skills centres contribute best by fostering close collaboration amongst clinical teachers and by complementing and enhancing the other components of the curriculum. They should not develop an alternative form of clinical teaching.

Models and manikins

Although by no means universally suitable, realistic anatomical models and manikins are now available to facilitate training in a wide range of clinical simulations including physical examination, and diagnostic and therapeutic procedures.

Some of the present simulators have limitations and are variably effective in demonstrating pathology e.g. those used for vaginal and rectal examinations.

High-level simulators

Recent exciting additions to the tutor's toolkit are the various 'high-level' simulators. Cardiac models, such as 'Harvey' (Gordon et al 1999), provide an unrivalled learning resource for comprehensive examination of the heart and vascular system. The ultimate sophistication is the human patient simulator, which is essentially a whole-body manikin capable of being programmed to reproduce a variety of clinical presentations and respond appropriately to diagnostic and therapeutic interventions on the part of the student. These models can be used for small or large groups as required.

"The expanded use of simulation for training and certification is inevitable"

Gordon et al 1999

Video recordings

The opportunity for video recording of individual student performance is highly rated by student and tutor alike and provides valuable feedback on the acquisition of clinical skills. A bank of pre-recorded videos provides a valuable resource for demonstrating aspects of clinical examination.

Telecommunications

Telecommunication links are particularly valuable in allowing live clinical sessions (e.g. a patient consultation, physical examination, procedural demonstration or operating theatre activity) to be relayed to larger groups of students, either from elsewhere in the centre or from a distance.

Computers and the World Wide Web

The role of the computer to enhance clinical skills learning has yet to be clarified but its value has been demonstrated in interactive PC-based tutorials and formative assessment programmes. The strength of this teaching medium lies in its ability to provide instant interactive feedback involving a range of rich media resources, e.g. high-quality medical images, video files, sound clips and access to the World Wide Web and its attendant resources.

Human resources

In addition to models and manikins clinical skills centres make extensive use of the human resources at their disposal. These include the students themselves, simulated patients and ultimately real patients. Each resource group has its advantages and care is required in making the appropriate choice.

Student colleagues

In communication skills training, for example, role playing by students may be a useful experience, particularly prior to exposure to simulated patients. Similarly, in the context of history-taking and physical examination valuable lessons may be learned not only by the student performing the interview or examination but by the role-playing 'patient'. It is important to remember that different cultures respond in different ways to examining and being examined. Intrusive examinations need to be handled with discretion. Experience of peer group activities in one centre (Ledingham & Harden 1998) suggests that once initial reluctance on the part of the students (and some staff) is overcome the situation is readily accepted and even appreciated.

Students from other disciplines

Some activities may be shared with nursing or dental students, e.g. oral cavity examination or measurement of pulse and blood pressure.

Simulated patients

Members of the lay public may be trained to act as patients and reproduce a clinical history in a consistent manner. Standardisation of performance is particularly important during 'high-stake' examinations.

A moderate amount of training is required for simulated patients to feel comfortable in their role and to help them understand more of the background of their simulated illness. They also need guidance on how to handle the student group and to know how to ask for 'time out' of their role if they become uncomfortable at any time during the interview. During teaching sessions the use of simulated patients offers certain advantages. It:

- controls the complexity of the learning situation
- allows repeat consultations and physical examinations
- permits mistakes to be made within a safe environment
- encourages direct feedback
- is independent of 'real' patient availability
- directly involves members of the local community in the health-care learning process.

In the early stages of the undergraduate medical curriculum simulated patients are a very important bridge between structured clinical skills instruction and actual clinical experience in conventional practice settings.

Real patients
Patients with stable clinical features have always played an important part in clinical examinations. Nowadays their role is being substantially extended and they may be rehearsed in several modifications of their history as part of the regular teaching sessions. They may also receive instruction in objective and constructive feedback. In some centres, particularly in North America, real patients with appropriate educational backgrounds have been recruited as 'patient instructors' and can become as effective clinical skills teachers as clinicians.

How do we teach clinical skills?

Educational strategies
Clinical skills tutors need to be aware of the overall learning outcomes of the course to which they are

"Patients can be useful to students in a number of different ways. Consider how they can contribute to teaching in the clinical skills facility. There are advantages in involving the community in the development of the next generation of health-care professionals"

Ledingham & Harden 1998

contributing. Careful consideration must then be given as to how best to address the specific objectives of the clinical teaching session for which they are responsible. In general terms, these are likely to reflect current trends in educational strategy, such as those summarised in the SPICES model (Harden et al 1984):

Student-centred. Students are given more responsibility for their own learning. More emphasis is placed on meeting the needs of the individual student.

Problem-based learning. Clinical skills instruction may be part of an overall PBL strategy or may introduce this approach to learning.

Integration. Clinical skills learning affords an excellent opportunity to unite the different subjects and disciplines, and promote the concept of the scientific basis of clinical practice.

Community-orientated. Although clinical skills centres are often for convenience sited within hospitals they should reflect the totality of health care and involve input from all relevant professionals.

Electives. Competency in clinical skills is a core curricular requirement but students may choose to study the subject in more depth either in elective programmes or special study modules, e.g. as a multidisciplinary learning aid.

Systems-based. By means of clearly defined sessional commitments all students should experience an adequate range of clinical skills instruction and achieve an adequate level of performance throughout their course.

Teaching methods

Clinical skills teaching may vary from the relatively straightforward didactic demonstration of individual skills to quite complex, case-based scenarios of which clinical skills learning is an integral component.

The usual approach to learning in clinical skills centres is by small group, student-centred, interactive sessions (see Chapter 7) in which tutors act as facilitators rather than information-givers. A typical undergraduate learning session lasts 2 hours and may involve tutors from all the health-care professions, working in an integrated, collaborative manner. Skill acquisition is always in context rather than in isolation. Role-playing in loosely structured and relevant scenarios prepare students for subsequent exposure to the 'real thing' in both hospital and community settings.

Example 1   Communication skills
In a plenary session students view two videos illustrating good and bad examples of the doctor–patient interview and make notes of the good and bad points in each. In small groups they are then individually videoed as they begin a simple interview with a simulated patient. The video they have just made is then discussed in the group with reference to the points observed in the initial session.

Example 2   Integrated clinical skills teaching
Each week of the systems-based course is devoted to the study of one core clinical problem. During the neck and shoulder pain week in the musculoskeletal system students learn how to take an appropriate history to differentiate between the various possible causes of the presentation. They learn how to examine the neck and shoulder and during general practice or outpatient attachments have the opportunity to see a variety of patients with related conditions. In the wards they have opportunities to see pre- and post-operative patients with shoulder surgery.

Previous reference has been made to the importance of staff development in relation to the structured teaching of clinical skills. Equally important is to observe certain basic rules:

- to arrive for the teaching session in good time (preferably 15 minutes before the session starts)
- to be suitably prepared (tutor instructions are invariably provided beforehand)
- to behave courteously to colleagues, students and support staff.

"The clinician as role model exerts a potent influence – either good or bad"

Maintenance of clinical skills necessitates continued relevant exposure and application.

A visit to the clinical skills centre at least the day before generally improves the smooth running of the session.

Assessment

Assessment of student performance is an integral part of clinical skills learning and plays an important role in determining students' behaviour. The clinical skills centre can contribute to assessment in a variety of ways. Regular formative assessment may be incorporated into the learning programme and the associated direct feedback has been shown to be highly appreciated. Students also have the opportunity to experience at first hand and prepare themselves for the challenge of the summative OSCEs at the end of the course. Student learning of clinical skills may also be facilitated by the completion of clinical skills checklists and case presentations, the latter being particularly useful in developing written communication skills.

Clinical skills centres and their staff are commonly involved in the preparation and delivery of the summative OSCEs. This includes not only assisting in the design and organisation of the OSCE stations but also providing a setting for the examination itself. Computers are playing an increasingly important role in the conduct of the examination and in the marking of the individual stations. The latter facilitates the development of personal assessment profiles, which are helpful in subsequent student counselling, and the preparation of further specific learning programmes.

Summary

Students' training in clinical skills is moving away from being exclusively dependent on ad hoc experiences with hospital patients to a structured programme of learning in a clinical skills centre. In this stress-free environment students can practise communication and examination skills without embarrassment or negative criticism and without interfering with patient management or well-being. Models, manikins and colleagues, as well as simulated patients and volunteer real patients, may be progressively available to facilitate training and in some cases provide constructive feedback. The programme of clinical skills training can be constructed using a mixture of educational input from dedicated skills centre staff and clinical input from systems tutors.

The whole programme can be integrated with other clinical exposure in primary care, wards and outpatient clinics and by telecommunication links with other resources or centres.

References and further reading

Bligh J 1995 The clinical skills unit. Postgraduate Medical Journal 71:730–732

Bradley P, Bligh J 1999 One year's experience with a clinical skills resource centre. Medical Education 33:114–120

Bullimore D W 1998 The clinical skills learning centre. In: Study Skills and Tomorrow's Doctors. W B Saunders, London, pp. 126–134

Chin D, Morphet J, Coady E, Davidson C 1997 Assessment of cardiopulmonary resuscitation in the membership examination of the Royal College of Physicians. Journal of the Royal College of Physicians 31:198–201

Dacre J, Nicol M, Holroyd D, Ingram D 1996 The development of a clinical skills centre. Journal of the Royal College of Physicians 30:318–324

General Medical Council 1993 Tomorrow's doctors. General Medical Council, London

Gordon M S, Issenberg S B, Mayer J W, Felner J M 1999 Developments in the use of simulators and multimedia computer systems in medical education. Medical teacher 21:32–36

Harden R M, Sowden S, Dunn W R 1984 Some educational strategies in curriculum development: the SPICES model. Medical Education 18: 284–297

Ledingham I McA, Harden R M 1998 Twelve tips for setting up a clinical skills teaching facility. Medical Teacher 20:503–507

Scherpbier A J J A, van der Vleuten C P M, Rethans J J, van der Steeg A F N 1997 Advances in Medical Education. Kluver, Dordrecht

Remmen R, Derese A, Scherbier A et al 1999 Can medical schools rely on clerkships to train students in basic clinical skills? Medical Education 33:600–605

Williams S, Dale J, Gluckman E, Willesley A 1997 Senior house officers' work related stressors, psychological distress, and confidence in performing clinical tasks in accident and emergency: a questionnaire study. British Medical Journal 314:713–718

Chapter 9
Hospital wards

J. A. Dent

Introduction

The clinical application of knowledge acquired in lectures and the clinical skills required for practice have traditionally been acquired by apprenticeship in a hospital ward. Fundamental to this experience has been the consultant-teaching ward round, but this has not been without its shortcomings. Late starts and inappropriate comments may discourage and alienate students, and lack of preparation and an absence of student orientation may mean that this valuable resource is not used to maximum advantage. In addition, the smaller number of in-patients now to be seen in hospital limits the number suitable for student teaching, while the increased size of the student group attending puts further pressure on all resources and on the curriculum timetable for ward-based teaching.

Despite these problems ward-based teaching provides an optimal opportunity for the demonstration and observation of physical examination, communication skills and interpersonal skills and for role modelling a humanistic approach to the patient. Not surprisingly, therefore, bedside teaching and medical clerking were deemed the most valuable methods of teaching by a survey of medical students (Ward, Moody & Mayberry 1997). Nevertheless, the role of bedside teaching has been declining in medical schools since the early 1960s from 37% to 16% (LaCombe 1997) as interest in technology, imaging and laboratory investigations has increased at the expense of direct contact with patients.

"To study the phenomena of disease without books is to sail an uncharted sea whilst to study books without patients is not to go to sea at all"

Sir William Osler (1849–1919) quoted by Nair, Coughlan & Hensley 1997

"Most medical students are taught by a system of negative reinforcement in the form of sarcastic remarks and derogatory comments"

Newton 1987

"Bedside teaching is the only site where history taking, physical examination, empathy and a caring attitude can be taught and learnt by example"

Nair, Coughlan & Hensley 1997

The 'Learning Triad'

Ward-based teaching brings together the 'Learning Triad' of patient, student and tutor.

Patients

Although for various reasons fewer patients are now available in hospital, the hospital ward still provides an important venue for clinical teaching. Suitable patients for clinical teaching should be selected with care and must be sufficiently well to be seen by students. For inexperienced students it is best if patients can communicate easily and succinctly and if possible have uncomplicated clinical histories and physical findings. It may be helpful for junior students to have access to 'healthy' patients who will provide valuable experience of normal anatomy and physiology.

Patients should be invited to participate and have the opportunity to decline to take part without feeling intimidated. They should be adequately briefed so that they know what will be expected of them, feel a part of the discussion and even give feedback to students afterwards. The majority then enjoy the experience and feel they have helped the students to learn. Concerns about breach of confidentiality and about provoking increased anxiety have been shown to be unfounded (Nair, Coughlan & Hensley 1997). Depending on the model of ward teaching to be used, a variety of patients will be required for varying lengths of time but consideration should be given to patients' needs and the possibility that phlebotomists, radiographers and visitors may also need to see the patient.

Students

Usually between two and five students are quoted as the optimal number for bedside teaching. They must be appropriately dressed with white coats and name badges. They should expect to behave professionally on the ward in a manner appropriate for student doctors, introducing themselves to staff and patients and clearly stating the purpose of their visit.

"Learners think that BST is an effective method for teaching professional skills and that most patients enjoy it"

Nair, Coughlan & Hensley 1997

Before beginning, students should be briefed so that they understand the purpose of the session and the goals to be achieved. Any warnings about the patient conditions to be seen should be given and checks made on students' level of initial understanding. When reflecting on their experiences students have found ward-based teaching the most valuable way of developing clinical skills. However, initially, some may feel intimidated by an unfamiliar environment and the proximity of nursing staff and be embarrassed when putting personal questions to a stranger. In addition they may feel anxious if unsure of their knowledge base or clinical abilities and fearful of consultant criticism of their inadequacies (Moss & McManus 1992). As a result some students position themselves towards the back of the group round the bedside to avoid participation while in contrast confident students can monopolise conversations with patients and tutors. An observant tutor is required to redress the balance and ensure that all students participate and anxieties are allayed.

Tutors

Whether they acknowledge it or not tutors are powerful role models for students, especially for those in the early years of the course. It is therefore important that they demonstrate the knowledge, skills and attitudes appropriate for a doctor.

Appropriate attitude

Tutors responsible for timetabled ward teaching must arrive punctually, introduce themselves to the students and demonstrate an enthusiastic approach to the session. A negative impression at this stage will have an immediate negative effect on the students' attitude and on the value of the session. Tutors must show a professional approach to the patients and interact appropriately with them and the students.

Not only permanent members of staff but also trainees and junior doctors may be involved in ward teaching. Each brings a different perspective of patient care which is valuable for student learning, but often they will have received no specific preparation for the teaching session

"The essential feature is enthusiasm on the part of the teacher"

Rees 1987

If you don't know the answer to a student's question be honest and say so.

and will not know how any particular session fits into the totality of the students' clinical experience at a particular stage of the course. Tutors' individual approach to clinical examination will also differ as examination technique is not usually standardised within the medical school. While it may be of benefit for more confident students to observe a variety of different approaches to clinical skills, weaker ones will find this lack of consistency confusing. Ideally, tutors should be briefed so that they are familiar with the approach to physical examination taught in the clinical skills centre and be conversant with the levels of expertise required of students at the various stages of the medical course.

Appropriate knowledge

Six domains of knowledge are required for the clinical tutor to function effectively (Irby 1994):

- Knowledge of medicine – involving integrated background knowledge of basic sciences, clinical sciences and clinical experience
- Knowledge of patients – a familiarity with disease and illness from experience of previous patients
- Knowledge of the context – an awareness of patients in their social context and at their stage of treatment
- Knowledge of learners – an understanding of the students' present stage in the course and of the curriculum requirements for that stage
- Knowledge of the general principles of teaching, including:
  — getting students involved in the learning process by indicating its relevance
  — asking questions, perhaps using the patient as an example of a problem-solving approach to the condition
  — keeping students' attention by indicating the relevance of the topic to another situation
  — relating the case being presented to broader aspects of the curriculum
  — meeting individual needs by responding to specific questions and providing personal tuition

You can maintain your relation with patients while talking to the students by keeping your hand on their shoulder or wrist.

"Well, that's something we should both look up this evening"
A senior clinician in answer to a student's question during a teaching ward round

— being realistic and selective so as to choose relevant cases to be seen

— providing feedback by critiquing case reports, presentations or examination technique

- Knowledge of case-based teaching scripts – the ability to demonstrate the patient as a representative of a certain illness; the specifics of the case are used but added to from other knowledge and experiences in order to make further generalised comments about the condition.

Appropriate skills

If demonstrating clinical tasks to students on the ward tutors must ensure that they are competent in performing them, that they are conversant with any new equipment and that they do not display inappropriate 'shortcuts'.

The ward

The learning triad requires a learning environment in which to function. Wards are not always ideal places for teaching but with some thought they can be made more suitable.

Ward teaching should not take place when meals, cleaners or visitors are expected. It helps if the staff and patients are expecting the teaching session at a certain time so that X-rays and case notes can be ready and patients do not have to be retrieved from the day room or X-ray department.

The use of a side room for pre- or post-ward round discussion provides a useful alternative venue for discussion once the patients have been seen. Occasionally a member of the nursing staff may be present in the teaching session to add multiprofessional input to the patient care discussion.

A teaching ward round deals with patients not diseases. It develops students' thinking processes and introduces an approach to patients that they will follow for the rest of their working lives as doctors (Rees 1987).

Educational objectives

Many of the educational objectives of the medical course can be practised to different extents by students at different stages of the course while they are working in the wards:

- Clinical skills. For junior students there are opportunities to become proficient at normal physical examination while more senior students gain practice in eliciting abnormal physical signs.
- Communication skills. Many and various opportunities exist for students to practise communication skills.
- Clinical reasoning. Students can observe this in practice by junior and senior staff.
- Practical procedures. Venepuncture, bladder catheterisation and cannulation of a peripheral vein are procedures which are readily available on most wards for students to practise.
- Patient investigation and management. There are many opportunities for students to observe and discuss aspects of both of these.
- Data interpretation and retrieval. Interpretation of laboratory reports and accessing scientific papers for reference are examples.
- Professional skills. The observation of both junior and senior doctors in their working relationship with other health-care professionals should help students develop role models for professional behaviour.
- Transferable skills. Many of the abilities acquired in the ward setting will be of value in other doctor–patient situations.
- Attitude and ethics. It is hoped that appropriate attitudes and ethics can be observed by the students in their ward attachments.

All these aspects can be seen in the context of the patient as an individual rather than in a purely theoretical context as seen in lectures. Students should be encouraged to return to the ward in private study time to practise clinical skills further. There is unlikely to be sufficient time for the session to be used formally for

"A good consultant is accessible, approachable and friendly, with the power of a god, the patience of a saint and the sense of humour of an undergraduate"

Lowry 1987

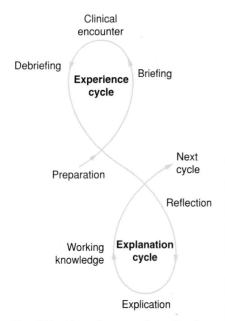

Fig. 9.1 Experience and explication cycles (redrawn from Cox 1993, with modifications)

formative assessment but the session can be used to check on individual students' competencies in small tasks.

Strategies

Planning bedside teaching

A plan of two linked cycles has been described (Cox 1993) to maximise the students' learning from each patient contact. The first, the 'experience cycle', involves student preparation and briefing to ensure that they are aware of what they are going to see and the opportunities available for learning. This is followed by the clinical experience of interacting with their patient, which may include discussing the illness, examining physical signs and thinking about management. The 'experience cycle' concludes with debriefing after leaving the patient when the data is seen and interpreted and any misperceptions or misunderstandings are clarified. The 'Experience cycle' maximises the value of time spent with the patients. It is followed by the 'Explanation cycle'. This cycle begins with reflection when students are encouraged to consider their recent clinical interaction in the light of previous experiences. This is done by explication as the clinical experiences are understood at different levels and finally a working knowledge is synthesised which prepares the students for seeing a subsequent patient. (see Fig. 9.1)

Logbooks and portfolios

The variety of clinical conditions available for a teaching session at any particular time will inevitably vary so ward-based teaching will of necessity be opportunistic. Some form of documentation is required to ensure that all students see a comparable mix of patients. Logbooks or palmtop computers can be used to document patients seen and to keep a record of the learning points (Davis & Dent 1994). These can be reviewed periodically and future sessions directed to making good any deficits.

Students' formal documentation of full case presentations can be collated as required and submitted for formative assessment later.

Task-based learning
A list of tasks to be performed or procedures to be observed and carried out is usually a course requirement.

Problem-based learning
The patient's complaint can be used as the focus of a problem-based learning exercise in which basic sciences and clinical sciences can be integrated.

Study guides
A prescribed list of conditions to be seen in the ward may be laid out in the study guide with the learning points to be achieved documented for each.

Models for managing learning in the ward

Shadowing a junior doctor
This model of learning has been formally adopted as part of the final year by some medical schools. Students spend a block of 4 or 6 weeks sharing the work and experiences of a junior doctor. Ideally this takes place in the unit that the students will work in themselves on qualifying. Opportunities exist to share in carrying out ward tasks, formulating management plans and prescribing.

Patient-centred model
Students attached to a ward for a period of time can be allocated a certain number of patients each who they initially admit and then follow throughout their time in the hospital. They are made responsible for presenting them on ward rounds and should be able to comment on their current investigations, laboratory results and present status. Opportunities exist for practice in examination and communication skills. Patients can be followed for X-ray and to surgery and even visited at home so the student can assess the impact of illness and convalescence on the patient in the context of their home environment.

Apprenticeship model

The student joins a normal working ward round but does not work as a team member. There are opportunities to observe the input of all those taking part, and to practise presentation skills and possibly practical procedures. Students' confidence is increased by interaction with senior doctors and other professionals, by observing the working practice of junior doctors and by seeing patients individually. There may be opportunities to practise decision-making. However, if there is no formal teaching the details of the ward round discussion are unlikely to be understood and weaker students may be ignored. Students may find that the only activities available for them are mundane ward chores although others may have opportunities to perform some practical procedures.

Grand rounds

In this traditional model a student group tags along at the end of an extensive consultant-led ward round which may include other senior clinicians, trainees, junior doctors and other health-care professionals such as nurses and therapists. There are opportunities to observe multiprofessional interaction and exposure to a variety of patients. However, students remain remote from the decision-making and are unlikely to understand the reasons considered as there is no opportunity for interaction with clinicians or patients in this model.

Business ward round

If a group of students is attached to a routine business ward round there is little opportunity for talking to patients but opportunities to ask and be asked questions exist to a varying degree.

Teaching ward round

This specially created ward round is aimed at taking students to a small number of selected patients to provide opportunities for them to see physical signs and hear aspects of the case history.

Reserved students may have little opportunity to interact with patients individually compared to their

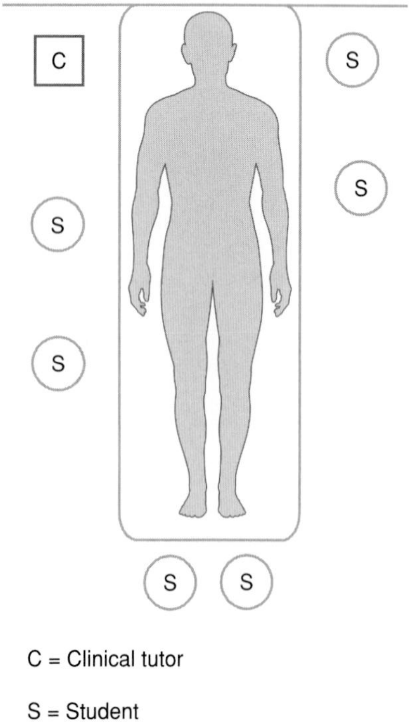

C = Clinical tutor

S = Student

Fig. 9.2 Demonstrator model

more self-confident counterparts' but opportunities to
ask and be asked questions exist to a varying degree:

- Demonstrator model (see Fig. 9.2). The clinical tutor
  demonstrates aspects of the case history and physical
  examination to the students
- Tutor model (see Fig. 9.3). The clinical tutor stands to
  the side and critiques each student in turn as they
  enquire into aspects of the history and carry out
  aspects of the physical examination.
- Observer model (see Fig. 9.4). The clinical tutor
  distances him or herself from the student–patient
  interaction and observes a single student or pair of
  students in a longer portion of history-taking or
  examination, providing feedback to them all at the end
  as they discuss their findings and clinical
  interpretation.

Report-back model

Working singly or in pairs, students take a history and
examination without supervision and subsequently report
back to the tutor in a tutorial room or side room to present
the case and receive feedback on content and delivery.

Opportunities are given for students to practise their
communication skills in their own time and to
demonstrate their presentation skills and knowledge of
the case but their bedside technique has been
unsupervised so no feedback on this can be given.

Clinical conference

A patient from the ward is presented in a side room at a
conference of senior clinicians which students attend.
Diagnostic and management problems are discussed by
the group once the patient has left. Students have the
opportunity to observe the multifaceted management of
difficult cases and the spectrum of professional opinion
which may be displayed.

Summary

Ward-based teaching offers unique opportunities for
student learning which, for a variety of reasons, are

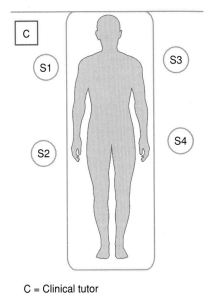

C = Clinical tutor

S = Student

Fig. 9.3 Tutor model

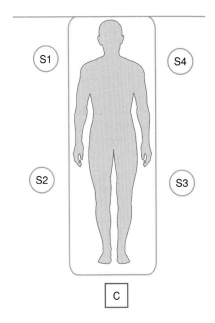

C = Clinical tutor

S = Student

Fig. 9.4 Observer model

becoming less efficiently utilised than previously. To attain maximum benefit from ward-based teaching, patients, students and tutors must each be appropriately prepared and the educational objectives to be attained acknowledged. Various strategies can be used to advantage in both the planning and organisation of ward teaching. A variety of styles of ward-based teaching have been described illustrating the advantages and disadvantages of each for the students involved.

References and further reading

Cox K 1993 Planning bedside teaching. Medical Journal of Australia 158:493–495

Davis M H, Dent J A 1994 Comparison of student learning in the out-patient clinic and ward round. Medical Education 28:208–212

Irby D M 1994 What clinical teachers in medicine need to know. Academic Medicine 69:333–342

Kroenke K, Omori D M, Landry F J, Ludcey C R 1997 Bedside teaching. Southern Medical Journal 90:1069–1074

LaCombe M A 1997 On bedside teaching. Annals of Internal Medicine 126:217–220

Lowry S 1992 What is a good consultant? As the junior doctor sees it. British Medical Journal 294:1601

Moss F, McManus I C 1992 The anxieties of new clinical students. Medical Education 26:17–20

Nair B R, Coughlan J L, Hensley M J 1997 Student and patient perspectives on bedside teaching. Medical Education 31:341–346

Newton D F 1987 What is a good Consultant? 'A worm's eye view'. British Medical Journal 295:106–107

Rees J 1987 How to do it: take a teaching ward round. British Medical Journal 295:424–425

Ward B, Moody G, Mayberry J F 1997 The views of medical students and junior doctors on pre-graduate clinical teaching. Postgraduate Medical Journal 73:723–725

Chapter 10
Ambulatory care

J. A. Dent

Introduction

When teaching in the ward today a clinician will find an environment quite different from that of a few years ago. Fewer patients are available as more conditions are treated on an outpatient basis and the duration of in-patient stay has been reduced by changes in surgical practice and rehabilitation. Current in-patients may be unavailable for bedside teaching if they are acutely ill or undergoing immediate pre-operative investigations. Finally the student group attending may be larger and more junior than previously seen for ward teaching. A more difficult burden of clinical teaching therefore falls on a smaller, sicker group of in-patients and ward-based teaching has become less suited to the undergraduate programme than it used to be.

Consequently facilities have been sought elsewhere and recent interest has shifted to the development of clinical teaching in ambulatory care.

Why teach in ambulatory care?

In contrast the ambulatory care setting offers a variety of clinical situations and a range of clinical conditions not now managed by in-patient care. The role of other health-care professionals and support services can more readily be appreciated here as patients are seen in an environment more closely resembling their home situation and more closely linked with primary care. With adequate numbers of patients available student/patient interaction can take place in a

"More medicine is now practiced in the ambulatory setting, making the inpatient arena less representative of the actual practice of medicine and a less desirable place for students to glean the fundamentals of clinical care and problem solving than in the past"

Fincher & Albritton 1993

non-threatening environment where sufficient time and appropriate supervision can be made available to maximise learning opportunities.

Where should ambulatory care teaching take place?

A number of frequently underutilised venues may be used:

- general outpatient clinics
- specialist or tertiary referral clinics
- multiprofessional clinics where staff from a variety of disciplines see patients together (e.g. hand clinic)
- combined clinics where different specialists consult together on a combined management problem (e.g. rheumatoid clinic)
- 'drop-in' clinics where patients may seek advice from a variety of health-care workers (e.g. diabetic foot clinic)
- clinical investigation unit (e.g. endoscopy suite)
- day surgery unit
- dedicated ambulatory care teaching centre (ACTC).

Self-help groups or community services who have bases in the outpatient department may also be available.

When should ambulatory care teaching be timetabled?

Teaching in the ambulatory care setting may take place throughout the curriculum. In the earlier years of study, when communication and examination skills are still being developed, visits to the ACTC act as a bridge between practice with simulated patients and manikins in the clinical skills centre and clinical exposure in a routine outpatient clinic. In the later clinical years, when more extensive clinical experience is required, students can be timetabled either for periodic visits or for extended attachments to different venues in ambulatory care.

What educational objectives can be realised?

In ward-based teaching the acquisition of expertise in certain competencies or outcomes is usually emphasised:

- knowledge
- clinical skills
- clinical reasoning
- patient management
- investigations
- information handling.

In the outpatient setting patients are seen nearer to the context of their own social circumstances and are therefore understood to be retaining individual responsibility for their own health. Their attendance at the clinic is part of the continuum of the management of their illness. Opportunities are therefore available for students to practise additional competencies or outcomes including:

- attitudes and ethics
- resource allocation
- health promotion and disease prevention
- practical procedures
- transferable skills.

How to facilitate learning in ambulatory care

Learning strategies

It is important to organise the content of an ambulatory care session so that these specified educational objectives can be met. Strategies are required to regulate the types of clinical condition to be seen. A structured logbook (Dent & Davis 1995) may be used to prescribe the conditions or tasks of core importance to be seen during the attachment and to document the content of each patient contact. The acronym EPITOME has been used:

- **e**nquiry into symptoms
- **p**hysical examination
- **i**nterpretation of investigations

Be sure you know the educational objectives which the students should be able to achieve. Identify which of these can be illustrated by the learning opportunities your clinic can provide.

Ensure that students recognise opportunities to relate the educational objectives of their course to the experiences provided in the outpatient setting. Do they have a logbook to complete?

"The variability and potentially worrisome gaps in the students' experiences in the ambulatory care settings studied are probably representative of students' experiences in such settings"

Gruppen et al 1993

Decide which model you are going to use in your clinic depending on how many rooms are available for you to use and how many members of staff are available to help with the clinic. Don't be afraid to change models during the clinic to vary the session for the students and yourself.

It appears that in most cases students have been fitted into existing clinics or patterns of teaching, with insufficient effort given to achieving the maximal educational benefit of the student"

Feltovich, Mast & Soler 1987

- **t**echnical procedure undertaken
- **o**ptions of diagnosis
- **m**anagement
- **e**ducation of the patient.

Managing student/patient interactions in a routine outpatient clinic

A variety of management models can be used to ensure that students maximise the opportunities to attain educational objectives without disrupting the delivery of the patient service. Students may take part to a variety of extents ranging from full participator to pure observer, but without satisfactory models their interaction with patients may become either unrestricted and prolong the clinic or inhibited and lead to passivity.

The choice of model depends to some extent on the number of rooms and staff available and on the number of students but in each model the student should be encouraged away from passive observation towards active learning and participation.

One student/one clinician

'Sitting-in' model
This model works well either when there is only one student, or when the student is inexperienced in clinical skills, or in specialist and multidisciplinary clinics.

An individual student's requirements are met by one-to-one teaching and students can interact confidently with the clinician and patients. However, student/patient interaction may become limited if the clinician conducts the interview without involving the student, while a reserved student may feel vulnerable in this setting and participate minimally (see Fig. 10.1).

Apprenticeship model
The student assumes the role of clinician and interviews the patient while the clinician acts as observer.

Active student/patient interaction is provided which reinforces the learning experience. Some students may feel intimidated when performing under observation and aspects of the consultation may have to be repeated by the clinician if relevant points have been overlooked. The duration of the clinic may be prolonged.

Team-member model
If a separate room is available the student can interview and examine a patient alone before presenting the findings when joined by the clinician or when reporting back to the main consulting room. The student has the freedom to interview and examine the patient without constraints and the clinician can proceed with the remainder of the clinic as usual. However, the student will miss other patients attending in the meantime.

Several students/one clinician
It becomes more difficult to organise teaching in a routine outpatient clinic when several students are present.

Grandstand model
Often four or more students are in the consulting room together and crowd around the clinician in an attempt to observe and hear the consultation. Interaction with both patient and clinician is limited and, as patients feel threatened by the large audience, the clinician's interaction with the patient may also be inhibited.

Supervising model
If several rooms are available the clinician can select a patient for each student to see individually in a separate room. After a suitable time, during which the clinician can see other patients, it is possible to go to each room in turn to hear each student report on the interview (see Fig. 10.2). The students have time and space to interview and examine their patient at their own pace and benefit from individual feedback on their performance. However, only a limited number of patients are seen by any one student and patients' time may be wasted while waiting for their turn. The clinician's time is heavily occupied hearing the presentations from each student so inevitably the clinic is prolonged.

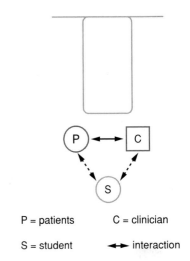

P = patients   C = clinician

S = student   ◄─► interaction

Fig. 10.1   Student/Clinician and student/patient interaction is variable

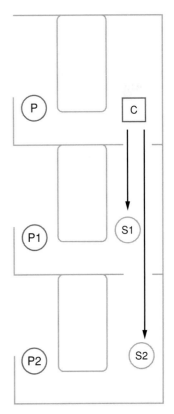

Fig. 10.2   Students practise consultations under supervision

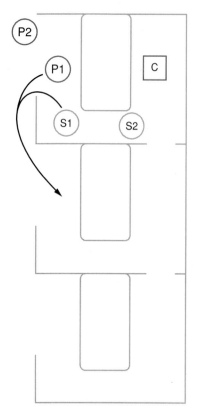

Fig. 10.3   Students see patients individually after initial consultation

"By using this model I found I could easily manage a group of students with varied abilities"

A senior clinician

Report-back model
Patients are distributed to students as described above but at an appointed time each student returns to the main consulting room to present his or her patient in turn. Students have time and space to interview and examine their patient at their own pace and subsequently see something of several other patients. Unfortunately patients may have to wait twice, first to be seen by the student and secondly for the presentation to the clinician.

Breakout model
All the students sit in with the clinician and observe the whole consultation. This model is particularly appropriate with inexperienced students or in a specialist clinic when particular clinical skills can be demonstrated. Each student then takes a patient in turn to interview or examine at his or her own pace in another room. Laboratory or radiological request forms may be completed at this time and side-room procedures observed. The clinic can be kept to time as the clinician is saved from completing routine forms. The students have opportunities to interview or examine patients individually and to practise transferable skills. Students see something of most patients attending but miss others while occupied with their own (see Fig. 10.3).

Several students/several clinicians
If two clinicians are available the task of organising students becomes easier.

Division and 'flip/flop' models
The student group can be divided between the clinicians in the clinic who then follow the 'sitting-in' or 'grandstand' models as before and interchange the group at half-time. In this model a variety of styles of clinical practice may be observed.

Shuttle model
The clinicians see patients simultaneously as usual and call the students in to see selected cases as they present

(see Fig. 10.4). This model maintains student involvement in the clinic and interesting cases are not missed. There may be insufficient time for individual student/patient interaction as patients are often only seen as 'demonstrations'.

Tutor model

If several rooms are available the student group may remain with one clinician who may then use any of the previous models as appropriate for the abilities of the students attending. Selected patients are seen while the remainder are seen by the other clinicians present. The opportunity now exists for students to see only appropriate, selected patients and the tutor is freed from the time constraints of the routine clinic to concentrate on teaching.

Managing students in day case surgery

Although currently underused, attachments to day surgery units can provide opportunities for students to interact with patients following the familiar in-patient ward approach or a skills-based approach (Seabrook et al 1998). As well as experience in general, pre-operative assessment and a variety of minor surgical conditions will be seen which are not now managed as in-patient procedures. Experiences in diagnosis, simple operations and rehabilitation are available together with multiprofessional teaching opportunities. As the numbers of patients attending is usually large and patients of necessity are otherwise well it is relatively easy to structure a teaching session to maximise the educational objectives to be achieved without impeding the throughput of patients.

Managing student/patient interactions in an ambulatory care teaching centre (ACTC)

A specific area in the outpatient department can be developed as an ACTC. This provides appropriate space and serves as a focus for student contact with both patients and the other members of the health-care team.

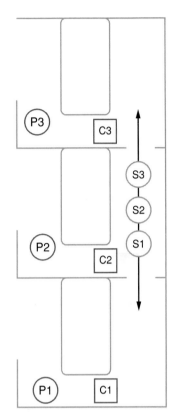

Fig. 10.4   Students see interesting patients but have little opportunity to relate to them

Appropriate space should be available for small group activities, for individual student/patient interviews (with or without observation by the tutor) and for patient demonstrations by other health-care workers. In this protected environment privacy is guaranteed and students feel comfortable to practise and make mistakes free from embarrassment or time constraints.

The tutor coordinating the session may follow any of the previous models for managing student/patient interactions and students may be interchanged between different tutors supervising various activities such as practice at history-taking, examination or patient demonstration. A store of video tapes to illustrate communication skills and clinical examination provides a useful backup resource.

Who is available for teaching?

Patients

Referred patients
Appropriate patients can be invited to visit the ACTC after their outpatient consultation. Clinical histories or signs relevant to the students' stage in the curriculum can then be demonstrated by the tutor in the 'grandstand' format, or students may be given the opportunity to interview patients either independently or under supervision as in the 'report-back' or 'supervising' models. Learning opportunities can be developed to focus on particular educational objectives. The cooperation of clinicians and nurses working in adjacent clinics is required if patients are to be referred for teaching and the willingness of patients both to be seen by students and to add further unexpected time to their outpatient visit is required. There is little control over the nature of the patients referred and their complaints may be inappropriate for the students' stage of learning; consequently it may be difficult for the tutor to utilise them efficiently. If no patients are referred the model cannot work and backup resources are required.

> *"Medical education in general is characterised by the paradox of students' need to learn by trial and error without the luxury and opportunity of making mistakes"*
>
> Woolliscroft & Schwenk 1989

> *"Many patients have actually enjoyed their interactions with students and have been glad to take part in their education"*
>
> Krackov et al 1993

Invited patients

Patients with good histories or stable clinical signs or those who have already taken part in teaching sessions are invited to join a 'bank' of real patients willing to attend on future occasions. In a systems-based course patients with relevant conditions can be invited at the appropriate time. An administrator is required to facilitate this system-sensitive group of patients for optimum advantage. In this model a patient is guaranteed to be present at the beginning of the session. The tutor has therefore had time in advance to select a management model for the session and to prepare the content for maximal educational advantage.

Simulated patients

Occasionally simulated patients can be introduced amongst the real patients. Working from a previously arranged script these volunteers can provide the students with opportunities to practise a particular competence in such fields as attitudes or ethics in a more realistic environment than the clinical skills centre (see Fig. 10.5).

Staff

Tutors

Tutors with a particular aptitude for clinical teaching who are not under constraint from a concurrent service commitment are required. Effective teaching is facilitated if this person actively involves students in the learning process and sets a good example of patient care skills. In the philosophy of teaching only factual knowledge designated as being of 'core' importance, a 'content expert' is not required but the tutor should be able to direct students to appropriate educational objectives and additional learning resources.

Junior staff

A senior tutor can help junior staff unfamiliar with teaching in this venue by demonstrating the approach required in the ACTC. Formal staff development sessions are also needed.

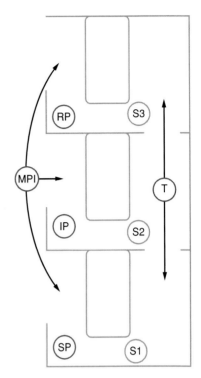

SP = simulated patient
IP   = invited patient
RP = referred patient
T   = tutor
MPI = multi professional input

Fig. 10.5   ACTC model

Multiprofessional staff

Other health-care professionals working in the ambulatory care setting can contribute to the teaching programme so in addition students can have the opportunity to observe the contribution made to patient care by professions allied to medicine:

- occupational therapist
- physiotherapist
- dietitian
- speech therapist
- chiropodist
- social worker.

Students

Medical students at different stages of the curriculum can be timetabled to a variety of venues in ambulatory care. Student nurses may also benefit from learning opportunities in the protected environment provided and some sessions there may be structured for multiprofessional learning. Dental students learning aspects of general medicine can also be included.

Advantages of teaching in the ambulatory care setting

The ambulatory care setting provides opportunities for undergraduate teaching which are not now so readily available in traditional ward teaching:

- A wide range of clinical conditions of both minor and major severity may be seen.
- Large numbers of both new patients and those undergoing a course of treatment or post-operative rehabilitation are available.
- Students have the opportunity to experience a multiprofessional approach to patient care.
- Expanding student numbers can be accommodated without exhausting the patients available.
- Students' attention can be focused on learning objectives.
- A 'bank' of patients can be built up to facilitate the delivery of a systems-sensitive programme.

Decide when the teaching session will end! Announcing this at the beginning will help the students to concentrate and pace themselves. No one can teach or learn indefinitely and the students may have seen as much as they can absorb without staying to the very end of the scheduled session.

- Multiprofessional education may be possible in some settings.

However, faculty must recognise the role ambulatory care teaching has in relieving pressure on ward-based teaching and provide appropriate resources for its implementation and development.

Summary

The ward setting has become less suitable for clinical teaching as in-patients are now fewer in number and more often acutely ill. Transferring the emphasis of teaching to the ambulatory care setting provides a new venue for student/patient interaction and for experiencing multiprofessional aspects of patient care. The educational objectives to be achieved in this setting are different from those traditionally emphasised in ward-based teaching.

Strategies required to facilitate learning in this setting include a structured logbook and a variety of models to regulate student/patient interaction to maximum advantage.

The educational opportunities available can be developed further by a clinical tutor working in a dedicated teaching area who can draw not only on the patients attending the clinic and on a bank of invited and simulated patients, but also on colleagues in other health-care professions who can all contribute to the student's experience of health-care delivery in the ambulatory care setting.

"Ambulatory education is timely and needed, and, to a large degree, ambulatory programmes are being rated highly by the students and physicians who participated in them"

Krackov et al 1993

References and further reading

Dent J A, Davis M H 1995 Role of ambulatory care for student-patient interaction: the EPITOME model. Medical Education 29:58–60

Feltovich J, Mast T A, Soler N G 1987 A survey of undergraduate internal medicine education in ambulatory care. Proceedings of the Annual Conference on Research in Medical Education 26:137–141

Fincher R M E, Albritton T A 1993 The ambulatory experience for junior medical students at the Medical College of Georgia. Teaching and Learning in Medicine 5:210–213

Gruppen L D, Wisdom K, Anderson D S, Woolliscroft J O 1993 Assessing the consistency and educational benefits of students' clinical experiences during an ambulatory care internal medicine rotation. Academic Medicine 68:674–680

Irby D M 1995 Teaching and learning in ambulatory care settings: a thematic review of the literature. Academic Medicine 70:898–931

Krackov S K, Packman C H, Regan-Smith M G, Birskovitch L, Seward S J, Baker S D 1993 Perspectives on ambulatory programs: barriers and implementation strategies. Teaching and Learning in Medicine 5:243–250

Seabrook M A, Lawson M, Malster M, Solly J, Rennie J, Baskerville P A 1998 Teaching medical students in a day surgery unit: adapting medical education to changes in clinical practice. Medical Teacher 20:222–226

Woolliscroft J O, Schwenk T L 1989 Teaching and learning in the ambulatory setting. Academic Medicine 644–648

Chapter 11
Primary care

J. S. Ker   D. Snadden

Introduction

Primary care medicine means different things to different people depending on the structure of their health-care system, but it can be broadly defined as the care delivered at a patient's point of first contact with the official health-care services.

Why bother with primary care medicine?

The majority of patients who consult the health-care services do so at primary care level; 90% of people accessing health-care services present in the primary care setting.

Since the World Health Organization's Alma Ata Declaration of 1978 nations have been trying to achieve 'Health for All by 2000' by emphasising the delivery of health care through their primary care medicine strategy.

With the implementation of this strategy has come the need to train more primary care health professionals. As choice of medical specialty can by positively influenced by the nature of the educational experience (Reid 1993), the development of an attractive primary care curriculum has become an essential component of recruitment.

The World Federation for Medical Education (WFME) have also recognised the need to reorientate medical education to meet the health-care needs of individuals and their communities. In 1993 they recommended the use of a wider number of clinical settings for learning

"Doctors find themselves unaccustomed to assess and evaluate the health care needs and priorities of their own country and people. They are incapable of providing or implementing preventative programmes. They are unprepared to work in the slums of the cities or to manage a rural health care team"

Alma Ata 1978

"The number of weeks in family practice showed the strongest association with specialty choice"

Bland 1995

"We are not graduating the kind of physician most needed by society"

AAMC 1990
Alma Ata 1978

"Teaching Primary care in hospital is like teaching forestry in a lumber yard"

A general practitioner

to ensure adequate experience with an increasing emphasis on primary care.

In 1979 the Network for Community Oriented Educational Institutions for Health Sciences was established to encourage more relevance in health professional education to reflect individual and community needs.

What does this mean for teaching primary care medicine?

The changing trends in the delivery of health care and the explosion of knowledge in medicine and related areas have had implications for medical education particularly in relation to teaching primary care medicine. Primary care medicine can offer educational opportunities for all members of the health-care professions at undergraduate, postgraduate and continuing education levels.

The uniqueness of the primary care setting is that it can offer:

- generalist experience
- exposure to continuity of care
- opportunities to learn to cope with uncertainty
- experience of a wide spectrum of disease
- patient-centred practice.

Medical schools in the US for example have undertaken major change in the preclinical phase of educating future physicians following the GPEP Report (Muller 1994). They have been inspired by the increase in understanding of the educational process, which emphasises learning methods centred on students and problems (Barrows & Tamblyn 1980) and the role of primary care.

In the UK the General Medical Council's 'Tomorrow's Doctors' (1993) also recognised the need to encourage more training of undergraduates in primary care as one of their main recommendations.

To meet these aims and trends all medical schools need to address how they can include primary care effectively in their curricula.

What is the difference between primary care medicine and general practice?

The Nature of General Practice, published by the Royal College of General Practitioners in the UK (1996), attempted to clarify the role of the general practitioner as the diagnostician in primary care with both scientific and humanitarian responsibilities. Secondly it pointed to the need for practitioners to remain in charge of their own professional standards.

In many countries modern general practice is now evidence-based with a healthy research and audit culture.

Primary care on the other hand, in the words of Heath (1998), is predominantly concerned with the socio-economic and environmental determinants of health. It tries to resist the medicalisation of health.

Many countries have an excellent network of primary care services led by village health workers or nurses.

The move towards a primary care focus for the delivery of health care, with the need for health interventions to be relevant, of high quality and based on priorities to achieve cost-effective results, makes it imperative for all health-care professionals involved in the delivery of care to have an awareness of their roles and responsibilities within primary care.

In addition to this a recent survey of research activity in the UK amongst junior academic general practitioners demonstrated a variable research activity score (Lester 1998), reflecting the small size and relative weakness of departments of general practice and highlighting the need to strengthen the academic basis of general practice in order to support a greater emphasis on teaching and research.

These are important aspects to consider when setting up teaching and learning opportunities for students in primary care.

What are the practical challenges in teaching primary care medicine?

Seven challenges have been identified for you to address in order to provide teaching and learning opportunities in primary care medicine:

1. What can you learn in primary care?
2. How can you establish/improve a primary care programme?
3. Which teaching method should you use?
4. What learning opportunities can you create in primary care?
5. What resources are required?
6. What staff development is required?
7. How should you evaluate the programme?

What can you learn in primary care?

Primary care medicine is about continuity of care, following patients through their illness experiences throughout their lives. It is about understanding the social background of patients and how this affects attitudes to illness and life events. It is essential to determine early what the preferred learning outcomes will be. The following is a suggested list of key and potential areas to consider:

- key areas
  - development of clinical skills
  - communication skills
  - patient illness in a lifestyle context
  - collaboration and teamwork
  - exploration of health beliefs
  - ethical dilemmas
  - health promotion
  - prevention programmes
- potential areas
  - interface with self-help groups
  - health education
  - technology-based skills
  - epidemiological experience
  - personnel management skills.

Learning in primary care medicine can be focused around the 'five Cs':

- care – practical aspects of illness and disease
- combination – prevention with cure
- continuity – in chronic diseases
- communication – with patients
- collaboration – with colleagues

Depending on the other facets of your curriculum, including the length of your primary care programme, several learning outcomes can be addressed simultaneously.

University of New Mexico, USA
This primary care programme focuses on the first 2 years of training. A large part of the week is left unscheduled for students to pursue clinical electives in which they participate in the care of patients under the guidance of a primary care physician. In the latter part of year one, students live and work in rural communities with regular links to the school.

How can you establish/improve a primary care medicine programme?

The challenges to face depend on whether a primary care programme is already in place in your curriculum or not.

In the current climate debates often focus not so much on whether to introduce primary care into the curriculum but on how and when it should be introduced. Levine (1980) identified five steps in establishing a change, which can be adapted to the development of a primary care programme:

- Establishing the diagnosis
  — Do you need a new primary care programme or change in an existing programme?
  — What are the barriers?
  — What are the advantages?
- Initiating change
  — Identify key people in primary care to form a steering group.
  — Neutralise the barriers.
  — Negotiate the change from within the faculty structure.
  — Ensure the change is understood by staff and students.
  — Encourage opinion and dialogue to promote ownership of the changes.
  — Determine the learning outcomes of the programme.

There is a tendency to develop too many learning outcomes for each session so students become defocused.

Determining your learning outcomes will enable you to determine your assessment criteria.

Be ready to accept and share responsibility for the programme.

"any change process must go through a phase of instability, the unfrozen state before leading to a new stable state"

Lewin 1968

- Tailoring the situation
  - — Develop an implementation plan of the teaching programme.
  - — Recognise the local constraints.
  - — Identify the resources.
  - — Commence staff development.
  - — Develop an assessment strategy.
- Implementing the solution
  - — Adopt the plan within the existing faculty organisational structure.
- Evaluating the product
  - — Assess the impact of change.

In the following two examples we can identify how primary care teaching was incorporated into the faculty programmes.

Cambridge, parallel tract programme
The department of general practice at the University of Cambridge have organised a programme where students in their clinical undergraduate programme have gained the majority of their clinical methods teaching in primary care. This runs in parallel with the more traditionally based hospital programme. A comparative evaluation has shown no disadvantage to either group at undergraduate level (Oswald 1993).

Linkoping, Sweden
The entire curriculum has been altered to promote teamwork through the design of a common curriculum in year one, with students then diversifying in their own professional tracts but having shared learning opportunities as appropriate. Primary care medicine has been introduced to promote learning of generic skills.

Which teaching method to use?
This is often dependent on your staff development programme and what your facilitators or teachers feel comfortable with in the context of their own experience as a trainer.

One of the strategies that helps to develop the most appropriate teaching method is to implement one which promotes life-long learning.

In many academic institutions primary care physicians are contributing more and more to the implementation of the undergraduate programme, bringing a breadth of experience and balance to the overall curriculum.

Problem-based learning has been used in Linkoping in Sweden to incorporate learning in primary care early in the curriculum.

Other programmes have used study guides to direct the student learning primary care and as a way of sharing expected outcomes with staff and students in the context of the whole curriculum. At the University of Dundee, students in year two have shared learning outcomes highlighted for their clinical programme in their study guide. The learning outcomes in primary care are therefore reflective of students' needs and change as they progress through their training.

Holding a preparatory session at the beginning of a primary care programme can promote understanding.

Primary care medicine can be taught in one-to-one or in small group settings. Sessions can be arranged as a block attachment or as a part of the longitudinal programme.

Longitudinal attachments

University of Newcastle, Australia

Sixty to seventy students per year participate in a 4-year programme. In year two, 8 half-days are spent in two general practices, shadowing the GP. Students are asked to document their observations of eight tasks as a series of one-page commentaries carried out by the GP in order to focus their understanding of different consultation techniques compared to hospital practice. The list of tasks is provided by faculty and may include the observation of a limited examination or use of time as a management tool.

University of Illinois, Chicago, USA

This longitudinal programme pairs every first-year medical student with a primary care physician for 3 years. It can be piloted and evaluated initially once the outcomes have been agreed with the curriculum committee or equivalent faculty group. The learning outcomes focus on:

- recognising the art of communication through early patient contact and role modelling
- developing a panel of patients to follow over a 3-year period
- developing a relationship with a primary care facilitator who can act as a mentor.

Block primary care attachments
Block attachments can be organised for students in urban and rural settings. One or two students can be attached to a health centre or live as part of the community as described below.

Community-based programme, University of Gezira, Sudan
Students are introduced to a rural health programme through an 11–step approach. They commence the programme following a 1-month integrated systems course:

Step 1: Communities are selected for students to go and stay with in the rural areas.

Step 2: Identification of investigative instruments.

Step 3: Students are exposed to real-life health issues at both community and individual levels.

Step 4: Students analyse the data.

Step 5: Identification of problems for the community.

Step 6: Students prioritise problems liaising with the community.

Step 7: A plan of action is written and funding is accessed.

Step 8: Students implement their plan with the community's cooperation.

Step 9: The Plan is followed up through regular visits.

Step 10: Evaluation of achievement.

Step 11: Submission of written report.

What learning opportunities can you create in primary care medicine?

Determining what learning opportunities are available in primary care is normally constrained only by the predetermined learning outcomes.

The following are some interesting examples of practical programmes of teaching in primary care medicine.

Project activity

At the University of Leeds students working in groups of three to five immediately following their primary care attachment are given a 2-week research module in their fourth year linking general practice and public health medicine.

Adopt a family

Students are given a family to visit during their undergraduate programme, either during each block of their course or when they are on primary care attachments. Students on a first-year programme in Wales were attached to a mother and her newborn baby for a year. A similar programme has been implemented in Newcastle-upon-Tyne, which in addition focuses on a family survey linking individual and epidemiological perspectives.

Role playing

This is a useful strategy to use as part of a preparatory session early on in the student's clinical experience but must be run by experienced supportive tutors.

First contact programme, University of Dundee

In order to integrate and make basic and clinical sciences relevant to clinical practice, students are introduced to the practice of medicine in the first year of their course. Students meet to discuss learning outcomes and to role-play scenarios based on real practice before going out into the community to meet patients in their own homes.

Multiprofessional uni programme

The Kellogg Foundation in South America has funded a joint primary care educational initiative in Cotia, Brazil. The educational programme coordinates all the training programmes in continuing education at primary and secondary care levels for all health-care workers. The focus of the educational programme is on the development of generic skills such as teamworking.

Health promotion poster development
The production of materials that can be utilised in primary care can give students the opportunity to collaborate with other professionals and to recognise the difficulties of health promotion in practice. Students in their second year in Dundee worked in collaboration with graphics students to produce a health promotion poster for the GP waiting room related to gastroenterology.

Simulated surgery
Simulated surgeries enable the consultation process with trained patients to be assessed by video, listening facility or one-way mirror. This limits the effect of an observer being present.

What resources are required?
Resources are crucial to the success of your primary care programme. A coordinator can be responsible for the administration of the programme.
Sites can include:

- health centres
- practice premises
- university health facilities
- voluntary agencies
- non-government facilities
- school welfare institutions.

Specific specialist clinics may also be available in primary care:

- nurse practitioner clinics
- physiotherapy clinics
- cottage hospital in-patient facilities
- midwifery-led clinics
- child health surveillance
- nurse-led asthma and diabetes clinics
- counselling services

What staff development is required?

There are many real barriers to recruitment of facilitators to implement primary care curricula. Many practitioners require financial compensation for their educational input to training at all levels.

Organising a preparatory workshop for facilitators can be beneficial in terms of both transfer of information and in addressing potential problems with implementation.

Try to offer a wide range of opportunities for staff to discuss programmes.

The University of Newcastle, Australia
The 5-year programme is an integrated problem-based course where general practitioners are involved in the delivery of the curriculum through:

- facilitating learning around biomedical problems that focus on stages of disease
- acting as tutors
- facilitating learning on specific primary care-focused topics
- focusing on the roles and responsibilities of GPs in the overall care of patients in a multidisciplinary setting.

How should you evaluate the primary care programme?

Evaluation of educational innovations and changes is often difficult. However, many of the examples identified use student opinion as part of their evaluation process. Questionnaires using a Likert scale and open-ended questions can give a balanced view.

Assessment of the students using the objective structured clinical examination (OSCE) to examine competence in discrete skills can contribute to the evaluation process.

Summary

Primary care medicine has much to offer in the teaching and learning of health-care professionals at all stages of career development.

Nursing homes often provide students with a rewarding experience in an area of increasing social need.

Ask each of your facilitators to keep a dossier of his or her teaching experience.

It is a setting that reflects the current needs of the patients at both individual and community levels.

Through this series of practical challenges you can maximise teaching and learning in primary care and provide opportunities for learning.

References and further reading

Barbero G 1995 Medical education in the light of the World Health Organisation Health for All strategy and the European Union. Medical Education 29:3–12

Barrows H S 1985 How to design a problem-based curriculum for the clinical years. Springer, New York

Colin R, Des Marchais J E 1996 Successful strategies in reforming medical education. Education for Health 9:3

General Medical Council 1993 Tomorrow's doctors. General Medical Council, London

Heath I 1998 Primary care values. British Medical Journal Publishing, London

Lester H E 1998 Survey of research activity, training needs, departmental support, and career intentions of junior academic general practitioners. British Journal of General Practice 8:1322–1326

Oswald N T A 1993 Teaching clinical methods to medical students. Medical Education 27:351–354

Reid L A 1993 The contribution of general practice to the medical curriculum. Annals of Community Oriented Education 6:115–123

Royal College of General Practitioners 1996. The nature of general medical practice. Report from General Practice 27

Chapter 12
Distance education

J. M. Laidlaw   E. A. Hesketh

Introduction

Distance education as an approach to learning is not a new concept but it has rapidly developed since the pioneering days of simple correspondence courses.

This decentralised, flexible method of learning is likely to expand in tandem with new technologies such as the Internet and multimedia initiatives. The increasing emphasis being placed on the concept of life-long learning will also give distance education a higher profile.

Defining distance education

There are several definitions of distance education in the literature. Here are two of them:

> *'Distance education consists of all arrangements for providing instruction through print or electronic communications media to persons engaged in planned learning in a place and time different from that of the instructor or instructors'*
>
> Moore 1990

> *'The term "distance education" covers the various forms of study at all levels which are not under the continuous, immediate supervision of tutors present with their students in lecture rooms, or in the same premises, but which nevertheless benefit from the planning, guidance and tuition of tutorial organisation'*
>
> Holmberg 1977

Oxford University had 'correspondence' courses as early as 1870.

The actual distance between learner and tutor is irrelevant.

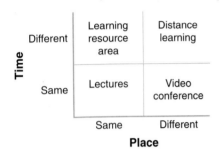

Fig. 12.1   Time/place window

Two key factors distinguish distance education from other types of learning. These are time and place. Distance education allows learners to study in their own place and at a time of their choice. This can be seen more clearly from the time/place window in Figure 12.1. For example, a self-study module in a learning resource area would lie in the window of 'same place' (i.e. to be studied at a fixed place) and 'different time' (i.e. study at any time), whereas distance learning lies in the 'different time and different place' window.

What then distinguishes distance learning from, say, studying a textbook? As alluded to in the definitions, in distance education there is an on-going responsibility to build into the learning experience teacher/learner interaction.

Why distance education?

The popularity of distance education lies in its ability to overcome many of the barriers that face traditional education. The Health Bulletin (1998) states that access to CME activities depends on factors such as geography, funding, time constraints, service pressures and specialty-specific problems. Distance education can certainly address some of these constraints if not all! For example learners may have work patterns that prohibit them from attending a specific course at a particular time; learners may simply be too busy to attend; the location of the course may not be convenient and result in considerable travel time and expenses for the learner. Other barriers may also concern finance; for example, from the employer's perspective it can be costly to release someone from work during the day to attend a course. In addition there may be educational barriers inherent in traditional learning. Distance education can allow learners to study a topic to the depth they desire and at a pace that suits them. After all, not everyone has the same learning needs or the same preferred learning style. Distance education therefore can cater for individual needs with regard to both content of the topic and method of study.

Doctors would like to know their strengths and weaknesses provided no one else knows their deficiencies.

In the medical profession distance education has been used extensively in the field of continuing education particularly to keep health-care professionals up to date with new techniques and therapies. The University of Dundee's Centre for Medical Education has been one of the main providers in the UK of distance learning programmes for doctors.

The educational approach

Although no global theory of distance education exists the following models do provide a basis for a theory: Rothkopf's (1965) model for written instruction, Skinner's (1954) behaviour-control model, Ausubel's (1960) organiser model and Gagne's (1970) teaching model.

As far as main educational principles are concerned, there really is very little difference between designing a course for face-to-face participants and one for those learning at a distance. Indeed Shale (1990) makes a plea for theoreticians and practitioners to 'stop emphasising points of difference between distance and traditional education but instead to identify common educational problems'.

"Distance Education is an applied field and, as such, borrows from a variety of theoretical frameworks"

Dillon & Walsh 1992

The components of distance education

In designing a distance education programme the following key areas need to be addressed:

- the educational needs of the learners
- the design of the materials
- the support mechanisms for students.

The educational needs of learners

Preparing distance education programmes for the medical profession or indeed the health-care professions is a challenging task. Rowntree (1994) suggests a variety of facts which should be known about distance learners before you start to design a course. These include a range of educational, social and economic facts such as:

Knowing some of these facts if not them all from the outset may help you better understand your distance learners and perhaps prevent 'drop-out' if things get too tough.

- Age, sex, place of study, occupation – you need to know and 'understand' the type of person for whom you are writing.
- Motivation – reason for enrolling on the course. For example, are learners wishing to gain a higher qualification or simply studying for interest? This will have implications for the content of the programme. Someone studying for a qualification is likely to do only what is required for the assessment/assignment, whereas someone studying purely for interest may engage with the optional activities.
- Learning factors – preferred learning styles, learning skills, experience of distance learning. Ideally programmes should offer learners a choice of study methods. For example, some learners prefer a problem-based approach while others like the more traditional information approach.
- Subject knowledge – attitude to the subject, prior knowledge/skills, misconceptions, relevant interests. When producing, for example, a programme for general dental practitioners on fissure caries it was found that dentists fell into three categories: those that were not up to date with the recommended sealant techniques; those that were aware of the techniques but needed their attitude to using them changed; those who were familiar with the techniques. The design and content of the programme had to cater for all three groups.
- Resources – available time for study, access to media/facilities, access to human support, funding. These factors have implications for your programme. For example, if your learners do not have access to library facilities or specific journals, they should be able to access the basic information from the core text(s) provided in the programme. Further references would be for optional reading only.

The design of distance learning materials
The main players in any distance education development, however, are the content expert, the education expert, the instructional designer and an editor. The design, development and production of

distance education programmes are therefore very much a team effort. Team members vary depending on the method of delivery which is chosen. For example, if you are intending to make use of CD-ROMs or the Internet then it would make sense to have a computer expert on your team. If you intend to use video then someone with expertise in that area would be a key member. It is also common practice to have a member of the target audience in the team. This helps to ensure that the programme is relevant and appropriate for that audience and is not written by a subject expert remote from the 'real world'.

In addition to Gagne's principles, the CRISIS model (Harden & Laidlaw 1992) is of value to those developing educational programmes for study at a distance. CRISIS is an acronym for the following criteria, all of which can contribute to the effectiveness of continuing medical education:

- convenience
- relevance
- individualisation
- self-assessment
- interest
- speculation and systematic.

Convenience

Voluntary participation must be easy. It has long been recognised that doctors educate themselves at home through reading books and journals. The role of the self-directed learner is therefore not really new to them. A distance education approach offers busy doctors the opportunity of studying in their own home or workplace and at a time best suited to them.

Relevance

The user's day-to-day role in medical practice must be reflected. The presentation of facts alone is of little use. It is how these facts are applied to the learner's everyday practice that is important. It is important therefore to identify precisely the target audience's educational needs and present the material in a context with which

"Distance education can only be designed and delivered with the highest quality by teams of specialists"

Moore 1997

the learner can identify. Patient management problems and everyday scenarios are often used to make the link between theory and practice.

Individualisation

Learners must have a say in what is learnt and be able to adapt the programme to their own needs. Individualisation therefore refers to building into the programme the ability to cope with the different levels of detail/study required by the target audience. After all, learners are likely to have different starting points on the topic as well as wanting different end points. It is also about offering a choice of learning style. We all learn in different ways and as adult learners bring our own experiences to the job in hand (Newble & Entwistle 1986). How distance learning can cater for the needs of individuals and provide them with different learning pathways is best illustrated by the following two examples.

Firstly, a distance learning programme on management produced by the Centre for Medical Education is aimed at doctors and nurses working in hospitals and in the community. It is designed to encourage multidisciplinary learning and can be used as a teaching resource for individuals or groups. The management package contains three booklets which are all interlinked. The distance learners can start learning about the topic with any booklet depending on their preferred method of study. If they are seeking a quick practical insight into the subject they commence with the booklet entitled 'I wish I had the answer!' If they wish to study the topic in greater depth then they are advised to read 'Facts not fiction'. For a problem-based approach they can start with the booklet 'Have you a better answer?'

Another of the Centre's distance learning programmes, entitled 'Moving to audit', used a different format to enable distance learners to study the subject in a way which best suited their needs. They could, for example, systematically read through the entire core text which contained the principles of audit. Of course a learner may wish only to skim through the core text selecting the sections of particular interest. Skimming is facilitated by the use of icons and headings. Alternatively, if learners preferred, they could learn about the topic through a series of challenges which were designed in the format of a doctor's diary.

Self-assessment

Self-assessment encourages doctors to evaluate their understanding of the subject and to remedy any gaps identified. As far as distance education is concerned it is a key component of programmes as it motivates learners and enables them to plot their progress. To a large extent the interaction of receiving feedback alleviates the isolation that some distance learners experience.

With regard to providing the feedback there really should be an element of choice by which distance learners can assess themselves. Feedback can be contained within the programme, it can be mailed, or it can be given by telephone or e-mail, or via audio/video conferencing. This list is by no means complete.

Self-assessment should enable learners to identify their strengths and weaknesses and suggest ways of resolving any learning problems. It is of help to learners to receive feedback not only from the 'experts' but, as we can see from the feedback sample sheet in Figure 12.2, from their own peers.

The computer can be used very successfully to generate tailored responses to individual distance learners, but of course this necessitates the computer being programmed in advance to store information on every possible option that a participant might choose.

One of the most effective forms of feedback and perhaps the most educational is to offer explanations not only to the response given by the learner, but to all the options that might have been selected.

Interest

Attention should be aroused, encouraging learners to participate in the programme and sustaining the learner's motivation to complete the course.

There is now a wide choice of media other than print to deliver distance learning. These include audio and

"Written feedback should be friendly"

Race 1994

"Learner feedback is listed as one of the five most important considerations in course design and instruction"

Rosenow 1976

Option	You	Your colleagues (%)	The authors
(a)		05	
(b)	*	40	
(c)		42	*
(d)		08	
(e)		05	

Fig. 12.2 Feedback sheet sample

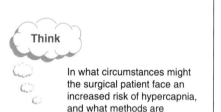

"for the distance educators the Internet is a land of infinite possibility"

Colyer 1997

Think

In what circumstances might the surgical patient face an increased risk of hypercapnia, and what methods are available to this risk?

Make a point of familiarising yourself with relevant monitoring systems in the operating theatre and intensive care unit

Fig. 12.3   Use of icons

video cassettes; interactive video; computer-assisted learning (CAL), CD-ROMs and the Internet; audio, video and computer teleconferencing; television and radio. All can add interest to a programme and encourage interaction providing they have been designed on sound educational principles.

Despite this technological revolution distance education in the printed format is still popular, but the trend is to augment and enhance it with electronic support materials. Desktop-published materials can look very professional providing the principles of good layout and design have been applied. Text can also be made more stimulating by applying various educational strategies such as using advance organisers, headings, illustrations and summaries. Also by introducing colour and various print styles you can create a programme with impact. Even the style of writing is vitally important. The most effective materials have been written in a conversational style.

Icons too are being used more in printed materials, to enable learners to select various types of activity that are flagged up, and in a distance education programme activities are a main feature. An example from the Royal College of Surgeons of Edinburgh's distance education programme 'SELECT' shows how effective the use of icons can be (see Fig. 12.3).

Competition, shrinking resources and the demand for more cost-effective education have, according to Mowen & Parks (1997), motivated academic administrators to adopt strategic marketing approaches. To entice a potential distance learner to enrol on a course you have to 'put on your Marketing hat'. A 'trigger' leaflet, usually the smallest component of any distance learning package, is often the key to its success (Hesketh & Laidlaw 1997). It helps raise awareness of your distance learning programme and encourages people to become interested in it. Spending time and money on the design of the triggers is well worth the effort.

Speculation and systematic

Speculation is about recognising controversial and grey areas in medicine and making it clear that sometimes everything is not always known about a subject. It is important that such areas of uncertainty are addressed and not glossed over. In distance learning self-assessment can be used to highlight grey areas. For example, where the correct answer to a multiple choice question is not clear, the learner can be shown the spread of responses from a team of experts.

The systematic element is about offering a planned programme with coverage of a whole subject or an identified part of it. The distance learning teacher needs to consider the topic areas to be studied, identify these for learners and show them how their studies will cover these areas.

Support mechanisms

There are a variety of mechanisms which can be used to provide the distance learner with support. Even although Knowles (1984) describes the adult learner in distance education as relatively independent and internally motivated, support for learners is crucial and can often determine whether a learner will continue with a programme of study or drop out. The support you can provide much depends on your funding and the technologies available to you and your learner. Here are just a few support mechanisms worth considering:

- Offer support when needed by the learner. This is usually in a one-to-one situation where the learner seeks tutor support.
- Offer a planned session between a tutor and an individual or a group of learners, or simply between a learner and his or her peers. If a group of learners are conveniently situated near each other, a face-to-face peer group meeting may be organised – one in which learners are encouraged to support each other.
- Offer a planned summer school or series of face-to-face workshops which are part of the distance learning course.

Remember you can also build in support through 'embedded support devices' within the distance learning materials.

If a learner is not able to allocate enough time to a distance education programme it is better to advise the learner to postpone participation to a more appropriate period.

A study on 'embedded support devices' such as margin texts, summaries, examples, questions with feedback, text in italics etc. has shown they assist learning.

Guard against making your study guide too voluminous or it will become a less effective tool for the distance learner.

There is also a trend today to incorporate into a distance learning package a study guide, which is basically a management tool to help self-directed learners manage their learning more effectively and efficiently. Study guides are dealt with in more depth in Chapter 18.

Summary

Distance education continues to grow in popularity amongst adult learners and will expand further as technologies develop. In the medical profession a large percentage of doctors have used this approach to learning to keep up to date with new techniques and therapies. It differs from other approaches to learning in that the learner is separated from the tutor, and there is no fixed time or place for study.

There are three key areas to address when developing a distance learning programme. Firstly, find out the educational needs of the learners. If a distance learning course does not meet the learners' needs in terms of many aspects, of which relevance, content, depth of study, preferred learning style, cost and accreditation are just a few, then it will either fail to attract people to enrol or result in drop-outs.

The second key area involves the design. Although there is no recognised theory underpinning distance education, designers have leaned heavily on Gagne's principles of learning, as well as on the CRISIS model to create innovative educational programmes.

The last issue is that of learner support. Even if the programmes are educationally sound, distance learners need additional support to help them in their self-directed role. These support mechanisms can vary from simply incorporating embedded support devices into the programmes, through to planning scheduled tutorial sessions using electronic media, organising kick-start or face-to-face courses, making use of study guides or providing tutor support on demand.

As the demand for life-long learning increases, the number of distance learners is likely to increase and, more importantly, be valued by institutions world-wide.

References and further reading

Ausubel D P 1960 The use of advance organisers in the learning and retention of meaningful material. Journal of Educational Psychology 51:267–272

Colyer A 1997 Copyright law, the Internet and distance education. American Journal of Distance Education 11(3):41–57

Dillon C L, Walsh S M 1992 Faculty: the neglected resource in distance education. American Journal of Distance Education 6(3): 5–21

Gagne R M 1970 The conditions of learning, 2nd edn. Holt, Rinehart and Winston, New York

Harden R M, Laidlaw J M 1992 Effective continuing education: the CRISIS criteria. Medical Education 26: 408–422

Hesketh E A, Laidlaw J M 1997 Selling educational events to healthcare professionals: twelve tips on the function and design of trigger leaflets. Medical Teacher 19(4): 250–256

Holmberg B 1977 Distance education: a survey and bibliography. Kogan Page, London

Knowles M S 1984 Andragogy in action. Jossey Bass, New York.

Moore M G 1990 Background and overview of contemporary American distance education. In: Moor M G (ed) Contemporary issues in American distance education. Pergamon, New York and London

Moore M G 1997 Editorial – The study guide: foundation of the course. American Journal of Distance Education 11(2): 1–2

Mowen A J, Parks S C 1997 Competitive marketing of distance education: a model for placing quality within a strategic planning context. American Journal of Distance Education 11(3): 27–40

Newble D I, Entwistle N J 1986 Learning styles and approaches: implications for medical education. Medical Education 20:162–175

Race P 1994 The open learning handbook – promoting quality in designing and delivering flexible learning, 2nd edn. Kogan Page, London

Rosenow E C 1976 Self-assessment of the physician. Journal of the Royal College of Physicians 10:408–412

Roth Kopf E Z 1965 Some theoretical and experimental approaches to problems in written instruction. In: Krumboltz J D (ed) Learning and the educational process. Rand McNally, Chicago

Rowntree D 1994 Preparing materials for open, distance and flexible learning. Kogan Page, London

Scottish Office 1998 Scottish Joint Consultants Committee and representatives of NHS Trust Chief Executives. Continuing medical education for career grade hospital doctors and dentists. Health Bulletin 56(3):624–630

Shale D 1990 Toward a reconceptualization of distance education. In: Moore M G (ed.), Contemporary issues in American distance education Pergamon Press, Oxford, pp. 333–343

Skinner B F 1954 The science of learning and the art of teaching. Harvard Educational Reviews 24:86–97

SECTION 3
EDUCATIONAL STRATEGIES

Chapter 13
Independent learning

R. M. Harden

Introduction

Other chapters in this book look at how students learn in large group settings such as lectures and in small groups working with their colleagues. What matters, irrespective of the approach to teaching and learning adopted, is the learning achieved by the individual student. In both traditional and innovative education programmes, students spend a significant proportion of their time learning on their own. Indeed, the formal learning in the taught part of the course may represent only the tip of the iceberg (see Fig. 13.1).

After a lecture, students master the topic by reading their notes or the relevant sections in a textbook. Students prepare for small group work and follow up such sessions by studying on their own. In the clinical setting, too, students need to find out more about the underlying problems of the patients they have seen from further reading or the use of electronic information sources. The intensity of independent learning in the traditional curriculum usually increases before a formal examination, with students attempting to revise or master the contents of a course over a relatively short period of time, sometimes at the expense of attendance at other scheduled sessions. In distance learning, independent learning is the major or sole activity.

The importance of independent learning may not be fully appreciated – time for it is not formally scheduled in the curriculum and appropriate learning resource material and support for students are often not provided. The increasing emphasis on independent

"Self instruction may be an alternative to other forms of teaching, but it can also be combined with them"

Rowntree 1990

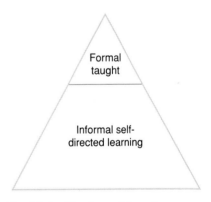

Fig. 13.1   The formal learning 'iceberg'

"a strategy that promotes self-directed learning is likely to be the most effective"

Spencer & Jordan 1999

learning acknowledges that learning is not something that someone else can do for students but that it must be done by students for themselves.

In this chapter we will consider:

- what we mean by 'independent learning' and related terms such as 'self-learning'
- why independent learning makes a key contribution to the curriculum
- some current trends in independent learning.

What is independent learning?

Six key principles

The concept of independent learning means different things to different people. It incorporates six key principles:

- Students learn on their own.
- Students have a measure of control over their own learning. They may choose:
  — where to learn
  — what to learn
  — how to learn
  — when to learn

  They take responsibility for:

  — deciding the context for learning
  — diagnosing personal learning needs
  — identifying resources
  — deciding time for learning and the pacing of learning.
- Students may be encouraged to develop their own personal learning plans (Challis 2000).
- The different needs of individual students are recognised and appropriate response is made to the specific needs of the individual learner.
- Student learning is supported, to a greater or lesser extent, by learning resources and study guides prepared for this purpose.
- The role of the teacher changes from a lecturer or transmitter of information to a manager of the learning process – a more demanding but a more rewarding role.

Independent learning is based on discovery-guided mentoring rather than on the transmission of information.

Terms used

A number of terms have been used to describe this approach to learning. These terms are often used interchangeably although different meanings may be implied.

- Independent learning – emphasises that students work on their own to meet their own learning needs.
- Self-managed learning, self-directed learning or self-regulated learning – emphasises that students have an element of control over their own learning with responsibility for diagnosis of learning needs and identifying resources. Implicit in this approach is that students have a clear understanding of the intended learning outcomes.
- Resource-based learning – emphasises the use of resource material in print or multimedia format as a basis for the students' learning, and the freedom this gives to the student.
- Flexible learning – emphasises the wide range of learning opportunities offered to students and a flexibility in responding to individual student needs and aspirations.
- Open learning – often used interchangeably with flexible learning. It emphasises the provision of greater access for students to their choice of education.
- Distance learning – emphasises that students work on their own at a distance from their teacher. Implicit in the approach is that the teachers interact with students and facilitate the students' learning.

  The two ideas underpinning the above concepts are:
- Students study individually on their own.
- Students have charge of the learning process.

Both features are absent in the lecture and present in distance learning where students direct their own studies to achieve the prescribed learning outcomes (see Fig. 13.2). In many education programmes, students work on their own, e.g. reading prescribed texts, but have little control of their learning. In other situations, students may control their learning, as in problem-based learning, but greater emphasis is placed on group rather than individual work.

"Flexible learning is a generic term that covers all these situations where learners have some say in how, where or when learning takes place"

Ellington, in Bell et al 1997

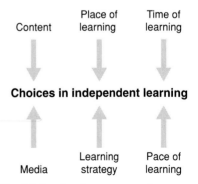

Fig. 13.2 Students can make choices in independent learning

"Self directed learning enables progressive educators to give greater expression to their philosophies"

Collins & Hammond

The Importance of independent learning

There are many reasons why independent learning has become more fashionable as a paradigm of learning in medical education.

A Modular and flexible curriculum

There has been a trend to modularity and flexibility in curriculum planning. Students, individually or in small groups, may rotate round a series of attachments. In electives or special study modules, they can choose to study areas in more depth. Independent learning has a useful role to play in these situations and can help to avoid unnecessary repetitive teaching by staff. Different groups of students may use the same resource pack and study guide, leaving the teacher free for one-to-one contact with students.

Different contexts for learning

Distance learning has increased in popularity (see Chapter 12). Here students are remote from the teacher and have to rely more on working on their own. Distance learning is particularly appropriate in postgraduate and continuing medical education. The CRISIS criteria for effective continuing education, developed in the context of distance learning, recognise the potential advantages implicit in independent learning (Harden & Laidlaw 1992):

- Convenience for the student in terms of time, pace and place
- Relevance to the needs of the practising doctor
- Individualisation to the needs of each learner
- Self-assessment by the student of his or her own competence
- Interest in the programme by the student
- Systematic coverage of the topic or theme for the programme
- Speculation – the grey areas where there may be uncertainty.

Active learning

Independent learning, if planned appropriately, encourages a more active approach to learning. Students adopt a deep rather than a superficial approach to learning and search for an understanding of the subject rather than just reproducing what they have learned. Students are encouraged to think and not just recall facts they have learned.

The needs of individual students

Students are not a homogenous group – they have different needs and different aspirations and learn in different ways. The adoption of an independent learning approach encourages these needs to be recognised and allows for student choice in terms of content, learning strategy and rates of learning (see Fig. 13.3).

Students can choose the learning method or approach which suits them best. They can skim learning material rapidly if they already understand it and spend more time with what is new or challenging to them. In mastery learning, students work with appropriate resource material until they reach the level of mastery required.

Student motivation

Independent learning gives students more responsibility for their learning and greater participation in the learning process. It allows them to choose the appropriate level for their studies. This in turn gives them a sense of ownership of their learning which has a positive effect on student motivation.

The role of the teacher

The teacher's role as a manager of the students' learning is well accepted and consistent with an independent learning approach. This facilitative role leaves teachers to develop new relationships with students and may result in greater trust between teacher and student. While many teachers feel most comfortable in the traditional role of information provider, others have discovered talents in developing resource material, a role which is also being recognised and rewarded.

"Their aims have been to promote greater active learning, more experiential learning and to encourage reflective learning"

Hudson et al 1997

Technophobes may choose to minimise contact with the computer. Encourage them to try computer assisted learning.

	No	Yes
Yes	Small PBL group	Distance learning
No	Lecture	Prescribed reading or study

Working on own

Fig. 13.3   Control of learning

Do not settle only for learning experiences with which the students are comfortable. Stretch the students both individually and personally.

"There is no right way to develop self-instructional materials. But there are lots of wrong ways"

Rowntree 1990

Cost-effectiveness

There are pressures on academic staff to provide coherent and effective teaching and learning programmes despite increasing student numbers and decreasing units of resource. There is strong opposition to these pressures and there are concerns that quality may suffer.

The justification for the introduction of independent learning lay previously with improved quality of learning rather than with cost savings. Independent learning can now, if used appropriately, contribute to cost savings. This is likely to require the sharing of resources between institutions. Careful timetabling is also required. If all students are scheduled to use a learning resource at the same time, then many copies may be required. If the period of time when students are 'ripe' for a resource is extended fewer copies are required and the exercise is more likely to be cost-effective. In an integrated endocrinology course made up of four modules and based on the use of resource material, for example, the timetable was so arranged that only a quarter of the students studied a module at any one time. This greatly reduced the need to duplicate resources.

Areas of controversy

The traditional curriculum emphasises the views on a topic of the teacher or lecturer with whom the student is in contact. The student may be seduced into the notion that there is one right answer or one approach to a problem. Independent learning allows him or her to be exposed to the rich environment of many visions and interpretations.

Outcome-based education

There is a move away from a process model of curriculum planning to a product one where the learning outcomes are made more explicit and where outcomes influence decisions about teaching and learning and about assessment.

"Uncertainty should not be hidden away as an embarrassment"

Alderson & Roberts 2000

With the destination to be reached clearly charted, students may wish to plan their own route. Independent learning thrives in such an environment.

The development of self-learning skills

The acquisition of the skills of self-learning and the ability to be able to keep up to date with developments in medicine are learning outcomes about which there is general agreement.

Traditional teaching methods do not emphasise the development of these skills. In contrast, independent learning encourages not only mastery of the content area being studied but also the development of generic skills of self-learning.

Trends in independent learning

Independent learning is not new. To a greater or lesser extent, students have always worked independently. One can identify, however, a number of changes in the approach to independent learning being adopted.

An increasingly important role

It was clearly demonstrated three decades ago in a randomised controlled trial (Harden et al 1969) that medical students learn as, or more, effectively when they work independently using learning resources prepared for the purpose, compared to students who attend lectures. Until recently, however, teachers have been slow to move away from an emphasis in the curriculum on lectures. There has been a significant change and independent learning is now playing an increasingly important role in the curriculum:

- Time previously scheduled for lectures or small group work is often rescheduled for independent learning.
- Independent learning is now an explicit planned part of the learning activities and protected time allocated for it is scheduled in the timetable.
- The role of the lecture is changing. Lectures are used to support independent learning rather than independent learning being used as an adjunct to support the lecture.

"The only man who is educated is the man who has learned how to learn"

Rogers 1983

"Medical faculties should examine critically the number of lecture hours they now schedule and consider major reductions in this passive form of learning"

Association of American Medical Colleges 1984

"If students are to learn effectively in resource-based learning courses, then they need more and better learning skills than those currently exhibited by students on conventional courses"

Brown & Smith 1996

Technology should enrich teaching not substitute for it.

To develop learning resources, expertise is needed in the content area, in the delivery medium and in instructional design.

A planned and supported programme

Independent learning, it is now appreciated, has to be carefully planned and not left to chance. The choice is not between a planned programme of lectures and other activities on the one hand, and on the other, students being left to fend for themselves.

Planning by the teacher for independent learning includes:

- recognising the role of independent learning in the curriculum, making this explicit to students and scheduling it in the timetable
- ensuring students have the necessary study skills with which to engage in independent learning in the first instance. Study skills training needed may include:
  — how to assess needs
  — how to plan learning
  — how to manage time
  — how to locate and use appropriate resources
  — how to evaluate outcomes of learning
- identifying the tools to be used by students in their studies, including library facilities, personal textbooks, multimedia programmes and the Internet.

A wide range of tools available

An increasingly wide range of tools to support independent learning has become available. Regrettably, however, the technical sophistication of the resources available is often not paralleled by their educational sophistication. Many lack the basic principles of educational design such as the incorporation of meaningful interactivity and feedback.

Too often computers have been used merely as mechanical page turners and the Internet has been abused, encouraging passive learning rather than a deeper understanding and reflection. The need is now recognised to incorporate proven effective educational strategies into the instructional design for self-learning.

Multimedia programmes are of particular value in supporting an integrated curriculum. They bring together and integrate in various ways the views of experts from a range of fields.

The provision of student support

The adoption of independent learning does not imply that the teacher abandons the student to work on his or her own. The role of the teacher as a facilitator in independent learning is an important one. This is achieved through interactions between student and teacher, face-to-face, by telephone or on the Internet. The teacher can also prepare study guides to support the student's learning as described in Chapter 18.

Study guides can:

- provide information not readily available to students in the information sources to which they have access
- provide guidance for students on the management of their learning, with advice on what they should learn, how they should learn it and how can they assess whether they have learned it
- suggest activities for students which reinforce their learning and relate it to clinical practice.

Study guides vary in the extent to which they emphasise each of these facilities, and the relative importance of each in a guide can be indicated by placing the guide in a triangle (the study guide triangle), with each function identified at one of the three points of the triangle (Harden, Laidlaw & Hesketh 1999). A guide placed equidistant from each of the points has all three functions equally represented.

Study guides may be in print or electronic format.

Students may also get support from their colleagues. This concept of collaborative learning has gained increased recognition. Students may be helped by:

- their peers
- students in the later years of a course assigned to help more junior students
- working in pairs as a basis for their studies.

The range of contexts

The wide range of contexts in which independent learning can occur is now recognised. These include:

- at home

"A study guide can be seen as a management tool which allows teachers to exercise their responsibilities while at the same time giving students an important part to play in managing their own learning"

Harden, Laidlaw & Hesketh 1999

"A peer support website can broaden student interest in learning independently and is especially pertinent to the needs of less confident students seeking to improve their academic performance"

Baker & Dillon 1999

- in areas in a learning centre or teaching institution developed for this purpose
- on the job or in the workplace (e.g. in task-based learning).

A focus for assessment

Portfolios prepared by students as part of their independent work serve not only as an aid to learning but as a powerful tool for assessment alongside more traditional tests based on written examinations and/or objective structured clinical examinations (OSCEs) (Challis 1999). This emphasises the importance of independent learning. What the students are intended to achieve and how they will record this should be documented.

Summary

Independent learning should occupy a key role in the curriculum. The twin aims are mastery of the topic under consideration and the development of the skills of self-learning. Teachers and curriculum planners should decide:

- how much time should be scheduled in the curriculum for independent learning? It is unlikely to be less than 25% or more than 75%.
- how to recognise and institutionalise the position adopted with regard to independent learning through:
  — protected time in the curriculum identified in the timetable?
  — provision of appropriate learning resources/recognition in the assessment procedures?
  — a staff development programme to orientate staff?
- what range of methods or tools will be offered to the student, e.g. printed material, videotapes, multimedia presentations, the Internet?
- how will students be supported as they work through the programme? Study guides can be seen as a tutor to which they have constant access.

"Traditional exams cannot test many of the skills and abilities developed by resource-based learning"

Brown & Smith 1996

"Having students acquire skills as active learners will require considerable effort and increased dedication to this goal of faculty members"

ACME-TRI report Association of American Medical Colleges 1993

References and further reading

Alderson P, Roberts I 2000 Should journals publish reviews that find no evidence to guide practice? British Medical Journal 320:376–377

Association of American Medical Colleges 1984 Physicians for the 21st Century: report of the project panel on the general professional education of the physicians and college preparation for medicine. Journal of Medical Education 59, Part 2:1–208

Anderson M B, Swanson A G 1993 Educating medical students – the ACME-TRI report with supplements. Acad Med 68(Suppl):S1–46

Baker J, Dillon G 1999 Peer support on the web. IETI 36, 1:65–70

Brown S, Smith B 1996 Resource-based learning. Kogan Page, London

Challis M 1999 Portfolio-based learning and assessment. Medical Teacher 21(4):370–386

Challis M 2000 AMEE Medical Education Guide no .18. Personal learning plans. Medical Teacher 22:3,225–236

Collins R, Hammond M 1987 Self-directed learning to educate medical educators: why do we use self-directed learning? Medical Teacher 9(4):425–432

Ellington H 1997 Flexible learning – your flexible friend! Keynote address in: implementing flexible learning. Aspects of educational and training technology volume XXIX. Kogan Page, London

Harden R M et al 1969 An experiment involving substitution of tape/slide programmes for lectures. Lancet 1:933–935

Harden R M, Laidlaw J M 1992 Effective continuing education: the CRISIS criteria. ASME Medical Education Booklet no. 4. Medical Education 26:408–422

Harden R M, Laidlaw J M, Hesketh E A 1999 AMEE Medical Education Guide no. 16. Study guides – their use and preparation. Medical Teacher 21(3):248–265

Hudson R, Maslin-Prothero S, Oates L 1997 Flexible learning in action: case studies in higher education. Staff and Educational Development Series. Kogan Page, London

Rogers C R 1983 Freedom to learn for the 80s. Out of print

Rowntree D 1990 Teaching through self-instruction: how to develop open learning materials. Kogan Page, London

Spencer J A, Jordan R K 1999 Learner-centred approaches in medical education. British Medical Journal 318(7193):1280–1283

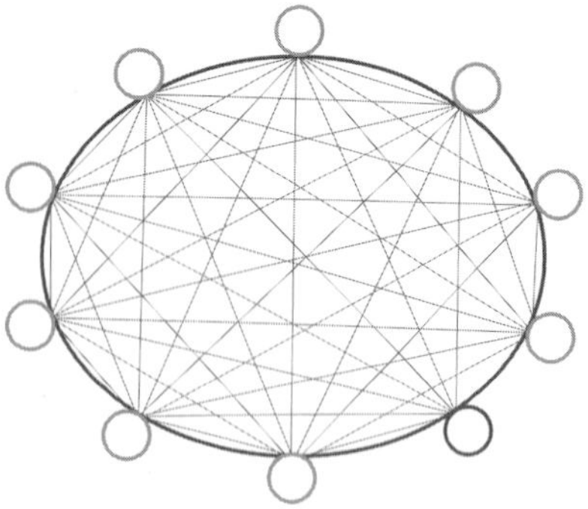

Chapter 14
Problem-based learning

A. Sefton

Introduction

What is problem-based learning?

Problem-based learning is student-centred and either represents the core method of learning or supplements didactic teaching. It is most often implemented early in medical programmes, although variants are now being introduced into clinical years.

The initiating problem stimulates students to explore basic scientific and clinical mechanisms and frequently social, psychological, ethical or professional issues. Knowledge is integrated and applied. Because of the potentially open-ended nature of the process, staff have an obligation to design well-structured problems that meet explicit goals.

Different, well-established medical examples are described in Neufeld & Barrows (1974), Henry, Byrne & Engel (1997), Kaufman (1985) and Tosteson, Adelstein & Carver (1994).

The problem stimulates students to reason, think critically and to weigh evidence; they seek out and share relevant information. Groups do not need prior knowledge to generate lively ideas as they identify areas for further collective and personal learning. Each student brings individual experience, thus making a distinctive contribution (see Figs 14.1 and 14.2).

An effective group provides a safe environment for sharing and testing new knowledge. Students practise the language of science and medicine, evaluate ideas and receive feedback from peers and tutor.

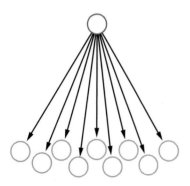

Possible interpersonal communication links for nine students and a tutor. These complex interactions must be facilitated and managed.

Fig. 14.1   A problem-based group

A typical didactic session with one-way communication.

Fig. 14.2   A didactic session

If clinical exposure is introduced concurrently, intellectual and practical skills develop in parallel. Clinical experiences enrich tutorial discussions.

In preparing students for professional practice, problem-based learning:

- encourages independence as they identify and meet individual learning needs
- stimulates reflection and self-direction for life-long learning
- supports on-going self-assessment
- introduces clinical reasoning, later refined with clinical experience
- enhances critical thinking and evidence-based decision-making
- ensures that knowledge is transferred, applied and retained by providing a relevant, integrated context
- offers practice and experience in introducing professional concepts and medical language
- supports effective teamwork and peer communication.

Developing a sequence of learning problems structures a modern, relevant, integrated curriculum, capable of progressive change and of minimising redundancy, overload and gaps (Field & Sefton 1997).

Experiencing a problem-based tutorial

Observing an effective tutorial group in action provides an opportunity to experience the basic characteristics. The initial impression is usually of an open, lively and free-flowing discussion in which all participate. The atmosphere is friendly and informal.

The local structure and sequence of tutorials may vary in style, even within established frameworks. With experience, groups become more targeted and efficient.

Effective tutors do not dominate or instruct. Indeed, who actually *is* the tutor may not be immediately apparent. She or he quietly monitors the process, ensuring that all are included and interactions focus on relevant issues.

"A particular goal of this student-centred, problem-based approach is to develop physicians who practice 'science in action' rather than attempting to apply learned formulas to clinical situations"

Tosteson, Adelstein & Carver 1994

"the key for problem-based learning is . . . to use a problem to drive the learning activities on a need-to-know basis"

Woods 1994

Trust the collective curiosity and motivation of the group to identify the issues arising from the problem and determine their learning goals.

Frameworks and sequences for problem-based learning

Well-designed problems are underpinned by a structure for reasoning, equally explicit to tutors and students. Typically:

- A trigger initiates the problem (on video, paper, computer).
- Groups brainstorm to identify cues and key issues.
- Broad thinking produces a rich array of possible explanations or mechanisms.
- Hypotheses are critically explored through reasoning and organised by priority or likelihood.
- Hypotheses are tested and refuted or supported by further information sought from the tutor or progressively revealed.
- A conclusion is reached on diagnosis and/or management.
- The group reviews the process.

Throughout, students identify learning issues to be pursued in the breaks between tutorials.

If there are three tutorials per problem, the first usually concludes during step 4, the second after 5. If two, the break is often during step 5.

Characteristics of an effective problem-based learning group

An effective group is cohesive, motivated, mutually supportive and actively engaged in learning. The group understands and energetically pursues its task.

Members respect each other's contributions but examine them critically. Discussion flows as students cooperate rather than compete. Quieter members are encouraged while the more confident restrain their tendencies to dominate. Individuals are supported during times of personal stress.

The atmosphere is friendly and good-humoured. Discussion is open but tactful and constructive. Difficulties that arise are not ignored, but dealt with sensitively in a climate of mutual tolerance.

Making explicit the underlying framework as well as the sequence and structure of the tutorials encourages groups to work efficiently.

"I thought the group I sat in with was doing really well for second year students – their collective knowledge and understanding was impressive. Then I found out that they were actually only a few months into first year!"
Visitor from UK to Graduate Medical Program, University of Sydney

Members are proud of their successful group. They look forward to tutorials and may spend time together outside sessions. Successful groups induct new tutors and restrain excessive interference from overly directive teachers.

Roles are shared; all take turns in scribing, leading discussion or accepting responsibility for acquiring information. If the tutor is delayed, well-established groups confidently start the tutorial and proceed effectively.

Groups often share food and drink – inside the rooms if permitted or by taking 'time out'.

Staff development

The importance of tutor training to equip teachers for their new roles cannot be over-emphasised. Indeed, basic training is usually mandatory. Some teachers find it hard to relinquish more didactic roles and opportunities to display content expertise, yet most enjoy the new experience.

Before starting as a tutor, it is usual (and may be required) to observe a group in the same school. In new programmes, tutors who initially observed programmes elsewhere must be aware of any differences in goals, expectations or organisation in their own school.

The nature of staff development and on-going support varies. Initial training may involve observation and practice with a group from the programme or recruited for the purpose. Alternatively the process may be modelled amongst the trainees themselves.

Effective training ensures that the necessary background, goals and local strategies are considered, together with information on assessment and evaluation. Specific issues of institutional emphasis (e.g. evidence-based medicine or information technology) require explanation and practice. Tutors need skills in monitoring the process and giving feedback.

In addition to materials supplied to students, tutors are usually issued with handbooks or guides, highlighting issues for each problem. They may also contain essential information to be revealed progressively.

Relax! Students in problem-based groups *will*:

- learn and understand content
- think critically
- use scientific and medical language
- correct errors
- learn how to learn.

One important source of on-going support is engagement with other tutors. Frequently a meeting is scheduled to discuss the current and upcoming problems, ideally with case writers or subject experts present. Issues of content and process are discussed, and difficulties or confusions resolved; experiences are shared and strategies reviewed. Such meetings encourage tutors to contribute to the quality control of the programme. To summarise, participants in a tutor training session attempt to:

- seek answers
- review the goals
- understand the role
- clarify local practices
- acknowledge and share concerns
- know resources and support
- practise new strategies
- meet fellow tutors
- participate enthusiastically!

Starting as a problem-based learning tutor

Would-be tutors need some crucial information before embarking on teaching:

- Are the students beginners or 'old hands'? What have they learned already?
- What model of problem-based learning is used? How many tutorials? What are the reasoning steps?
- Are guides or handbooks supplied to tutors?
- What is the tutor's role in guiding the breadth and depth of learning?
- What additional learning activities are provided? Are other resources available? What support is offered to students in difficulties?
- How are students assessed? Do tutors assess?

Nervous new tutors generally find it easier to take established groups than to initiate inexperienced groups. Helping students to form a new group requires particular skills; some experienced tutors prefer that role.

Seek information about the characteristics of your group from previous tutors and get to know the individuals as quickly as possible.

Make sure that you can communicate directly with your group for messages (e-mail, phone call, bulletin board, mailbox). Plan ahead and be prepared:

- Understand the model used.
- Know the students' level.
- Review the goals.
- Read tutor information.
- Identify key discussion points.

Who makes a good problem-based tutor?

Good tutors encourage appropriate interaction by maintaining an open and trusting environment. They reflect on their own performance.

Most problem-based teachers enjoy facilitating learning and enhancing reasoning skills. With training, undergraduates, research students and staff at all levels of appointment have become effective tutors.

Although successful tutors may be drawn from diverse disciplines, the majority are most comfortable tutoring in areas related to their own expertise. Some prior knowledge or experience may allow tutors to enhance a group's effectiveness, provided that they facilitate and do not dictate. Relevant experience leading to a sense of comfort may come from prior research, teaching or clinical practice or from previous tutoring on the same problems (Wilkerson 1994).

Does subject expertise matter? Any trained tutor who facilitates group learning is appropriate. Thus individuals with educational, scientific, health professional or humanities backgrounds have been effective medical problem-based tutors. By contrast, subject experts who deliver mini-lectures or interrupt the free flow of a group's discussion are inappropriate since they circumvent the essential exploration and interaction that underpin the success of problem-based learning.

However expert in a particular subject teachers may be, not all will easily adopt the facilitatory practices needed. Such a shift in role requires an understanding of the goals of problem-based learning, flexibility and an awareness of students' needs.

Good tutors encourage behaviours that enhance the sessions, ensuring that all participate appropriately. They help set expectations and provide thoughtful insights to the group.

At the end of the session a tutor should reflect on the following questions to formulate an impression of his or her performance:

- Are we achieving our goals?
- Could I have done better?

When difficulties arise, it is better to deal with them than let them fester:

- Tactful directness is appropriate.
- Seek support/solutions from the group.
- Offer practical assistance where possible.
- Deal with personal issues in private.
- Know sources for student assistance.
- Do not be tempted to undertake a counselling role.

- Were there high or low points?
- Did I intervene appropriately?
- Should I have a word with…?
- Is the time well balanced?
- Did everyone participate?

Dealing with difficulties

Encourage the group to articulate concerns, make suggestions and own the solutions.

Examples of difficulties and solutions are:

- Dominant students, confident and perhaps wrong
  Encourage the group to examine all statements critically and maybe have a quiet word with the student outside the tutorial.

- Silent students – personality or failure to keep up?
  Sensitise the group to the needs of the shyer or less confident; make 'space' for contributions, suggest particular roles.

- Uncooperative, disruptive students
  Encourage group discussion and solutions; interview the student privately; in extreme cases consult the course director.

- Students who persistently seek information from the tutor
  Respond with open questions; encourage others to contribute.

- A group that fails to 'gel', or in which personality clashes develop
  Raise the issues; elicit suggestions for diagnosing the problem(s) and developing practical solutions.

- A group that bogs down, reporting information retrieved rather than advancing the discussion (common)
  Suggest that the group exchanges information beforehand by e-mail, in paper summaries or in a separate meeting.

What is the tutor's role in assessment?

Tutors must know local assessment strategies. Individual students and/or groups may be assessed summatively (determining progress) or formatively (for feedback).

The group

At the end of each problem, groups usually review their processes, encouraging self-reflection and enhancing their collective performance. Some students, however, are uncomfortable with self-assessment and personal discussion; differences reflect national characteristics, cultural backgrounds, fluency in the local language, confidence and personality. Overall, the comfort of students with the method, as well as trust in the tutor and fellow members, affects their willingness to engage in meaningful reflection and revelation.

The skills of the tutor are tested when a group is unwilling to take responsibility for the process or to participate effectively. The essential trust must be established early; students who fear a penalty or negative outcome are unlikely to commit themselves honestly and openly. Useful questions to discuss would include:

- How did we go as a group? What went particularly well?
- What could I have done better?
- Were there difficult situations?
- Was anything particularly helpful?

Facilitatory strategies include posing open-ended questions or inviting comments on particular situations.

Formative group assessment can occur when tutors are exchanged for one problem in order to provide independent feedback to the group and tutor. More formal reviews require expert observation or the use of group assessment instruments.

Individual students

Tutors may be expected to provide formative feedback to each member. One useful device is a self-assessment student questionnaire reviewing appropriate

Compared with didactic methods, problem-based learning:

- is active and self-directed
- is enjoyed more by staff and students
- offers 'safe', cooperative learning
- introduces early clinical reasoning
- includes scientific, social, ethical issues
- knowledge is integrated, readily applied
- encourages use of medical language

but:

- students are more anxious about the boundaries of knowledge expected.

behaviours; the tutor returns it with comments and may interview each individual privately.

Individual students are assessed using a variety of written, oral and/or clinical tests in order to determine their progression and ultimate graduation. If they are competitively graded in examinations, students may avoid sharing and contributing to the group process. In that circumstance, tutors need particular skills to encourage cooperation.

Tutors are usually expected to note absences and to assist and perhaps report on students experiencing difficulties. They may be required to judge each student's performance summatively. Most tutors and students find that task uncomfortable and somewhat unreliable, even when criteria are established and training is provided.

Evaluating problem-based learning tutorials

Students enjoy commenting on the effectiveness of teaching and learning, providing that the demand is not excessive, their views are taken seriously and consequent action is evident. At the end of each problem, and particularly in the final tutorial of a term, time is usefully allocated for evaluation.

Both the process and the learning in problem-based tutorials are evaluated against explicit goals. Thus the tutor's overview of the effectiveness of group processes offers insights for the members. In addition, specific questions of content or confusions can be noted. Tutors can pass on their group's views to curriculum managers who should then notify students of any resulting changes.

Students normally complete an evaluation of the tutor. The explicit skills considered most important for effective facilitation should be identified so that constructive feedback is provided to teachers and managers.

Sample issues for tutor evaluation include:

- tutor characteristics: helpfulness, interest, enthusiasm
- support of clinical reasoning

- encouragement of independent learning
- enhancement of group process
- provision of feedback.

Summary

In this chapter, the characteristics of teaching in problem-based learning tutorials are outlined. The tutor is a facilitator, rather than a source of information, a role that requires training. Broad goals of problem-based learning are indicated, and include the encouragement of self-directed learning, clinical reasoning and teamwork. Implementation varies, so tutors must clarify local expectations and practical details. They need to know what supporting teaching activities are offered, the students' previous learning experiences and resources available for students and staff. The roles of tutors differ, so local expectations in terms of assessment and evaluation must be understood.

Acknowledgement

I am grateful to Jill Gordon who made helpful comments on a draft of this chapter.

References and further reading

Albanese M A, Mitchell S 1993 Academic Medicine 68:52–81

Field M J, Sefton A J 1998 Computer-based management of content in a problem-based medical curriculum. Medical Education 32:163–171

Henry R, Byrne K, Engel C 1997 Imperatives in medical education, University of Newcastle, Faculty of Health Sciences, Newcastle, NSW

Kaufman A 1985 Implementing problem-based education. Lessons from successful innovations. Springer, New York

Moore G T, Block S D, Style C B, Mitchell R 1994 Academic Medicine 69:983–989

Neufeld V, Barrows H 1974 Journal of Medical Education 49:1040–1050

Sackett D L, Richardson W S, Rosenberg W, Haynes R B 1997 Evidence-based medicine: how to practice and teach EBM. Churchill Livingstone, New York

Tosteson D C, Adelstein S J, Carver S T 1994 New pathways to medical education. Harvard University Press, Cambridge, MA

Vernon T A, Blake R L 1993 Academic Medicine 68:550–563

Wilkerson L 1994 Academic Medicine 69:646–648

Woods D R 1994 Problem-based learning: how to gain the most from PBL. D R Woods, Hamilton, Ontario

Chapter 15
Integrated learning

J. S. Ker

"The best way to create interest in a subject is to render it worth knowing – to make the knowledge usable in one's thinking beyond the situation in which learning has occurred"

Bruner

Introduction

Why is there a need for integrated learning?
Medical practice begins with learning from the scientific literature and ends with learning to care for patients. Every health-care practitioner has to be able to apply the relevant knowledge, skills and professional attitudes in order to resolve each individual's health or disease concern.

Although there are many common presentations of health and disease, every individual presents his or her illness or health concern from a personal perspective. In other words, there is no finite number of patient presentations that can be taught or learnt. All practitioners must therefore:

- develop the ability of being able to access relevant knowledge, skills and attitudes when presented with a health-care problem
- have the ability to reconstruct their understanding of health-care problems based on their experience
- be able to adapt their understanding in the presence of a new problem.

This process of developing flexible, changing and adaptable knowledge can be described in educational terms as integrated learning.

Within the medical curriculum the process has previously been mainly left to chance. It was assumed implicitly that all practitioners would eventually be able to integrate their knowledge from the experience they encountered in their clinical practice. The curriculum easily divided into two parts: a preclinical course of basic medical science and a 3-year clinical programme. In many schools this divide was compounded by physical separation between the university campus and the teaching hospital and by the tension between the academic and vocational requirements of the profession.

However, increased patient turnover and decreased in-patient stay have shifted the focus for student placements away from the teaching hospital environment to the community and ambulatory care settings where students now gain their clinical experience.

Increased expectations from patients and increased accountability to funding authorities have also influenced the pressure for change to ensure all practitioners are able to integrate their learning.

The explosion of knowledge in biomedical sciences and the rapidity of change make it essential that physicians should know how to link basic science concepts with their practice to enable them to continue learning. The challenge for clinical teachers is how to provide students with the necessary facilitated support to integrated learning which will enable them to practise a high standard of relevant medicine.

An integrated curriculum is a strategy to achieving life-long learning skills. Integration is a learner-centred strategy recognising that we all learn at different paces and that health-care practitioners spend the majority of their practising life being responsible for their own educational development.

Identify the local barriers to increased integration as an initial step.

What implications does integrated learning have for medical education?

Integration in medical education has therefore been a major feature of recent reforms (World Federation of Medical Education Edinburgh Declaration 1993, General Medical Council 1993). As a result many undergraduate medical schools introduced curricular changes in the 1990s; however, many developed an integrated curriculum which assessed the curriculum instead of the learner.

"What is integration? A way of making the theoretical practical"

Blum 1973

The purpose of an integrated curriculum is to produce a graduate who 'becomes his/her own educator' (Connelly 1972).

An integrated teaching approach helps students learn through:

- active rather than passive learning
- self-assessment
- individualisation
- self-learning.

What is the educational rationale?

The theory of integration in relation to adult learning is linked to life-long learning theory.

There are many different theories of integration adapted from general education:

- In the SPICES model for the development of educational strategies curriculum integration is described along a continuum between integration and discipline-based teaching (see Fig. 2.4). In 1998 the concept was further described as a series of 11 rungs on a ladder from isolation to transdisciplinary integration. Subjects are the product of integrative processes in themselves; what is for discussion is how far along the integration ladder you are (see Fig. 15.1).
- Skillbeck (1972) described three levels of integration:
  — Level 1 Subject
  — Level 2 Interdisciplinary
  — Level 3 Loss of separate disciplines
- Kooi (1975) described integration in terms of a conceptual approach versus a process approach.
- Lynch (1977) defined integration as a means of interrelating various subjects, having commenced with a global concept.

In practice a curriculum committee has to agree on a definition and determine how much integration is desirable over a time period. At a systems level in the delivery of the curriculum each system has to determine how much vertical and how much horizontal integration will be presented. Horizontal integration describes

"a way of making education purposeful"

Acland 1967

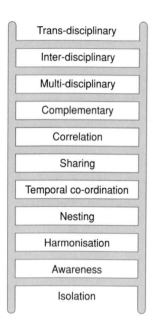

Fig. 15.1 Integration ladder

Trans-disciplinary
Inter-disciplinary
Multi-disciplinary
Complementary
Correlation
Sharing
Temporal co-ordination
Nesting
Harmonisation
Awareness
Isolation

Form a consensus understanding of integration for your school.

integration across topics or subjects. (see Fig. 15.2). Vertical integration describes integration throughout the course (see Fig. 15.3). In practice integrated courses have elements of both.

It must be noted that the teaching staff, the faculty structure and the departmental organisation will all help to determine the integrated learning environment for students.

What are the educational advantages of integrated learning?

There are many advantages to integrated learning. An integrated curriculum:

- presents a coherent picture of knowledge
- facilitates integrative learning.

However these are not mutually exclusive. Presentation of integrated material should encourage integrative thinking and such learning experiences should facilitate the development of useful knowledge structures in the learner.

Curriculum integration can help the learner:

- cope with changes in knowledge
- deal with outdated knowledge
- understand knowledge.

Coping with changes in knowledge

Integration enables the curriculum to be organised around key concepts and principles and encourages higher-level thinking.

Example: The life cycle

This is a central concept of reproduction, growth and ageing in which normal and abnormal structure, function and behavioural aspects can be presented. Knowledge is accessed from a more interrelated flexible structure.

When curriculum overload is highlighted it is often due to factual overload. Integration enables the learner to focus on the basic principles of the varieties of

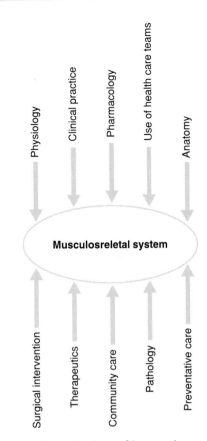

Fig. 15.2   Horizontal integration

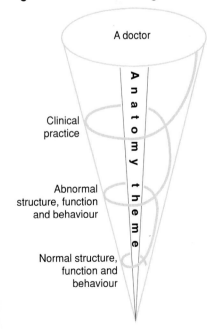

Fig. 15.3   Vertical integration

knowledge. Learning is then meaningful and the curriculum is not overloaded.

Dealing with outdated knowledge

When knowledge becomes out of date it is not the basic cognitive structures that are vulnerable but the factual content.

Example: Treatment of duodenal ulcer

1950 psychological
1960 surgical
1970–1980s H2 antagonists
1990s antibiotics.

Understanding the underlying pathophysiological processes of inflammation and infection has been essential for keeping up to date.

Understanding knowledge

Interrelating different areas of knowledge can be difficult for the learner and traditionally it has been assumed to have taken place in an ad hoc manner.

Passing from one subject to another provides the student with different perspectives of knowledge, and learning becomes fragmented; if the disciplines have different status within the school students will have an imbalanced exposure.

Example: Medicine and surgery

Traditionally medicine and surgery based in the hospital setting were perceived as disciplines with high status and paediatrics and primary care medicine perceived as being of lesser status.

Using an integrated approach has the following advantages. It:

- enables a unified presentation of a problem
- minimalises contradiction of concepts
- avoids repetition within the curriculum
- facilitates interdisciplinary cooperation
- provides opportunities for learning for staff
- identifies research problems
- motivates students.

Any of these advantages can be used in discussions at strategic planning meetings to convince the curriculum committee.

Many curricula which are traditionally subject-based depend on extrinsic forms of motivation such as examinations and competition. In contrast interactive learning stimulates interest by emphasising the application of theory by encouraging student participation and by providing opportunities for cooperative learning. The emphasis of integrated learning is on it being a dynamic process in which the learners take responsibility for their own learning.

What are the educational disadvantages of an integrated curriculum?

As with all aspects of education there are always some concerns in the development of an integrated curriculum. These include the following:

- the potential to miss out basic concepts
- time-consuming liaising with other staff members
- decreased expertise of teaching staff
- the need for more preparation by teaching staff.

In implementing an integrated strategy build in solutions which address these concerns.

Practical pathways to achieving integration

The concept of curricular integration incorporates many ideas e.g.:

- ways of organising a timetable to cope with expansion of knowledge
- characteristics of curriculum planning

The implementation of curriculum integration, however, needs to be considered at two levels:

- at a strategic level
- at an operational level.

How do you develop an integrated course or curriculum at strategic level?

Learning outcomes

The University of Dundee has developed 12 detailed learning outcomes which are addressed throughout the 5 years of the programme. These serve to provide an integrated and overriding set of purposes applicable for all the learning opportunities students encounter. The students are assessed throughout the curriculum on their abilities in all 12 outcomes.

Core curriculum
The concept of a core curriculum in the health-care context has been adapted from its use in secondary schools and is seen as a method of integration at a strategic level.

Systems-based approach
In a medical context fragmentation occurs due to the dichotomy between theory and practice, between hospital and the different types of health-care professional. A systems-based approach enables various perspectives to be considered at the same time as teachers from different disciplines focus on one topic at the same time.

Example: Gastroenterology system
A multidisciplinary group developed a balanced programme for second-year students covering admissions to hospital, review of pathology workload and an analysis of primary care consultations which reflected current clinical practice.

Integrated learning focus
Allocating time and resources within the curriculum can be a useful way of ensuring that integrated learning opportunities are available.

However, tutors often feel vulnerable when facilitating sessions which draw on experience and knowledge from other disciplines and clinical settings. A dedicated teaching area which can accommodate posters, pots and patients can be designed to enable students to bring together their learning from the week to solve new problems. It can be led by a multidisciplinary team which itself is a relevant role model as students begin to appreciate the reality of a team approach to patient care.

"to the young mind everything is individual, stands by itself. By and by it finds out how to join two things and see in them one nature; then three, then three thousand discovering roots running underground whereby contrary and remote things cohere and flower out from one stem"

Emerson

Problem-based curriculum

Problem-based learning is a very useful way of integrating learning (Barrows 1985). Students are presented with a problem just as a physician would be and then in small groups have to identify, with the help of a trained facilitator, what areas they need to be competent in to manage it (see Chapter 14).

How do you develop an integrated course or curriculum at operational level?

Integration by study guides

Study guides are a tool to help students manage their learning (Laidlaw & Harden 1990) and therefore can be a means of integrating student activities in relation to curriculum objectives at both strategic and operational levels.

Integrating basic and clinical sciences

The Principles of Clinical Medicine unit is a 2-year longitudinal course devised by the Oregon Health Sciences University, USA, and directed through an interdisciplinary steering committee. Large group sessions provide specific content but students participate in small group and self-directed study using both computer-assisted learning (CAL) and teaching laboratories. Students also have the same tutor for ambulatory patient care sessions.

Patient record books/logbooks

Patient record books and logbooks are seen as a useful integrative tool. Students in paediatrics in Bangladesh record their clerking but are required to generalise their learning from each patient through a series of questions discussed with their ward tutor. The questions attempt to bring the relevant theory to the bedside and so enable students to apply their theoretical learning in the clinical context.

At the University of Dundee, phase two students produce a structured therapeutic report based on the patients they have interviewed. Students then identify specific learning points in relation to each patient. This encourages the development of a reflective practitioner and also enables students to integrate history, examination and management skills across the systems.

How do you integrate different clinical settings?

Practice of medicine programme

Clinical teachers from different clinical settings have formed a working group at the University of Dundee to determine the clinical teaching and learning programme for phase two students.

A common set of learning outcomes based on the overarching curriculum outcomes has been constructed by clinicians from general practice, clinical skills and the wards. This enables teaching and learning in the different clinical settings to complement and reinforce each other. Programme posters in the wards, general practitioner surgeries and student areas alert all involved to the week's programme. Teachers' facilitation across clinical settings has occasionally been possible. A practising medicine booklet sets out a patient-centred model of consultation to be used in all settings and gives guidance on constructing an appropriate written record for each setting.

Condition diagramming

Condition diagramming has been used in Texas, USA (Russell 1985), to help students integrate clinical data. It uses a defined format to establish information required in the context of patient needs. The condition diagram consists of background information, prevention factors, induction factors, interventions, complications and pertinent data which determine the differential diagnosis and the possible outcomes. The diagram attempts to have both versatility and order and can be dynamic. A progress diagram would reflect the patient's progress.

How do you avoid major deficiencies in the curricular programme?

Some topic areas, which might otherwise be overlooked in the curriculum structure, are integrated into the programme using a variety of strategies.

A longitudinal programme

In Harvard Medical School, USA, a longitudinal programme has been developed which identifies areas in the course where primary, secondary and tertiary health promotion and disease prevention could be introduced to students in the early years to match their professional development at different phases. Students built on this in their clinical attachments to ambulatory care focusing on health promotion.

Early patient contact

Several medical schools have introduced patients at an early stage of the curriculum. The purpose of this is to increase the relevance of the basic clinical sciences and to help to identify any communication problems students may have at an early stage of their training.

'Doctoring' programme

At UCLA School of Medicine, USA, a programme on doctoring has been introduced to cover topic areas neglected within the curricular structure. Students follow and manage a panel of simulated patients over the course of the year and can focus on such diverse areas as continuity of care, nutrition, cost containment, family violence, law and ethics.

How can technology advance integrated learning?

Computer skills can be useful in helping students integrate their learning.

Integrating information technology

At King's College Medical School, London, the implementation of integrated academic and clinical studies was found to be particularly difficult.

Electronic reference material has been made widely available and students are required to use it to complete course material.

The provision of computer notebooks for each student and a dial-up network service from distant sites maximise the integration of technology into the curriculum but most importantly enable students to access material in order to make links across clinical settings and from basic science to clinical practice. Students then have the ability to develop flexible useful knowledge, which can be accessed when required.

Integrating medical decision-making

An integrated case studies and medical decision-making course at the University of Pittsburgh, USA, uses information science and computer technology to bridge the gap. The course consists of 13 problem-based learning exercises exploring clinical scenarios. Students working in small groups on networked computers progress through the scenarios with a facilitator. The juxtaposition of basic science and clinical material and the ability to alternate between materials were found to be major strengths of the programme.

Mind mapping

Mind mapping has been used by a group in a Master of Public Health programme in Switzerland which employs concept mapping using computer technology to enhance meaningful learning and to enable students to define their own learning outcomes.

How do you evaluate the process of integration?

Developing diagnostic competence

A Dutch study analysed results from three different medical schools comparing traditional discipline teaching with an integrated curriculum by assessing their diagnostic competence for 30 case histories.

The study reported that diagnostic competence was more accurate in the students from the integrated schools. However, this difference only became apparent in the clinical years.

Summary

In this chapter we have attempted to define integrated learning in the context of current clinical and educational practice and to demonstrate this through examples of practical pathways to integrated learning at both strategic and operational levels.

"Tell me and I will hear, show me and I will see, involve me and I will understand"

Adapted from WHO

References and further reading

Barrows H S 1985 How to design a problem based curriculum for the preclinical years. Springer, New York

Chastonay P H 1999. Use of concept mapping to define learning objectives in a Master of Public Health programme. Teaching and Learning in Medicine 11:21–25

Fields S A 1995 Principles of clinical medicine: an interdisciplinary 2 year longitudinal course. Medical Education 29:53–57

General Medical Council 1993 Tomorrow's doctors. General Medical Council, London

Laidlaw J M, Harden R M 1990 What is a study guide? Medical Teacher 12: 7–12

Russell I J 1985 Conditioning diagramming: a new approach to teaching clinical integration. Medical Education 19:220–225

Sivam S P, Iatridis P G, Vaughn S 1995 Integration of pharmacology to a problem based learning curriculum for medical students. Medical Education 29

Slavin S J, Wilkes M S, Usatine R 1995 Doctoring III: Innovations in education in the clinical years. Academic Medicine 70

Taylor W C, Moore G T 1994 Health promotion and disease prevention integration into a medical school curriculum. Medical Education 28

Chapter 16
Multiprofessional education

S. Cable

Introduction

Integration of education and practice

The trend within education and practice is currently towards integration, educational content and practice brought together on the basis of rules of relevance rather than traditional, professional knowledge boundaries. This move, in part, has been driven by a demand for closer working relationships between health professionals, on the part of both governments and patients, and by the increasing complexity of patient problems. Underlying this trend is the idea that multi-professional education will provide a foundation stone upon which multiprofessional working practices can be built. However, the fact of one resulting in the other remains a subject of vigorous debate.

Goals of multiprofessional working and learning

Success is a relative concept in the pluralistic arena of health care. The ideologies of clinician, patient, educator, accountant and manager may all highlight different perspectives of what multiprofessionalisation is expected to deliver, perspectives likely to elicit strong emotions amongst the different stakeholders. Table 16.1 shows goals, stakeholders and potential measures of multiprofessional working and learning.

"The Department of Health urges more interprofessional education presumably in order to generate effective collaboration between members of the caring professions. Can such a linear relationship be accepted without reservation?"

Engel 1997

"Hopefully we will be able to work together more efficiently once we've qualified. We've got a better idea now of how what each of us does links together for the patient"

Medical student

Table 16.1   Goals, stakeholders and potential measures of multiprofessional working and learning

Goal	Ideological orientation	Example of scope for multiprofessionalism
Improved quality of care	Clinical/Service	Monitor incidences of mismanagement
Increased patient satisfaction	Individual	Individually tailored care packages
Improved working relationships	Organisational	Regular team meetings attended by all professions
Integrated learning practices	Educational	Curriculum designed to encourage student interaction/teamworking
Economic efficiency	Financial	Reduction in duplication of activity/documentation
Greater centralised control	Managerial	Prescribed multiprofessional protocols

Consequently, developments need to be planned with agreement on evaluations and measurement of outcomes negotiated in advance, so that the on-going commitment of all parties is retained.

In much of the literature and numerous studies of multiprofessional education, the rationale for its implementation appears to be considered as self-evident: that bringing students together to learn will enhance their future collaborative practice. One of the few studies more explicitly outlining the underlying basis for multiprofessional education proposes that bringing together different groups is a tool for modifying attitudes. The approach adopted is based on the contact hypothesis of intergroup behaviour (Carpenter & Hewstone 1996). This hypothesis highlights the challenge for undergraduate teaching in that successful outcomes require a number of influential variables to be taken into account:

- institutional support
- equal status of participants
- positive expectations
- cooperative atmosphere
- successful joint working
- concern for and understanding of the differences as well as similarities

"we can characterize the traditional pattern of medical school training as one dominated by 'partition', associated with the development of high social distance, and cosmopolitan loyalties; while the traditional pattern of training in schools of nursing has been dominated by 'patronage', associated with a strong focus on task completion ('getting through the work') and local loyalties"

Beattie 1995

"Students perceived MPE to be of low priority in the eyes of school staff and teachers did not practice what they preached"

Davidson & Lucas 1995

Ensure realistic timescales in the development of multiprofessional programmes and pay scrupulous attention to the logistics. Students will be quickly turned off by a badly organised programme.

"It was interesting to get a different dimension; the nurses talked about difficulties that they faced that I hadn't considered before"

Medical student

- experience of working together as equals and perception that members of the group are typical and not just exceptions to the stereotype.

Such a list highlights the need for careful planning of the interactions between students and a consideration of the numerous factors that can result in success or failure of an encounter. For example, in gerontology Clark (1993) highlighted that introducing a multidisciplinary dimension can create problems because disciplines and departments, the organisation units of universities, are not generally conducive to multidisciplinary effort or integration. Barriers identified in other studies include lack of planning and lack of teacher commitment.

The teacher therefore needs to establish what outcomes it is hoped to achieve and the most effective strategy for their achievement. Potential goals of MPE might include:

- development of collaborative competencies
- modification of attitudes, perceptions and stereotypes of other professions
- financial and political expediency
- enhancement of motivation of students to collaborate through identification of common objectives, values and beliefs
- development of a common language and greater shared meaning for interprofessional communication.

However, there is currently little evidence to support the appropriate stage at which interprofessional integration through education should begin, with a field split between those who advocate contact from the outset of professional education and those supporting the need for establishment of a professional identity in order that assimilation rather than role confusion occurs. Teachers should therefore consider the delineation of their own underlying philosophies, rationale and learning objectives for the approach they propose.

Degrees of multiprofessional education

Numerous terms are used to define multiprofessional education. The underlying premise seems to be that it is an educational process involving two or more professional groups learning within a multidisciplinary context. Whilst the context often appears to refer to a classroom or practice situation it may be more appropriate to explicate the complexities of multiprofessional education at a range of different levels: interpersonal, interprofessional, interdepartmental, interinstitutional and intercultural. These are outlined below as ten phases of integration.

Phases of multiprofessional education integration
(Development of these levels acknowledges the original work undertaken by Professor Ronald Harden.)

Isolationism
Education is organised around content that is absolutely unique and core to the particular profession, the discipline or a pure subject. Courses are also organised without consideration of the content of other professional courses.

Acknowledgement
Education recognises the contribution made by other professions and the content and teaching strategies used in other courses. However, there is no cross-professional contact.

Content exchange
Educators from one professional group review the programmes of other professions and integrate the content into their own programmes. This may be in terms of such areas as subject matter, educational resources or assessment strategies.

Teacher exchange
Staff from one profession teach in the programme of another profession. This may be because they have particular expertise in a subject unavailable in another

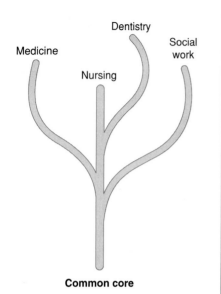

Fig. 16.1   Tree model

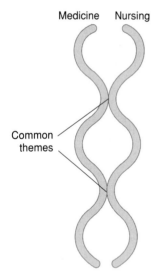

Fig. 16.2   Recurrent contact model

teaching team or in order to provide a different professional perspective on a subject or clinical discipline.

Shared premises

Programmes are timetabled in order to place students in the same classroom at the same time. This is largely for purposes of resource efficiency and little formal interaction occurs between students of different professions.

Joint teaching

Staff of different professions co-develop and deliver material providing different perspectives. This also creates an opportunity for modelling collaboration, which need not preclude conflict, but this should be constructive rather than combative.

Integrated activity

Students of different professions are brought together for joint projects, activities and assessments to which they all contribute and which are designed in a way that maximises interaction and promotes the sharing of responsibility in process and outcome. Problem-based learning may provide a useful framework for developing such activities and may take place in classroom or clinical settings.

Curricular overhaul

The curriculum of whole programmes is reviewed and consideration is given to the respective philosophies, learning objectives, modes of delivery and resources/logistics. Examples of frameworks for integrating complete programmes might include tree and branch-type or recurrent contact models (see Figs 16.1 and 16.2 respectively).

Organisational blending

Structures and frameworks are put in place to support collaborative cross-professional educational enterprise. Staff of different professions are encouraged to work together and the resources shared to achieve this goal.

Administrative activity is combined in common areas and there is a sharing of information within the organisation.

Cultural integration

There is acceptance of the need for integration and the richness of interprofessional exchange and sharing. There is a respect for both dependency and autonomy of different professions within educational preparation. Exchange between individual staff members occurs in a respectful and trusting context and the importance of this interdependence is evident in the practices and relationships within the institution.

Consideration of these phases may provide the individual teacher with an indication of the level to which a faculty or department has committed itself to multiprofessional education in a range of areas. It may also provide the framework for an audit tool for different modules or subjects or a facility for mapping the developments within particular programmes.

Creating a positive multiprofessional learning atmosphere

Considering the context: the 'five Cs'

Prior to developing multiprofessional education it is important that the teacher reflects upon demands and barriers that may influence the success of multiprofessional education initiatives. Consideration of the 'five Cs' of institutional, professional and personal development may provide one tool to aid this:

- Climate. Is this locally supportive of a move towards multiprofessional education? Developments may require redistribution of resources between schools or faculties, goals may be different and conspiracy theories as to motives for such a move rife. Thus considerable planning, consultation and information dissemination are required. Students who have had previous multiprofessional experiences may be positively or negatively influential on the success.

Involve all staff participating in the delivery in planning and the ethos of the approach. A single, cynical staff member can do much to undermine the development of a positive multiprofessional perspective in a student group.

- Curriculum model. Is this to be multiprofessionally integrated, are learning objectives clearly defined and is it sufficiently aptitude-responsive to cater for the diversity of student needs and abilities that integration may involve? Is this based on a planned curriculum model, a common core, recurrent contact at pre-defined times for specific content areas or opportunistic?
- Commitment. This is likely to be required at all levels. Thus there is a need for managerial support, a willingness to invest in staff development time, realistic timescales and an acceptance of failures as well as successes as developments are implemented and evaluated.
- Charisma. Charismatic enthusiasts appear to be the prime initiators of successful multiprofessional working in most studies. The ability to 'sell' the developments to both colleagues and students is essential, as in the plethora of educational developments the logistics of multiprofessional education may result in its demise without individuals prepared to drive it forward.
- Concrete examples. Examples that provide models of multiprofessional learning are a useful tool. What examples of implementation exist in practice? How can they be translated to your particular context? Examples that reflect 'real-life' practices may prove particularly popular, such as health-care students involved in joint exercises or, even more broadly, medical students and art students involved in the development and delivery of health promotion messages. Thus use of the available institutional expertise at the widest level is important.

Types of multiprofessional learning

Barr (1996) delineates a number of approaches that the teacher may consider in delivering multiprofessional education:

- Received learning. Lectures and written material might include work on the nature of teams, information on the roles of other health professionals or literature on intergroup dynamics and the nature and history of the professions.

- Exchange-based learning. Students should be encouraged to exchange information on experiences, practices, beliefs and values. This might involve workshops, debates or discussions on communication, ethics, clinical problems or case studies including the management of clinical conflict.
- Observation-based learning. This might range from students shadowing different health professionals to professionally mixed student pairs undertaking joint visits to patients in hospital and home and collaborating in the presentation of their findings.
- Problem-based learning. Trigger situations are developed around a clinical case study requiring a team, a professionally mixed group of students to undertake a joint task. The task will require the distribution of work between the different professionals and should encourage the establishment and understanding of the capabilities, skills and knowledge of different group members.
- Simulation-based exercises. Exercises are created that require students to take on a role to manage a problem. Simulation may include entire scenarios or may involve the subdivision of situations into parts in order to evaluate activity. One example may be the development of a team objective structured clinical examination (TOSCE). Simulation has been argued to provide more predictability of outcome because it is developed for purpose and variables are more likely to be controlled.
- Practice-based learning. Assignments may be undertaken on clinical attachments or site visits. They may comprise exercises that require students to recruit the views of colleagues, peers or mentors in order to complete an assignment. Alternatively, they may involve multidisciplinary ward rounds or meetings that encourage the active participation of students.

Whichever approach is adopted it is important that the teacher tries to focus on what learning outcome it is

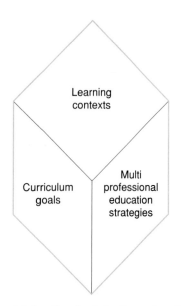

Fig. 16.3   Harden's 3–dimensional representation of multi-professional education

proposed to achieve. A structured focus is expressed diagramatically in the three-dimensional model proposed by Harden (1998) (see Fig. 16.3). This is based on the consideration of the curriculum goals, i.e. what we are trying to achieve (e.g. social contact, attitude change, shared goals, common language, greater role understanding in a professionally mixed student cohort); the learning contexts, i.e. where this is best achieved (in the classroom, clinic, hospital or community) and whether it is a skill-based subject or a value-based subject; and the multiprofessional educational strategies that are appropriate for achieving the defined learning objectives.

Preparing for a multiprofessional educational session

Content considerations

Having recognised the multiple influences upon implementation one must consider the specific requirements of the joint educational session. Barr (1996) suggests that multiprofessional education content should comprise three types: common, specialist and comparative.

Common content

Common content might include themes from health and social sciences that involve the same learning objectives for all groups of students. These may include common clinical skills or knowledge. However, it may quickly become evident that seemingly common content is often based upon different assumptions, language differences between professions and variations in learning styles amongst student groups.

Specialist content

Specialist content is essential to the maintenance of the individuality of professions. Thus multiprofessional education requires mutual understanding and respect between professions, not a common single framework of knowledge.

Comparative content

Comparative content is the bridge between common and specialist content. This provides the mechanism by which professionals come to learn about one another in terms of such matters as roles, functions, relationships and language.

Influences on learning

Location

Work-based initiatives tend towards specific tasks and often occur on an ad hoc basis. Tope (1996) has highlighted that students value the opportunity to interact in 'real life', that is, in patient-orientated situations. This, however, requires the teacher either to take educational responsibility for organising the education of all students within a unit, providing appropriate education to meet their particular learning needs, or to rely on opportunistic education, rounding up students as available for joint teaching. Such interventions may require negotiation with those responsible for the education of non-medical students.

University-based initiatives provide greater opportunity for more reflection and theoretical analysis of collaboration. However, they lack immediacy and are removed from the conflicts, personalities and tensions that may undermine multiprofessional working in practice.

Duration and frequency

All initiatives require clear objectives and the shorter they are, the more specific the objectives need to be. Many of the studies described in the literature are short and often one-off in nature and their value on longer-term behavioural change is almost impossible to verify. However, along with duration may go frequency; frequency of multiprofessional educational interventions might demonstrate a greater commitment to the concept than a single longer one-off activity.

Assessment

Students have to prioritise their work. The primary focusing factors are surely examinations. Work on

"The intent of interprofessional education is not to produce khaki-brown generic workers. Its goal is better described by the metaphor of a richly coloured tapestry within which many colours are interwoven to create a picture that no one colour can produce on its own"

Headrick, Wilcock & Batalden 1998

Known territory is important to student security. Programmes run in the camp of one particular professional group may be seen as being owned by that group and this may alienate other groups. Try to use a neutral venue or use different territory on different occasions.

Consider how students prioritise their work and use assessment formats which emphasise the importance placed by faculty upon developing a multiprofessional approach to practice, such as group presentations and assessment by multiprofessional teaching teams.

collaboration and interprofessional relations is difficult and arguably unsuitable for assessment by written examination. Students may see the subject matter in this area as soft-option material or of lesser value in working towards their ultimate goal of academic success. The teacher therefore needs to consider the assessment process in relation to the identified outcome. Care is also required to avoid competitive, individualistic assessments that might undermine a collaborative atmosphere that has been built up throughout a programme. Variations in learning styles and aptitude are likely to be wider in mixed professional groups and this should also be considered in the design of assessment.

Stage
Undergraduate initiatives must consider the issue of immature or ill-developed role identity and the effect the interprofessional education initiatives might have on this. Additionally the stage in the undergraduate programme is a significant factor. A student nurse in year two is likely to have considerably more practice experience than a medical student in traditional programmes. Whilst the practice/theory orientation of the two groups may be skilfully used to advantage by a well-prepared teacher, there is a danger that medical students may feel out of touch with the realities of clinical work and therefore alienated and even patronised.

Learning and teaching styles
Westberg & Jason (1993) highlight the importance of the learning relationship between student and teacher in order to create a relationship in which the student feels valued, safe enough to contribute, in control of his or her own learning and trusted to learn. Such a relationship, they propose, is conducive to developing the skills, attitudes and relationships that enable students to work collaboratively both inter- and intraprofessionally in practice. They define extremes of a spectrum highlighting at one end collaboration and at the other authoritarianism; the latter having been traditionally favoured in medicine.

Summary

Clinical practice is undergoing radical change. Technological and educational advances are enabling new roles to be developed and old roles to be renegotiated. Education can play a part in preparing students for collaborative and cooperative practice. These developments need to be supported at all levels of the organisation; however, for the teacher in practice or classroom, planning, commitment, enthusiasm and the modelling of collaborative practice with other educational colleagues are all essential elements of a successful initiative.

Strategies might include shared teaching, teacher exchange, shadowing or a more radical curriculum review. However, the lessons from a wide range of studies require teachers to take account of how this fits with students' notions of practice. Teachers from different professions bring different values, expectations and requirements to an initiative and these have to be thrashed out in advance of a course so that they do not surface as conflict and a reinforcement of interprofessional disharmony in action.

References and further reading

Barr H 1996 Ends and means in interprofessional education: towards a typology. Education for Health 9(3):341–352

Beattie A 1995 War and peace among the health tribes. In: Soothill K, Mackay L, Webb C (eds) Interprofessional relations in health care. Edward Arnold, London, ch. 2, pp. 11–30

Carpenter J, Hewstone M 1996 Shared learning for doctors and social workers: evaluation of a programme. British Journal of Social Work 26:239–257

Clark P 1993 A typology of interdisciplinary education in gerontology and geriatrics: are we really doing what we say we are? Journal of Interprofessional Care 7(3):217–228

Davidson L, Lucas J 1995 Multiprofessional education in the undergraduate health professions curriculum: observations from Adelaide, Linkoping and Salford. Journal of Interprofessional Care 9(2):163–176

Engel C 1997 Collaboration through interprofessional education? In: Vanclay L (ed) Interprofessional education: what, how, when? CAIPE Bulletin 13:19

Harden R M 1998 AMEE Guide no. 12 Multiprofessional education part 1 Effective multiprofessional education: a three-dimensional perspective. Medical Teacher 20(5):402–408

Headrick L A, Wilcock P M, Batalden P B 1998 Interprofessional working and continuing education. British Medical Journal 316:771–774

Tope R 1996 Integrated interdisciplinary learning between health and social care professions. A feasibility study. Avebury, Aldershot

Westberg J, Jason H 1993 Collaborative clinical education. The Foundation of Effective Health Care. Springer, New York

SECTION 4
TOOLS/AIDS

Chapter 17
Instructional design

A. Stewart

Introduction

Unless they operate on a totally ad lib basis, all medical teachers employ some kind of design process to put together the instruction they deliver in class. The instructional design (ID) process takes many forms; a review of the ERIC database reveals that there are over 60 models, and a comprehensive 800–page tome on the subject (Dills & Romiszowski 1997) suggests that there is no shortage of new ideas. At its most straightforward, instructional design is a process through which we can identify the nature of the learning that is intended to take place, work out an approach to teaching that will facilitate achievement of that learning, and administer some kind of assessment that will determine whether the intended learning has, in fact, taken place.

Learning outcomes

Identifying the nature of learning outcomes is a key aspect of the instructional design process. If we don't identify the learning outcomes clearly, then we might finish up working hard at doing very well what we should not have been doing in the first place!

Because teachers often tend to 'cover the subject' (usually because there is a content-centred curriculum) it is too easy to assume that the planned outcome is that the student will gain a sufficient grasp of the subject to be able to answer the questions raised in an examination. Since these examinations frequently require the recall of factual information, gaining a grasp of the subject

- Consider the outcomes to be achieved.
- Organise appropriate instructional events to facilitate learning.
- Determine whether learning has taken place.

finishes up as memorising a lot of information. When we cover the aetiology, epidemiology, pathophysiology etc. of any topic we can, in effect, be passing on factual information, the regurgitation of which is required in an examination which will probably be in multiple choice question format.

In recent years, however, there has been a move away from the 'sponge syndrome' where students were expected to absorb the information provided and, when squeezed at examination time, give it back – minus what had evaporated! It was not expected that there would be any transformation of the information. Now, instead, there is an emphasis on a so-called 'deep approach' to learning where students are expected to understand and apply the knowledge acquired. All the evidence regarding how students approach learning, together with our best understanding of how knowledge is built up, certainly suggests that students have to be able to construct their own knowledge, build on an existing knowledge base and find relevance and meaning in the process.

Relevance and meaning are found through trying to make connections between the ideas that are being encountered and the real world of the practice of medicine. Ideas and practices, the practical application of knowledge, therefore provide the basis for students' learning.

Knowledge

One of the features that characterise students who adopt the 'deep approach' to learning is that they try to get to grips with the ideas behind the words; they try to understand the concepts and principles that are involved, rather than merely to remember the facts. Concepts can be thought of as information about objects, events and processes that allow us to differentiate various things and classes, understand relationships between objects, and generalise about events, things and processes. A considerable amount of learning is concerned with the learning of concepts. Lack of understanding of concepts leads to lack of clarity in thinking.

Understanding concepts helps us to:

- differentiate between things
- understand relationships
- generalise about events, things and processes.

While concepts help us to classify diverse phenomena, principles enable us to predict, explain and control phenomena. Principles state relationships between two or more concepts. In general, principles can be converted into 'if-then' statements. When students have learned a principle they should be able to do more than simply state the principle; they should be able to make some predictions from it and use it to explain appropriate events.

In the structure of knowledge, concepts are combined into principles. A principle is not simply a number of concepts linked in the same sentence. A principle states a relationship between classes of event that enable us to predict consequences, explain events, infer causes, control situations and solve problems.

The acquisition of concepts and principles is therefore the key to acquiring knowledge.

Skills

Learning medicine, however, is not only about acquiring knowledge. Associated with that knowledge there has to be a practical ability to carry out procedures and utilise skills. Such abilities are also key learning outcomes.

Attitudes

Any task that a doctor has to perform will involve knowledge, skills and attitudes. Unfortunately, because attitudes are difficult to define and explain and because they are not easy to measure, they have until recently tended to be ignored.

Topic and task analyses

Because defining attitudes is so difficult the topic has only recently been included in the identification of learning outcomes. Identifying knowledge and skills outcomes is much more straightforward and is usually done through topic and task analyses.

Topic analysis

Reigeluth, Merrill & Bunderson (1994) examined the implications for instructional design arising from the

Understanding principles helps us to:

- predict consequences
- explain events
- infer causes
- control situations.

Focus on the concepts and principles and the facts will fall into place.

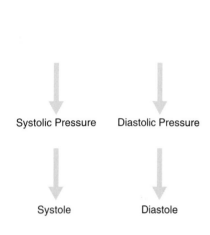

Systolic Pressure   Diastolic Pressure

Systole   Diastole

Fig. 17.1   Blood pressure

Procedural-prerequisite relations

- the performer must do X
before he can do Y.

Procedural-decision relations

- given condition A, the performer
must do X rather than Y or Z.

Fig. 17.2   Task analysis

structure of subject matter. By subject matter structure they meant the interrelationships among the components of the subject matter, and by components they meant the individual concepts, principles, facts etc.

They proposed that a content structure, in relation to a learning structure or learning hierarchy, can be represented by a diagram that shows the learning-prerequisite relations among the components of the subject matter. The learning structure describes what must be known before something else can be learned. For example, the concepts of systolic pressure and diastolic pressure must both be understood before the concept of blood pressure can be learned. Similarly, the concepts of systole and diastole have to be understood before the concepts of their respective pressures can be learned (see Fig. 17.1). A learning-prerequisite relation is characterised by the statement: 'A learner must know X in order to learn Y.'

Two points need to be noted here. Firstly, it is important to work out what the concepts are. Secondly, it is important to work out what their inter-relationships are. Since new knowledge has to be built on existing knowledge, absence of prerequisites can mean that new learning doesn't take place.

Although the term 'hierarchy' is normally used to describe the inter-relationships between concepts, other relationships such as those found in concept mapping might be more appropriate and will certainly be equally useful.

Task analysis

The term 'task analysis' is often used to cover what is, in effect, a learning hierarchy analysis. It is really most appropriately used, however, when referring to a job task analysis (Mager & Beach 1967) that requires the instructional designer to list all of the tasks in a job and the steps included in each task.

In relation to procedural tasks, Reigeluth, Merrill & Bunderson (1994) proposed that there should be two types of procedural relation (see Fig. 17.2). Procedural-prerequisite relations are the relations among the steps of a single procedure (specifically, the order for performing those steps); they can be shown in a procedural hierarchy:

Taking blood: simplified procedural hierarchy

Step 1 Expose venepuncture site.
Step 2 Palpate site.
Step 3 Attach needle to vacutainer holder/syringe.
Step 4 Apply tourniquet.
Step 5 Cleanse venepuncture site.
Step 6 Anchor vein with thumb.
Step 7 Insert needle bevel up by direct puncture at angle of 45°.
Step 8 Insert vacutainer tube.
Step 9 Withdraw filled vacutainer tube.
Step 10 Loosen tourniquet.
Step 11 Withdraw needle and vacutainer holder.
Step 12 Cover insertion site with gauze and apply pressure.

The procedural-prerequisite relation is characterised by the statement: 'The performer must do X before he can do Y.'

Procedural-decision relations are the relations between alternate procedures and they describe the factors necessary for deciding which procedure, or sub-procedure, to use in a given situation. A flow diagram is one way of portraying a decision structure, and the relation is characterised by the statement: 'Given condition A, the performer must do X rather than Y or Z.'

Creating the conditions for learning

In the process of instructional design, the identification of the nature of the desired learning outcomes alone is insufficient; it must be followed up by designing the kind of teaching that is going to take place so that these learning outcomes are likely to be achieved.

Successive editions of Gagne's influential book on instructional design (1985) have followed the evolution from behavioural to cognitive perspectives on learning and have indicated how the student has to construct knowledge rather than merely respond to the stimulus of teaching.

Conditions for learning involve arranging external events (external to the mind) that support internal processing (internal to the mind).

Cognitive Outcomes (Gagne 1985)

- *Intellectual skills*
  - *— discrimination*
  - *— concrete concepts*
  - *— defined concepts*
  - *— roles*
  - *— problem-solving*
- *Verbal information*
  - *— memory recall*
- *Cognitive strategies*
  - *— learning how to learn and think*
- *Motor skills*
  - *— Goal-directed muscular movement*
- *Attitudes*
  - *— mental state influencing action*

Gagne's model is basically concerned with the kind of learning outcome to be achieved and the arrangement of specific instructional events which are tailored to the achievement of those kinds of outcome. The instructional events provide information and interaction that enhance the possibilities of learning.

In essence, creating the conditions for learning is concerned with arranging events external to the mind of the student that support processes internal to the mind of the student. It means that teachers have to organise what they do when teaching in order to influence appropriately what goes on inside learners' minds so that they can learn.

The learning of concepts and principles comes into a category of cognitive outcome that Gagne calls 'intellectual skills', a category that is concerned with complex or procedural knowledge. Other cognitive categories are 'verbal information' which is concerned with memory or recall, and 'cognitive strategies' which is concerned with strategies for learning how to learn.

Intellectual skills include five subcategories that range from the basic skill of recognising similarities and differences (discrimination) to skills in the application of learned rules or principles (problem-solving). For each of these kinds of learning outcome, a particular strategy of instruction is required.

Gagne's 'events of instruction'

The set of events in Gagne's approach consists of nine activities carried out by a teacher and learners during instruction. These are based on an information processing model of human cognition and correspond to the internal mental processes required for learning:

1. gaining attention
2. informing the learner of the objective
3. stimulating recall of prerequisite learning

These prepare the learner for the instruction. The student's attention is stimulated and focused on what is to be learned. Expectations of what is to be learned are clarified by informing learners of the objectives. The basis on which learning is to be built is established by recalling relevant prior learning.

4. presenting the stimulus material
5. providing learning guidance

These are the core of the teaching/learning process, with the presentation of information and the provision of guidance about what is being learned helping the student to make sense of the topic and build up understanding.

6. eliciting the performance
7. providing feedback about performance correctness

Events 6 and 7 give the student the opportunity to check and enhance learning by presenting practice opportunities and providing feedback.

8. assessing the performance

An assessment is made of the outcome(s) to be learned and, therefore, a measure of the effectiveness of both teaching and learning.

9. enhancing retention and transfer.

Finally, enhancing retention and transfer is achieved through giving the student an opportunity to think about how what has been learned can be applied in other contexts.

The schema approach

Knowledge appears to be structured by individuals in meaningful ways which grow and change over time; the way in which it is stored is related to the way it is encoded when it is learned (Romberg & Carpenter 1986). New knowledge is constructed by the learner in a process of building new relationships essential to learning (Resnick & Ford 1981).

One model suggested as an explanation for this building process is the notion of 'schema' – the building blocks of cognition (Rumelhart 1980). Activating relevant prior knowledge is, essentially, a schema activation exercise. When new information is presented in an organised and structured way and appropriate explanations are given, the learner engages in a process of schema construction. In a time of summary at the end of the session, the student has the opportunity of schema refining; what has been learned can be checked against what is being summarised.

Schema activation

In schema activation existing knowledge relevant to the new material about to be presented is activated. It is unlikely that only one new idea is to be presented in the session. It might be that the new material to be presented will need activation of more than one set of existing knowledge structures. It might mean pulling together previously acquired knowledge from several different areas of experience. This schema activation exercise is probably sufficiently important in the learning experience that teachers need to consider much more carefully how to help learners prepare for the session and how to begin the session to ensure maximum readiness for the new material presented.

Schema construction

New information presented is likely to be accepted by the students in the form we present it and then built into their own cognitive structure. It is important, therefore, that it is presented in a structured and organised way. It is very difficult for students to take amorphous material and make any kind of structure of it! Some form of topic analysis should be carried out prior to delivery so teachers can see how the different parts of the material relate to each other – what needs to come before what, and where understanding of one concept is dependent on prior understanding of another. Having previously clarified one's thoughts on the topic it is possible to present it in a structured form which will enable students to assimilate it into their own knowledge structures.

In this process of schema construction it is important for the student to be thinking about the material. It is the responsibility of the teacher, as facilitator, to encourage students to be thinking about the material presented and attempting to relate it to what is already known, to work out what it means in their own context, or to think about

 Schema activation:

- helps learners to 'tune in'
- encourages learners to bring to mind relevant prior knowledge
- assists learners to prepare their prior knowledge to be the foundation on which new knowledge will now be constructed.

Schema construction helps the learner to make sense of the new material by:

- linking it to existing knowledge
- making it relevant to learning needs
- highlighting its significance to future practice
- presenting it in an organised and structured way
- providing appropriate 'explanations'

ways in which this might prove to be useful in future applications. In so doing, students are not only creating meaning and constructing knowledge but are actually strengthening their own learning skills.

The teacher needs to ensure that the teaching/learning session is not given over solely to the providing of information and the building up of knowledge; it is not only knowing *that* but knowing *how* which is important to the student. The objectives of the course will almost certainly involve higher-order thinking skills and it is these which have to be developed during the session. Students need to be encouraged and given the opportunity to apply acquired knowledge in activities such as analysis, synthesis, evaluation and problem-solving. Objectives relating to attitudinal and emotional aspects of the tasks to be performed also need to be remembered; interaction between students in an exchange of views often needs to be facilitated so that conflicting views can be considered and resolution achieved.

Schema refining

Towards the end of the session it is advisable to give students the opportunity to become involved in schema refining as the teacher reviews the material and key points covered. Students can then re-examine the nature of the knowledge which has been constructed in their minds and refine as necessary, perhaps modifying in the light of further consideration at that point. One of the most useful activities for students to undertake may be to make a summary in their own words of the main thrust of the session and to annotate this in relation to previous learning and possible future application.

The idea of a beginning, a middle and an end has been around for a long time, as has the advice to 'tell them what you're going to say, say it, and tell them what you've said.' What is different is an understanding of how such approaches can, in fact, work. The schema activation, schema construction and schema refinement model for teaching, coupled with encouragement of students to engage in deeper processing and thinking, give us a credible and robust basis for the design of our teaching.

 Schema refining involves:

- reviewing the topic to give learners a chance to check their constructions
- reviewing what has been presented to let the learner reflect upon what has been learned
- reviewing the topic and projecting forward to situations that let the learner make applications of what has been learned.

Summary

The instructional design process involves the identification of the nature of the learning that is intended to take place, the development of an approach to teaching that will facilitate achievement of that learning, and the provision of some kind of assessment that will enable teacher and student to determine whether the intended learning has, in fact, taken place.

The nature of learning outcomes is best identified in terms of the concepts and principles arising from an analysis of the topic or, in the case of tasks, in terms of steps or stages arising from an analysis of the performance of the task.

Gagne's 'events of instruction' approach provides a systematic way to prepare students for the learning experience, to present new material together with guidance in understanding it, and to check that they have understood the material and can apply the knowledge acquired. The 'schema' approach provides an alternative framework for activating relevant prior knowledge, building on existing knowledge, finding meaning and relevance in the new material, and checking that the new knowledge constructed is as intended.

References and further reading

Dills C R, Romiszowski A J 1997 Instructional development paradigms, Educational Technology Publications, Englewood Cliffs, NJ

Gagne R M 1985 The conditions of learning, 4th edn. Holt, Rinehart & Winston, New York

Mager R F, Beach K M 1967 Developing vocational instruction. Fearon, Belmont, CA.

Reigeluth C M, Merrill M D, Bunderson C V 1994 'The structure of subject matter content and its instructional design implications'. In: Merrill M D, Mitchell D G (eds) Instructional design theory. Educational Technology Publications, Englewood Cliffs, NJ

Resnick L B, Ford W W 1981 The psychology of mathematics for instruction. Lawrence Erlbaum Associates, Hillsdale, NJ

Romberg T A, Carpenter T P 1986 'Research on teaching and learning mathematics'. In: Wittrock M C, (ed.) Handbook of research on teaching, 3rd edn. MacMillan, New York, pp. 850–873

Rumelhart D E 1980 'Schemata: the building blocks of cognition'. In: Spiro R J, Bruce B C, Brewer W F (eds) Theoretical issues in reading comprehension. Lawrence Erlbaum, pp. 33–58. Lawrence Erlbaum Associates, Hillsdale, NJ

Chapter 18
Study guides

J. M. Laidlaw   E. A. Hesketh

Introduction

This chapter deals with study guides and in particular
the need for them, their various roles in the continuum
of medical education, and the features which can
be incorporated to help the learner study more
effectively.

A study guide is an aid, usually in the form of printed
notes, designed to facilitate students with their studies.
Not only does the guide give students an indication of
what they should be learning, it also informs them how
they should best learn and how they can recognise that
they have mastered the topic being studied. A guide can
also be seen as a management tool which allows doctors
to exercise their teaching and training responsibilities
while at the same time giving the students and trainees
an important part to play in managing their own
learning. Rowntree (1986) captured the idea well when
he likened a study guide to a tutor sitting on the
student's shoulder, available 24 hours a day to offer
advice on what to do at any stage of the student's
studies.

*"A study guide is not a tool
which constrains or unnecessarily
spoon feeds. Rather it is an
instrument which allows students to
take more responsibility for their
own learning"*

Laidlaw & Harden 1990

Why use study guides?

There are several reasons why study guides are
becoming more popular with students at either
undergraduate or postgraduate level. Doctors intent
on keeping up to date with new techniques and
therapies are also making use of study guides especially
when they accompany distance learning programmes.
We have highlighted overleaf some of the reasons for
the increasing interest in this educational tool. You

The knowledge required of a doctor is expanding at more than 14% per year.

can most likely add to the list from your own experience.

The problem of overload

Students are expected to learn more about medicine today than ever before, but within the same timespan. In postgraduate and continuing education the problem is much the same – doctors have to keep up to date with new treatments and management of diseases as well as trying to tackle new technologies. Clearly all students and trainees need to be selective about the essential information they take on board, and for this reason they need an educational tool that will point them in the right direction.

A menu of learning opportunities

There are new approaches to learning and a variety of learning opportunities on offer for students and trainees – but which route of study should a learner adopt? Bearing in mind that we all have different learning styles, it is important to try to match the styles and approaches as much as possible thus ensuring effective learning. No longer are students content to sit passively in the lecture theatre for hours on end to absorb information. Lectures, which can be most effective if they are interactive, continue to remain on most timetables, but the development of clinical skills units and the many resources in ambulatory care, as outlined in Chapters 8 and 10, all make up a large menu of exciting learning opportunities for undergraduate and postgraduate students.

A variety of educational approaches

Distance learning, problem-based learning, evidence-based learning, outcome-based learning, service-based learning and task-based learning are only a few of the approaches that are becoming more commonplace in undergraduate and postgraduate education. No matter which approach is adopted, learning requires to be facilitated and a guide can help ensure this happens. Harden et al (1996) remind us that 'educators are becoming more aware of the need to develop forms of learning that are rooted in the learner's practical experience and in the job they are to undertake as a professional on completion of training.' Learning on the job' for example, has much to commend it for the trainee doctor but too often learning in such an excellent environment is not always maximised due to heavy service commitment. It is a problem which can be addressed to some extent with the use of study guides as they can ensure that the doctor in training uses the tasks being carried out daily as the focus for further study. *Learning paediatrics: a training guide for senior house officers* (Mitchell et al 1998) was developed to support SHOs in new paediatric posts. It focused on everyday Clinical Problems and provided practical advice and a framework on which to base further study.

Roles for study guides

So how can study guides actually help learners? In facilitating learning they have three specific roles:

- assisting in the management of student learning.
- providing a focus for student activities relating to the learning
- providing information on the subject or topic of study.

Given these three roles, it is not surprising that the actual format and presentation of study guides can look very different. From the model shown in Figure 18.1 you can see that guides can be placed at any point on the triangle depending on their purpose. It is more likely, however, that you will find most guides located in the middle, as they will have incorporated to some extent all three roles. We will first look at some of the features of study guides designed to help students or trainees manage their own learning.

Managing learning

If the role of the study guide is to help students or trainees manage their own learning then it might contain the components described overleaf.

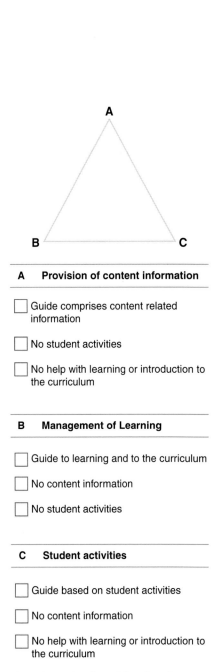

| A | Provision of content information |

☐ Guide comprises content related information

☐ No student activities

☐ No help with learning or introduction to the curriculum

| B | Management of Learning |

☐ Guide to learning and to the curriculum

☐ No content information

☐ No student activities

| C | Student activities |

☐ Guide based on student activities

☐ No content information

☐ No help with learning or introduction to the curriculum

Fig. 18.1 Study guide triangle

An overview

This might include the framework for the course, salient points in the study of the topic, some cross-referencing and a scene setter. The scene setter is used to put the topic being studied in the context of the 'bigger picture' so that learners recognise the relevance of the topic being studied. For example, undergraduate students using a study guide to learn more about the thyroid gland need to be aware that this is one of many topics being covered in the endocrine system block. Similarly in a study guide for SHOs learning paediatrics they need to be made aware that dealing with the breathless child is just one task that might be encountered when managing acutely ill children.

Prerequisites

You might wish to include a statement of the requirements expected of students before they commence with their new studies. Some study guides include a pre-test to help students assess their prior knowledge and identify any gaps which need to be revised.

Learning outcomes

All learners need to know what is expected of them – in other words, they need to be informed of the learning outcomes (or objectives). A clear statement of what you hope the learners will achieve on studying a particular topic is essential if you have to keep the learners on track. In specifying learning outcomes it is an added bonus if you can differentiate between the key outcomes and those which the student might wish to master, time permitting. It is certainly important that the outcomes set are achievable.

Learning strategies

Mention ought to be made of the approaches to learning that should be followed. If the student is expected to be a self-directed learner then this information should be highlighted. If the student has a choice in the problem-based learning mode then again this should be stated. There certainly should be a framework or structure for a course of study enabling students to build upon it and in so doing develop their learning en route.

Learning opportunities

Lectures, small group teaching, clinical skills teaching, demonstrations and many more opportunities are on offer to undergraduate and postgraduate students. They need to know how best to use these resources to maximise their learning.

A timetable

There is not always a timetable included in a guide but there should at least be some indication of the amount of time students should devote to a particular topic. Time is a precious commodity and running out of it does little for morale!

Assessment details

How to prepare for the examinations coupled with the type of assessment tool is perhaps the first page that a student will read. This is not spoon-feeding students; it is perhaps making life less stressful for them.

Staff contacts

Having a mentor or supervisor is information worth knowing about but not once the course is over. A name to contact and a note of available hours to make that contact are worth their weight in gold.

Tips or personal comments

It is so reassuring to be given a few words of wisdom from the 'expert' or at least from someone who has years of experience to their credit.

The majority of the components above very much aid the learning process; however, the self-directed learner also needs to be kept motivated throughout the period of study. This can be achieved by building into the guide some interesting features such as case studies, self-assessment quizzes or scenarios, or simply by highlighting the importance and relevance of the subject. Attention to details such as the layout and design and

"Where you refer to textbooks in your study guide you will help the students enormously if you add the chapter and pages which they should look at and in a sentence tell them why you want them to read the section"

Instructional designer

"Most of the 1,000,000 head-injured attenders at hospital in the UK each year do not need admission, but it is critically important to identify the 10% who do"

Consultant neurosurgeon

the style of writing can all help to make a guide a user-friendly tool – and something that will not simply collect dust on a shelf or be thrown in the wastepaper basket!

Providing the focus for learning

Where the guide has been prepared more as a workbook to be used in conjunction with various learning activities and opportunities, there may be instructions for students to summarise, interpret and apply principles to another context. The guide in this situation really becomes the focus for the learning activities to be undertaken. In addition, learners might also be asked to 'think' about an issue, reflect upon a point, and apply their new-found knowledge and skills to practice. In so doing, they are more likely to experience deep rather than superficial learning. This was exactly the approach adopted in a study guide for doctors starting their surgical training. While studying hypoxia, for example, doctors are invited to: stop and think about the drugs that affect the respiratory centre; reflect on case studies that are used to introduce the topic (Fig. 18.2); apply the knowledge gained to their own clinical situation. They are also encouraged in this particular study guide to keep a record of these activities in a portfolio. Diaries or logbooks are often used to document learning experiences that subsequently can be formatively or summatively assessed.

Providing information on a topic

To some extent you can say that all study guides provide learners with information about the topic(s) being studied, but if you think back to the model (Fig. 18.1) you will be reminded that the function of some guides is to give more core information than others.

It is likely that the type of information will fall into the following two categories:

- previously published information – for example, quotations from other texts, an article from a journal, further references

Think

Remind yourself of the drugs which affect the respiratory centre.

?

In case 3, why was Mrs. A. W. hypoxic?

Shallow respiration suggests:
- inadequate reversal of neuromuscular blocking agents
- inadequate recovery from anaesthesia
- opiate overdose

Fig. 18.2   Study guide example of 'think' and 'reflect'

"Portfolios can provide you with the evidence of a learner's ability to meet the standards of your course"

Medical teacher

- new information – for example, tips and comments from the teacher/trainer, a glossary, key points on the topic being studied.

You might find, for example, that a textbook does not adequately cover a topic, so by adding your own piece of text you can address the problem; or perhaps information in a textbook is outdated, in which case an up-to-date statement in a study guide might suffice. Then there is the situation where there are differing views on a topic. It is easier to document these views, including your own, in your study guide. Deciding how much core information should be incorporated into a guide much depends on the accessibility to the students of textbooks or journals. If these are scarce commodities then include the pertinent sections; otherwise you will end up with some very frustrated students who have joined the lengthy library queue.

Preparing a study guide

Time spent in the preparation of a study guide is well rewarded. Students are likely to make very good use of guides that really do facilitate learning. There are various strategies which can be adopted to make your guide an effective educational tool. Here are just some inclusions worth considering:

- Use advance organisers. Their purpose is to prepare the learners for new learning experiences. They should take on board what the learners already know and what they need to know to continue successfully with their study.
- Make use of headings which help to provide a structure to your writing and also ensure that the reader more easily assimilates the information.
- Build in some self-assessment exercises but try to make them imaginative and a challenge. Producing endless lists of questions that require a true/false response can thwart stimulation. Too much of a 'sameness' is boring! If you intend the learners to write their responses to the questions in the guide then make sure you leave adequate space for them to do so.

Be selective with your further references. It can frustrate the student if:

- they cannot easily access them
- they are given too many choices.

Remember inter-library loans are expensive.

- Incorporate some illustrations. Bear in mind that illustrations can have different functions – the most important being to help your learners better understand a given piece of text. This can be achieved in different ways. Illustrations can be used to break up text and make it less dense to read. They can be incorporated to add some light relief by providing a bit of humour hopefully to keep your learners 'switched on'. Then, of course, you can use illustrations for the sole purpose of helping learners better visualise a complex concept or remember key points. If you do decide to make use of them be sure that you do just that. Never go to the bother of incorporating an illustration just for the sake of it.

Faulkner (1984) gives good advice when referring to the compilation of training manuals and the same advice can be applied to study guides. Here are some of his ideas to get you started:

- Keep sentences short and simple – they tend to be more easily understood.
- Write in the active voice – text is more easily understood.
- Adopt a conversational style – it is much more user-friendly.
- Use familiar words – they are more easily understood and indeed read.

Once you have reached this stage in the preparation of a study guide your job is almost complete…but not quite. We have suggested that you build in features that will facilitate learning. We have highlighted the fact that by keeping sentences succinct and incorporating where appropriate some graphics – be these cartoons, charts, graphs etc. – you can better keep your learners motivated.

Attention to the layout and typography of the study guide are the final points to consider. For instance, it is not advisable to use type smaller than 10 point; otherwise you are in danger of the material not being read. If line lengths are too short you impair legibility. Captions divorced from the figures to which they refer frustrate the readers. Illustrations which appear as 'specks' on the paper are not worth using. This list is by no means complete.

Then it comes to the production phase. Here are some questions that should be addressed:

- How many copies of the study guide are required?
  This will help you to decide whether it is an in-house printing production or a commercial production.

- Is colour really necessary or is it just to make the product look nice?
  Think about your budget carefully here.

- What type of paper should be used?
  There is a wide range of paper available. Matt paper can give a very professional finish, and although a glossy look might give a good first impression, if you are expected to write on such a surface your attitude to it will definitely change.

- Are you planning to print on both sides of the paper?
  You need to think carefully about the opacity of the paper. There is nothing worse than an image from a previous page shining through as you struggle to read new information.

Summary

The best way to appreciate the key role which study guides play in the field of medical education is to produce a guide and introduce it into your own teaching situation. They are beneficial not only to the learners but also to those doing the teaching and training. They can better help you plan the learning; select topics for discussions; monitor the learners' progress; coordinate educational activities; plug gaps in content; and integrate theory with on-the-job learning.

So the first decision to make if you are going to produce a study guide is to decide on its role. Will it be designed to:

- assist students in managing their own learning?
- provide a focus for the educational activities relating to learning?

- provide information on the topics being studied?
- address all three of the above functions?

Once these questions have been answered think carefully about the features of guides and the educational strategies which can help to make learning more effective. Only then should you put pen to paper.

References and further reading

Faulkner L 1984 Designing training manuals for the business and industry classroom. Presentation at the Association of Educational Communications and Technology Convention, Dallas, TX

Harden R M, Laidlaw J M, Ker J S, Mitchell H 1996 Task-based learning: an educational strategy for undergraduate, postgraduate and continuing medical education. Part 1. AMEE Medical Education Guide no. 7, Medical Teacher 18:7–13

Laidlaw J M, Harden R M 1990 What is . . . a study guide? Medical Teacher, 12: 7–12

Mitchell H E, Harden R M, Laidlaw J M 1998 Towards effective on the job learning: the development of a paediatric training guide. Medical Teacher 20:91–98

Rowntree D 1986 Teaching through self-instruction. Kogan Page, London

Chapter 19
Computers

N. McManus

Introduction

Computers as an aid to teaching medicine are next to useless without the software designed to support learning and the content material supplied by subject matter experts. They can even be more of a hindrance than an aid. This chapter will outline some of the ways in which computers may be employed to enhance teaching rather than simply being used because they are there.

Background

It is possible to use a computer without knowing what is going on inside, but a basic understanding of the components will help if you encounter an unusual event.

Potted history

Computing is not a new subject; Charles Babbage designed the first programmable computer in 1833. Programmable electronic computers were first built in the 1940s. Their design was based on vacuum tubes that were fragile, bulky and expensive. A computer with the calculating power of one of today's simple calculators would have taken up an entire room.

Development accelerated in the 1960s with the introduction of transistors and integrated circuits. Magnetic tapes and disks followed, replacing punched cards storage devices, and since then the world of computing has developed at a phenomenal rate. If the motor industry had undergone the same scale of development we would now be driving cars

"I think that there may be a world market for maybe five computers"

Thomas Watson, Chairman of the Board, IBM 1943

capable of a million miles per hour, and running for thousands of miles on a spoonful of fuel!

Hardware

Computer systems can be thought of as modular in design, the basic modules being processing, storage and input/output devices.

Processing

The central processing unit (CPU) is where all program execution and arithmetic calculations take place. Some of today's CPUs are capable of executing more than 500 million instructions per second, but the range of speeds available is huge. There are many different makes of processor, and in general these are not transferable between different types of computer.

Storage

Computers have numerous levels of storage device available. The basic level is the hard disk. This is a permanent rewritable storage device where any data stored is retained when the power is turned off. The next level up from this are memory chips, which are typically 150 000 times faster to access than the hard disk. Memory is volatile, and anything not written back to disk is likely to be lost when the computer is turned off. Inside the processor, small amounts of data can be stored and retrieved about 50 times faster than from memory.

When you start running a program, it is copied from hard disk into memory and then executed. If there is insufficient memory available, sections allocated to other tasks which have not been used recently are temporarily copied to hard disk in order to free some space. This process is called 'virtual memory' paging, and is why you will sometimes notice an unusually high amount of disk activity. Adding more memory to your computer will reduce the need to do this, and therefore increase its performance.

If you are working on a file on a removable disk, e.g. a floppy, *always* save and close the document before removing the disk from the drive. Failing to do so can lead to anything from loss of your latest changes to the complete loss of the file.

Larger capacity floppy drives such as ZIP from Iomega Corporation can store the same amount of information as 70 floppy disks, and can be invaluable for transferring large files.

Input/output devices

Input/output (I/O) devices are needed to connect your computer to the outside world. The most common devices you will use are connections for the keyboard, mouse and monitor. Scanners and digital cameras can be connected for acquiring images, which can then be manipulated for use on-screen or sent to an attached printer. I/O devices are currently connected to computers by a number of different ports and sockets. The connection process can be simpler now thanks to the universal serial bus (USB), whereby many peripherals use the same type of connector and can be linked together.

Platforms

There are four main types of computer currently used in educational environments:

- PC
- Apple
- Unix workstation
- Palmtop computer.

A basic program must be installed on each of these to allow any tasks to be performed – this is referred to as the 'operating system'. The most common platform used currently is the PC, with the predominant operating system being Microsoft Windows. A new version of Windows is released every couple of years, and this can lead to problems and incompatibilities with any pre-existing software.

Some institutions use Apple computers, and most commercial packages are available for both PC and Mac. It is possible for a Mac to run PC software using an emulator. Unix workstations are less common in medical education, being restricted mainly to scientific departments or research projects. In general these

If you are transferring data using disks other than standard 3.5″ floppies, always make sure that the recipient has the hardware necessary to read the disk.

If your department is upgrading or buying new machines, you may also need to obtain updated versions of your software, which may not always be possible for CAL packages.

machines are more powerful than PCs or Macs, but not as simple to use.

Palmtop computers such as the Psion or Palm are handy devices that can fit easily into a lab-coat pocket. Good medical software for these can be hard to find but installing programs is straightforward. Packages are distributed typically on floppy disk or CD and are then transferred from another machine using an infrared connection or cable.

Choosing a new computer

If you are deciding on which specifications are necessary for a new machine, you should define what it is you will be using it for. A computer used primarily for graphical work will require a large monitor and fast video card, whereas one for simply reading e-mail and word processing will not.

Some points to remember:

- You can never have too much memory, and 64Mb would be the minimum specification for a new machine bought today.
- PCs are advertised primarily by their processor speed, but the other components are just as important to their performance.
- Hard disk capacities are rising, but large cheap disks tend to be quite slow to access. A slow disk will bring down the performance of the whole computer.
- There is no such thing as a 'future-proofed' computer, so don't rely on being able to upgrade all the components.
- If you run applications over a heavily loaded network, then buying the fastest computer available may make hardly any difference. The bottleneck in this case would be information being transferred over the network.

If you buy a top-of-the-range computer, you would typically expect it to last about 3 years before you notice everyday tasks take longer to perform. You will then wish to consider upgrading.

"640K ought to be enough for everybody"

Bill Gates, Microsoft 1981

Computer-assisted learning (CAL)

There are many different names used for this, including computer-based teaching (CBT) and computer-assisted instruction (CAI), but they all mean the same thing: teaching material delivered on computer. The form that material takes can be anything from basic text-only resources to immersive simulated environments, but the aim is the same in each case – to assist students' learning.

Styles of CAL package

There is a large range of styles of CAL package available, and more often than not the style is a reflection of the development tool picked by the CAL builders. Common styles are described below.

Basic text and images

Learning resources like this are common, and the layout is usually similar to a textbook page.

Progressive screen display and animations

It can be less confusing to the student not to be bombarded with a whole screenful of information at once, and to be able to see animated descriptions of a topic rather than pages of textual description.

Active approach

The previous methods are passive – the student reads what is on the screen and presses the 'next' button or follows a hypertext link. Alternatively, students can be made to take a more active role in the programme. By performing tasks such as constructing concept maps of the topic being studied they are actively thinking about and using what they are learning.

Simulation

Many simulators are not intended to be used primarily as learning packages. They are aimed at those who have already covered a topic and who are looking to put into practice what they have learned. If you do intend using a simulator as a learning tool, you should make sure that

"CAL packages are great. You can work at your own pace and hyperlinks are useful for finding associated information easily"

Medical student

the students also have access to resource material where they can locate textbook solutions to cases and conditions which may appear. This could range from course textbooks to online material included in or linked from the simulator package.

Course delivery

As an extension to the above, there are tools which allow tutors to gather their teaching materials and present them to the student in an integrated environment. These tools then automatically provide communications facilities for learners, allowing discussion and real-time chat sessions to take place. Tools such as WebCT (www.webct.com) can be used to quickly construct courses for delivery over the Web.

Using pre-built CAL

Defining what sort of package you need

There is a great temptation to use CAL simply because it's there and not because you have a need for it. You should not select a CAL package for use by your students simply because it is 'something like' the topic you are teaching. If only a small portion of it is connected with your topic then students feel they are wasting their time using the package. Students will quickly discover if this is the case, and spread the word to avoid it.

Locating possible packages

There are many sources for CAL packages, the most immediately accessible to academics being the World Wide Web (see Appendix). Some organisations such as the Computers in Teaching Initiative Centre for Medicine (http://www.cticm.bristol.ac.uk/) review CAL packages and rate them for their quality and applicability to courses.

Assessing the quality of CAL

Before allowing your students access to a package it should first be evaluated to ensure it meets your objectives in terms of content and pedagogical approach. The criteria you should be looking for in CAL are:

- **Compatibility**. Will the package run on the computers available to your students? If it does not, and there are no available versions that will, then there is no point assessing the package further.
- **Content**. Does the content of the package cover the topic to your satisfaction, and is the information correct? It is important to check that the content is appropriate to the level of study and that the practices described within the package are appropriate to your institution. It is especially important to check this if the package has been written abroad or was originally intended for a different type of learner.
- **Construction**. Has the package been written well and is the user interface intuitive and well explained? Your students must be able to navigate through the package easily and the route along which they move should be a logical approach to the subject that is being studied. If this is not the case it will result in, at best, a dislike of the package or, at worst, utter confusion.
- **Cost**. If there is a charge for the CAL consider if it is reasonable for the size and complexity of package and how it fares with regard to the previous points. Find out whether a CAL package has a one-off charge or if there is a cost-per-user fee when installed on a network.

When assessing simulation packages, the level of realism can be looked at in two ways:

- Realism of the simulation. The simulation engine modelling the physical system or patient can be assessed by how accurately and comprehensively it mimics the body's reactions to a variety of treatments.
- Realism of the environment. Virtual environments can be created with virtual reality 3D models and video footage showing patient reactions. Just as valid as this would be a simple text interface, where the actual visualisation of the scene is left to the user. Surprisingly, the latter can give a more realistic experience (provided the underlying simulation engine is accurate), in the same way that sequences in films can seem more life-like if you don't see directly what's happening.

It is possible to have simulations at either extreme, but the best case is to have a mixture of both simulation and environmental reality.

Constructing your own CAL packages

If you cannot locate a package to achieve your objective, then you may need to build one in-house. If you attempt to construct your own CAL package, there is the risk of 'reinventing the wheel'. You should view examples built by experienced CAL producers to get some ideas about interfaces and interaction styles before starting. You may also be able to obtain development templates, which will accelerate your development process. Suitable places to find examples are project Web servers such as those involved in the Teaching & Learning Technology Programme (http://www.tltp.ac.uk/), or you can search the Web for 'computer assisted learning development' to obtain up-to-the-minute information.

There are at least four kinds of expertise required for the successful production of CAL packages:

- Subject matter knowledge is required for the creation of content material.
- Computing skills are necessary to ensure that the final product will function as intended, at an acceptable speed, and not cause the computer to crash.
- You should think carefully about which pedagogical approach you want the package to follow, and organise the interface appropriately.
- An element of graphic design will be needed to produce a pleasant-to-use interface.

Popular choices for development tools include:

- Asymmetrix Toolbook
- Macromedia Authorware or Dreamweaver.

Assessment

Computer-based assessment packages such as Question Mark (Question Mark Computing Ltd.) are used widely. The possible types of question in these programs range from simple multiple choice questions to image-based or full-text responses. For self-assessment tests students can be given immediate feedback on their answers, explanations of the correct answers, and the option to study remedial material if their test score was not acceptable. Responses made by students can be logged and may be used to contribute to summative assessment if students are made aware of this before starting.

Computers rarely mark essay-style questions themselves; instead responses of this kind tend to be set aside for a tutor or expert to mark later.

Presentations

The use of computers in presentations has been commonplace in business environments for many years. It is possible to project the display from the computer on to lecture theatre screens. The data projectors required for this are now adequate to achieve a similar quality in image resolution and definition to that of 35 mm slides projected using conventional techniques.

Two types of data projection system are available:

- Flat liquid crystal display (LCD) panels. These are placed on top of a high-power overhead projector (OHP) unit. It is possible to use panels with normal OHPs but the image projected is dim.
- True projectors. These contain bulb, imaging module and lenses all in the one unit.

Slides are typically prepared in a presentation package like Microsoft PowerPoint on a laptop computer, which is then plugged into a projector in the lecture theatre.

Advantages
The main advantages of using computer presentation systems like this are described below.

Preparation
The turn-around time for creating new visual material is very short, as there is no need to print to film and develop as 35 mm slides. This means that it is possible to add sections to lectures covering recent developments

If you are using a flat-panel LCD, make sure you turn off the OHP *before* the panel. It is easy to overheat panels accidentally when using high-power projectors and this can ruin them.

Always try out your laptop connected to the projector before the day of the lecture. Unexpected complications are common and you may need time to obtain technical assistance and/or another machine for your presentation if there are incompatibilities.

or topical stories as late as a few minutes before presentation.

Content

The content of slides is no longer limited to static images and text. It is possible to embed sound and video clips in the same presentation, which makes presenting the material much simpler than having to switch to video recorders and tape decks. The fewer pieces of equipment you use, the less likely it is that something will fail.

Interaction

The students can be involved with the presentation by using interactive audience response systems. By distributing handsets (similar to remote controls) to the audience, the students can respond to slides containing specially prepared questions. This can be useful for finding out in which areas the students' knowledge is lacking, and tailoring the lecture to fill those gaps.

Access

After the presentation has been given, the file containing the slides can be made available to the students on your computer network. This means they can replay the slides themselves, obtain printouts or even transfer slides for viewing on their home computer.

Disadvantages

There are inevitably some disadvantages to using these presentation systems:

- You must have access to a data projector. Initially there may not be enough projectors to go round your institution but as more and more teachers use computer presentations more will be purchased. In many institutions data projectors are as common in lecture theatres as slide projectors.
- The temptation to change your slides at the last minute can lead to unusable presentations.
- You will need to find out in advance the resolution at which the projector is capable of running. If your laptop and the projector operate at different display

If you must make any changes just before your presentation, make a copy of the file as a backup, just in case anything goes wrong.

resolutions, then the image on the screen will be resized to fill the available screen. This can result in blocky and sometimes unreadable text and images. Similarly, if you need to change your laptop's display resolution to match the projector, any images contained within your presentation will be rescaled.

It pays to be paranoid when giving presentations electronically. You should always take an extra floppy disk containing your presentation and carry it separately from your laptop.

To avoid display problems, build your presentation with your screen display set to the same resolution as that of the projector you will be using.

Summary

When used appropriately, computers can enhance the learning experience. Some care must be taken in the choice of hardware and software to ensure that they will fulfill the function required. It is worth taking the time to evaluate any packages you are interested in using before buying them but if nothing suitable is available it may be necessary to build your own. If you need to produce your own materials use a package template to avoid unnecessary work. Finally always check your presentations in the location they will be used and take a backup copy on disk just in case.

References and further reading

Asgari-Jirhandeh N, Haywood J 1997 Computer awareness among medical students: a survey. Medical Education 31:225–229

McAuley R J 1998 Requiring students to have computers: questions for consideration. Academic Medicine 73:669–673

Microsoft Office 2000 for Windows for Dummies 1999. IDG Books

Petrusa E R, Issenberg S B, Mayer J W, Felner J M, Brown D D, Waugh R A, Kondos G T et al 1999. Implementation of a four-year multimedia computer curriculum in cardiology at six medical schools. Academic Medicine 74:123–129

Race P, McDowell S 1996 500 computing tips for teachers and lecturers. Kogan Page, London

Chapter 20
Audio and video recordings

A. Stewart

Introduction

The use of media technology in teaching has long been considered a way of improving the process of communication and the accompanying process of learning. However, although developments in media technology are opening up new possibilities for its use, doubt has been expressed about the efficacy of media technology and its indiscriminate use has been criticised in research findings. Nevertheless, there is an intuitive feeling that it can be made to work effectively. The question is, how?

Since the 1980s new understanding of how students learn has emerged and has provided a basis for both the improvement of teaching and the enhancing of learning through the use of media technology. This new understanding of the learning process has come from a number of different areas of investigation which, collectively, have provided a robust model of how students learn. If we know how students learn, we are in a much stronger position to discover how to teach more effectively and we are in a much stronger position to design and use media in our teaching to improve communication and facilitate learning. Media technology in the teaching process must contribute to the learning process by providing the stimulus or the explanation which triggers deeper cognitive processing on the part of learners, allowing them to build up their knowledge structure through what they are seeing and hearing.

"Media are mere vehicles that deliver instruction but do not influence student achievement any more than the truck that delivers our groceries causes changes in nutrition. . . . Only the content of the vehicle can influence achievement"

Clark 1983

Given our present understanding of the cognitive processes involved in learning, it seems plausible to suppose that what is seen and heard in the media becomes part of the student's internal processing and facilitates the construction of meaning.

Media has the *potential* to contribute to learning. Whether it does or not depends on the way it has been designed and the way it is being used. If the attributes of the media are applied within an instructional design process to facilitate the achievement of specific learning outcomes it is very likely that learning will take place.

It isn't the media *per se* which facilitates learning; it's what happens within the media.

Video in teaching and training

Video is potentially a very powerful medium for communication and learning, bringing colour, moving images and sound together. By exploiting the various cinematic techniques, image manipulation processes and time modification approaches, it can be used effectively in all three areas of learning – knowledge, skills and attitudes.

Research carried out in the 1940s and 1950s in relation to film in education, which is just as applicable today to video in education, indicated that it can be used to reveal the remote, the invisible and the inaccessible.

The nature of 'remoteness' depends upon local factors; it might mean using video to reveal what is happening next door, in another part of town or on another continent. Revealing what is 'inaccessible' also depends on local conditions and circumstances. It might mean having video cameras in an area where there is high risk of infection and where the presence of additional people would result in increased risk, or it might mean using a video camera with an endoscope to demonstrate abnormalities in the gastrointestinal system. The 'invisible' might mean, simply, using a video camera with a microscope, but it might also mean using animation to illustrate a process which it is impossible to see even under a microscope or to represent what is conceptual rather than physical.

 "Knowledge is structured by individuals in meaningful ways which grow and change over time"

Romberg & Carpenter 1986

To use video effectively:

1. Point out what can be learned.
2. Draw attention to specific points to look for.
3. Encourage viewers to think through issues raised.

Don't be persuaded by media research that makes extravagant claims for media effectiveness. It is probably without foundation.

These various characteristics of video, together with other characteristics associated with the process of video production (such as being able to zoom in on detail) have become known as 'attributes' of video. This concept arose from a movement away from the research of the 1960s and 1970s which concerned itself with which mode of delivery (i.e. methods and media) resulted in the highest levels of learning, towards a different approach which focused on unique media characteristics and their connections to the development or enhancement of students' cognitive skills. Each of the media was considered to possess inherent codes or symbol systems that engaged specific cognitive abilities among users. For example, does a 'fade' between scenes (i.e. fading down to black and then fading up again to the picture) help the viewer to infer that there has been a passage of time? Does a split-screen image help the viewer to discriminate and to contrast and compare?

While some attributes are associated with only one medium, others are common to several media. The attributes of video present only the potential for learning. It is how we, the producers of the video, exploit these attributes that determines whether the video will be effective in learning.

Video can be used in education for the teaching of concepts, principles and procedures. It can also be used very effectively in facilitating achievement of affective learning outcomes. The teaching, however, has to be within an instructional design framework (see Chapter 17).

Video in the teaching of concepts

A considerable amount of learning is concerned with learning concepts. When we are trying to facilitate the learning of concepts we can either give a definition of the concept then give examples of it, or we can present examples from which students are able to work out what the definition might be because they have had to think about the characterising features of the concept. Video can be used in both methods to present examples by normal videographic techniques or by specialised techniques such as animation. For example, the concept of meiosis might be illustrated by animation indicating the crossover between a pair of chromosomes.

Video in the teaching of principles

Principles state relationships between two or more concepts. In general, principles can be converted into 'if-then' statements. When students have learned a principle they should be able to do more than simply state the principle; they should be able to make some predictions from it and explain appropriate events using the principle.

In general, there are three phases in teaching a principle. Firstly, the student is motivated to find out the nature of a particular principle. Secondly, the principle is composed. Finally, the student practises applying the principle.

Video is useful in the teaching of principles in that it can be used to arouse interest in the principle by showing some phenomenon and raising the question of why this is happening. It can also be used within the explanation to provide the necessary elaboration. Sometimes this may be possible with normal videographic techniques, but at other times it might require animation.

For example, the principle of pupil reaction to light could be demonstrated by normal videographic technique if the camera is framed on a close-up of the human eye and a narrow beam of light from a torch is passed across the eye. The viewers will be able to see the constriction of the pupil and the speed of response.

Video in the teaching of procedures

When students are developing a procedural skill, three kinds of information have to be made available. Before attempting to perform the procedure they should be made aware of what the objectives are and the performance criteria which go with them; they also need to have an overview of the task and how it would be performed by an expert. During practice, there are often critical cues available to students which it is difficult for the novice to discriminate in the flood of information. Attention must be called to these critical cues and help

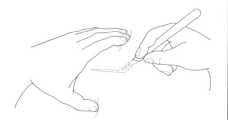

Fig. 20.1 'Over the shoulder' camera shot

given to discriminate between them. After practice, students need to be given feedback on particular acts and knowledge of results on the completed task.

One of the most important aspects of teaching a procedure is in giving an overview of the procedure as it would be performed by an expert. Obviously, video is particularly useful for this purpose. It is important, however, in demonstrating a procedure that the camera angle used should correspond to the field of vision which the person performing the task would have. This is called a 'subjective' camera angle and is usually achieved by shooting over the shoulder of the performer (see Fig. 20.1). An 'objective' camera angle would be a shot of the procedure from the point of view of an observer on the opposite side of the room from the doctor carrying out the procedure. This kind of shot unfortunately may create left/right disorientation for the observer.

Video in the teaching of attitudes

The education of medical students is frequently lacking in opportunities to acquire appropriate attitudes. We tend to concentrate on the knowledge and skills and ignore the attitudes. The problem for teachers is that attitudes are not easy to measure and are difficult both to define and to explain. They are very important, however, and teachers must try to make sure that students learn the right attitudes.

Although there are no guaranteed methods of teaching attitudes, there are five general approaches which can be used:

- providing information
- providing examples or models
- providing experience
- providing discussion
- using role-playing sessions.

Video is particularly useful in relation to attitudes because it appears to be able to convey the affective dimension of events with a power that other media do not have. Thus, in providing examples or models, video can not only inform but also provide vicarious experience; the viewer can learn the cognitive and procedural content within an attitudinal and emotional context. For example, when using video to teach nasogastric intubation, the knowledge and skills aspects of the procedure can be appreciated, but so, also, can the attitudes to be adopted towards the patient in explaining what is going to happen and empathising with the unpleasantness of the experience. Video can also be used to record the interaction between doctor and patient and the doctor can subsequently analyse the performance in respect of both skills and attitudes.

Using instructional video

Although the 'programme' idea dies hard, it is not always necessary to produce or to use a stand-alone video programme of 30 minutes' or so duration. Frequently, video clips are more effective, particularly in a classroom setting. Short illustrative clips of video, with or without sound, can be used very effectively to support the teacher's presentation to the class. The attributes of video in relation to the achievement of cognitive, psychomotor and affective learning outcomes can readily be exploited without the production of a stand-alone programme.

Using a short sequence of video is analogous to using a few slides; they are used to illustrate the point, to help explain the concept or principle, or to show how something is done.

Instructional video can be used in places other than the classroom. If it is a skill or a procedure that is being taught, it is frequently more appropriate to use the video in the setting in which the student is going to practise the skill or the procedure. This 'contextualises' the learning. However, it also suggests that the student is going to practise the skill or the procedure immediately after viewing the video or, perhaps, after viewing only a part of the video which demonstrates a component part of the skill or procedure.

If the video is being used to teach attitudes, it would be appropriate to use it in a small group teaching session where there can be discussion of the issues raised. A

"Learners are positively affected when persuasive messages are presented in as credible a manner as possible. Learners who experience a purposeful emotional involvement or arousal during instruction are likely to change their attitudes in the direction advocated in the mediated message"

Simonson 1995

classroom might be appropriate, but a smaller room where the group can sit in a circle for the discussion would usually be more desirable.

How and where video is used is less important than why it is used. What really matters is that the teacher who plans to use video has already identified the kind of learning to be achieved and is satisfied that the video in question can facilitate that kind of learning.

Instructional video can, of course, be used by the student in an independent way either in the library, in a resource centre, or at home. One of the advantages of video is that the cassette is relatively small and inexpensive, so copies can be made available quite readily. Also, many people have video replay facilities in their homes which can be used for learning.

Audio recordings

Audio recordings do not have the glamour of some other media, yet for some subject areas they are particularly useful. For years, audio tape has been the most effective medium for teaching languages. This is obviously because, in language learning, it is important that we are able to hear how words sound. So we could speculate that in any situation where the nature of the sound is important, audio recordings might be a useful medium to use. For example, when we are trying to help students identify the sounds associated with the heart and lungs, the use of audio recordings could be advantageous. Where sound discrimination is an essential learning outcome, any media system which can include recorded sound is obviously going to be valuable.

Research on the use of audio instruction in the 1960s and 1970s employed aptitude treatment interaction designs in which there was an attempt to explore the interactions between specific instructional materials and individual learners. Most of these have been in the area of self-paced or individualised instruction and audio-tutorial instruction, and from these and earlier investigations we can identify the key attributes of audio recordings for learning.

So what are the attributes of audio recordings? How can these attributes be exploited in the design of instructional experiences?

Remember that when we are looking at the attributes of a particular medium, we are considering those characteristics of the medium which, when exploited within an instructional design framework, are potentially capable of triggering cognitive processing on the part of the learner.

Obviously the most important characteristic of audio recordings is their ability to carry audible cues. These cues can be either verbal or non-verbal. Non-verbal cues in medical education would include things like heart and lung sounds. The purpose of having these recorded on tape or CD would be to help listeners to develop recognition and discrimination skills. Verbal cues are, of course, spoken language – the commentary. We need to ask ourselves, therefore, what it is about a spoken commentary that makes it different from a printed commentary. In a printed commentary, we are limited in the way we can highlight or emphasise words or phrases. In a spoken commentary, however, we can use intonation and inflection to achieve these purposes. In theory, therefore, we ought to be able to use the verbal cues very effectively to convey the message. Many CD-ROMs developed for teaching include a spoken commentary as well as a printed version that the student can read from the screen.

The ability to carry real sounds, i.e. sounds of actual phenomena, and the ability to convey a spoken message, become the two key attributes of audio recordings. It is these attributes which we must seek to exploit when we are considering the design and development of learning opportunities and learning materials.

Summary

Video and audio, whether recorded as analogue signal on tape or as digital signal on disk, or stored digitally in a computer, provide a useful resource for teaching in medicine.

"Research has evolved to emphasise learning with media and developing technology to support and optimise thinking, learning, and teaching process"

Hannafin et al 1996

Video is potentially particularly useful since it can be used to help facilitate learning in the three areas of human learning – knowledge, skills and attitudes – and, within the knowledge area, to facilitate learning of both concepts and principles. What affects its effectiveness, however, is the extent to which, in its production, the attributes of video have been exploited within an appropriate instructional design framework.

Audio is of more limited use since its attributes suggest facilitation of a relatively restricted range of learning outcomes. However, since video usually includes an audio dimension, video and audio together are potentially powerful for facilitating learning.

References and further reading

Clark R 1983 Reconsidering research on learning from media. Review of Educational Research 53(4):445–459

Hannafin K M, Houper S R, Reiber L P, Kini A S 1996 Research on and research with emerging technologies. In: Jonassen D H (ed.) Handbook of Research for Educational Communications and Technology. Simon & Schuster Macmillan, New York

Romberg T A, Carpenter T P 1986 Research on teaching and learning mathematics. In: Wittrock M C (ed.) Handbook of research on teaching, 3rd edn. Macmillan, New York, pp 850–873

Simonson M 1995 Instructional technology and attitude change. In: Anglin G J (ed.) Instructional Technology, Past, Present and Future, 2nd edn. Libraries Unlimited, Englewood, CO

SECTION 5
CURRICULUM THEMES

Chapter 21
Basic sciences

G. C. Leslie

Introduction

Historically the basic (preclinical) sciences for medicine were generally accepted as being:

- anatomy
- histology
- physiology
- biochemistry.

Integrated teaching of these preclinical subjects was the exception rather than the rule. Indeed the territorial rights to both subject quantity and timetable were strongly defended so that in one institution histology was taught within anatomy, in another as a separate subject by physiologists and in yet another by both! Biochemistry was in some institutes just a division within the physiology department. Notwithstanding these territorial 'arrangements' individual academics, on good personal terms, did make the occasional *ad hoc* attempt to run related courses in parallel, e.g. neuroanatomy with neurophysiology. This departmental based approach to the curriculum characterised both the preclinical and clinical years of the traditional medical course before the General Medical Council (GMC 1993) published its recommendations for UK medical schools.

The last few decades have seen an explosion of knowledge, nowhere more so than in the fields of: genetics, cellular biology and molecular biology. While fresh concepts in these – the new – basic sciences have emerged, much of the supporting data is in the detail. Academics stimulated by these ever-expanding fields have not surprisingly wanted to both excite and enthuse their students with the very latest findings. Not surprisingly the addition of new findings to 'old' findings over the past few decades has created an overload of information on medical courses. These two views were taken up by the GMC as it planned its recommendations for undergraduate training in the UK.

The challenge

Recent changes to medical education have set out both a strategy and a challenge to medical schools. The strategy embodied in the GMC recommendations was not mandatory but none the less demanded change: change to an integrated core curriculum and provision of special study modules (SSMs). The challenge, since the GMC chose not to discuss tactics, lay in the implementation of the recommendations. How is each medical school going to provide a core curriculum and integrate teaching in the basic medical sciences within such a curriculum?

Five challenging areas can be identified where progress may be made:

- identification of core material
- integration of core material
- delivery of core material
- assessment of basic sciences within the core
- basic sciences and SSMs

Critical path analysis in developing the management of a new curriculum could be used to identify times when these various strands might successfully be brought together.

Identification of core material

This topic is certainly one that generates many debates and it is probably one of the most difficult to resolve. Although this chapter is concerned with the basic sciences and their integration it is crucial that clinicians are involved with the basic scientists in these discussions *from the start*. Teachers within a single cognate subject area, e.g. physiology, or a subject topic, e.g. respiratory physiology, must not confer in departmental isolation but work in concert with clinicians, e.g. respiratory physicians. It may be prudent also to involve the professions allied to medicine. Physiotherapists can provide a different multiprofessional viewpoint in relation to the example of respiratory physiology. Each system group of contributors can 'brainstorm' to identify core basic sciences. All, individually or in concert, can do so at local, national and international levels.

Local enquiry

Intra- and interprofessional 'topic' meetings, formal and informal, can well establish a local viewpoint within a given subject. These collaborations will expose individual preferences or prejudices, but hopefully will resolve into a hard-core acceptance of fundamentals and principles. In addition it should be possible to identify the minimum of detail required to illustrate core and to acquire this information.

National Enquiry

The GMC's Education Committee is 'promoting the development of core courses relating to particular topics through various institutions and organisations' (GMC 1993). These core courses, many of which have yet to appear, will allow local groupings of teachers to run a cross-check on their own perceptions of core.

An alternative 'national' opportunity occurs at the meetings of the societies of the basic science specialties where the sharing of ideas can take place.

International enquiry

This may be regarded as an extension of the national level. The definition of core should be the same from one country to another. Who would argue against the fundamental that physiological control of arterial blood pressure is the same the world over?

Confirmations of these national and international approaches may increasingly be made through the World Wide Web, where it is possible to browse the curriculum content of many institutions. The greater the overlap of material, the more confident one can become of defining core material within a cognate subject area or topic. This has the further advantage of providing insight into the presentation of core in different schools.

Integration of core material

Horizontally, within the basic sciences
Integration of the basic sciences is attainable, but needs:

- cooperation
- consensus
- common sense
- commitment.

Integration of histological, physiological and biochemical aspects of cells, tissues, organs and systems is relatively easy, given the above four criteria. Integration of anatomy with the other basic sciences may seem slightly more difficult, given the nature of the subject with its specific relational requirements. The problem is highlighted in the systems-based approach. While physiology and biochemistry can readily adapt, the integration of anatomy which follows a 'regions approach' is more difficult. A common-sense resolution to integration can lie in a 'systems-sensitive' approach. For example, when studying the structures associated with the thorax it intuitively seems the time to consider the functioning of the respiratory and cardiovascular systems too. Likewise, neuroanatomy, neurophysiology and neurochemistry can well integrate systematically into 'the neurosciences', while the gastrointestinal system integrates largely with studying the anatomy of the abdomen. Using common sense to achieve cooperation and consensus results in commitment.

Vertically, within the curriculum
The basic sciences are just as relevant in later years of the medical curriculum and also in postgraduate medicine but they are not always as 'visible'. This is because the tendency is to focus on disease and illness. Every time a neurological examination is conducted, every time a blood pressure measurement is made or an enzyme

assay is requested, there are respective examples of the applications of anatomical, physiological and biochemical sciences. Good clinical teachers can, through the use of any task or problem, greatly assist students in self-learning by taking a few minutes to focus away from the patient and towards the basic sciences.

Examples of this good practice can readily be augmented during students' self-learning with specialised textbooks in which the authors devote space to those basic sciences relevant to the main content of the book.

SSMs can be offered in basic sciences both in early years or in the later part of the course when students are more able to integrate them with the clinical studies they have experienced.

Delivery of core material

Having achieved recognition of and agreement on both what core material is within the basic sciences and its integration into the curriculum, a number of questions arise.

When should it be delivered?

There seems little doubt that the classical basic sciences are a strong foundation upon which to build. Given this premise, it would seem logical to deliver them early within the degree programme (Harden, Davis & Crosby 1997). This does not of course preclude them from also being presented as appropriate later in the programme.

If presented by system then in what order should it be tackled?

The order in which systems teaching is delivered is an open question, whose answer may well depend on local circumstances of staffing and timetabling. Hopefully, however, the consensus will contain the notion that it is good practice to teach the 'easier' topics first.

Who should deliver it?

The professional basic scientist is probably the best person for the job. Such staff are active in their discipline and, through research interests, are well aware of current

- Reveal
- Recall
- Refresh
- Review
- Reinforce.

Build in flexibility.

When responsible for organising timetables, defend 'free study time' (for self-directed learning) vigorously, or else the process of generating curriculum overload will begin all over again!

"The clinical presentation on 'back pain' was greatly enhanced by the presence of an anatomist and physiologist 'recalling' the appropriate basic contributions from anatomy and physiology"

3rd year medical student

developments. Traditionally the preclinical teachers have been the staff first encountered by new entrants, who often suffer the stresses of arriving at and adjusting to university life and a different form of teaching. Over the years these staff have gained experience of how to support immature students and develop their confidence. These factors are both worthy of note if the curriculum is to be successfully presented.

Basic science core input to later years in the course can be the remit of either the scientist or the clinician, or both.

What methods should be used?

Alternative methods of curriculum delivery, such as problem-based or task-centred learning, call for a different ordered approach but still require the core component of the basic sciences. None the less, here also the caveat of not overfilling the timetable must be adhered to.

Assessment of basic sciences within the core

Any new educational development requires assessment. Assessment of the basic sciences and their integration may therefore include:

- students' core knowledge and its application
- their learning experience
- their development.

Evaluation of the benefits and drawbacks of the new venture include:

- When and how often to assess/evaluate?
- How to assess/evaluate and what methods to use?

Computer-assisted assessment

Computer marking software such as 'QuestionMark' provides a rapid response to the assessment of core knowledge using a variety of question formats. For example:

- multiple choice
- multiple response
- extended matching items (EMIs)

- calculations
- 'hot spot' diagrams
- true/false questions.

These formats allow teachers working in groups an opportunity to ask 'integrated questions' regarding core knowledge. However, the initial construction of quality questions can be anything but rapid. Well-constructed EMIs assess students' logical applications of core knowledge and its understanding but this new methodology currently requires student training, since few have experience of this mode of assessment. The requirement 'to train' can, however, be incorporated in the presentation of formative assessments, which consist of randomised presentations of a set number from a bank of relevant questions. We have arranged to give our students a formative test at the end of each block. The test is available on the local area network for 1 week following the end of a systems block of teaching.

Progress testing

In our first-year course there are three summative assessments, at about 3-monthly intervals. A selection of questions used in these first-year assessments could readily be repeated in later years' assessments – a move towards the concept in progress testing. In-depth analysis of student performance year on year could then lead indirectly to both appraisal of the learning experience and an individual's development.

Spot exams

It is not necessary to abandon all of the old and tried methods of assessment. Instead they can be reconstructed and made relevant for use in integrated assessment. Simple examples exist in the 'old' anatomy-type spot examination. Rather than ask the student to identify a structure or recall in detail its relationships, one may alternatively ask a question about its function and/or biochemistry. For example, with a pin marking the left ventricle the problem might be: 'Indicate the enzymes most likely to be elevated in plasma following an occlusion of the blood supply to this tissue.'

Invite colleagues external to the basic sciences to attend meetings when setting questions for assessments. In such meetings there are opportunities not only to reinforce agreements between basic scientists and clinicians as to what 'core' is but also to carry out an internal audit so that the boundaries of 'core' are not exceeded.

"some of the present day art and science of medicine is fundamental to its practice and will certainly endure"

GMC 1993

Orals

The oral examination, be it in first or final year, is another example of where it is possible to integrate assessment activity (along with communication skills) in the basic sciences.

Basic sciences and special study modules

Vertical integration of basic sciences throughout the 5 years of the medical course can be augmented by their inclusion within SSMs. This can be achieved in several ways. An SSM can be:

* basic science-specific, e.g. 'Physiology beyond core'
* integrated into a clinical attachment, e.g. revisiting anatomy when doing a surgical placement
* integrated into a laboratory-based attachment in clinical sciences, e.g. biochemistry within a clinical sciences attachment.

Course evaluation

As well as presenting the formative test a computer program can also be used to retrieve feedback. 'QuestionMark' can be used to acquire individual student responses about the course and about its delivery by the teaching staff. These data can be supplemented by convening meetings of a basic sciences staff–student committee, in which class representatives report class concerns and comments.

Change, challenge and control

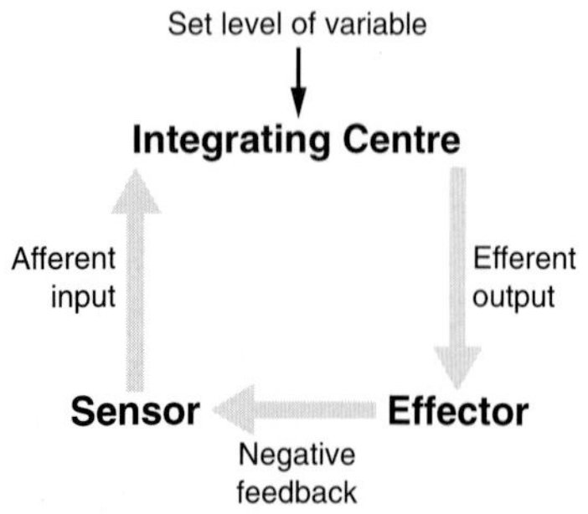

The innovations which have been put in place to implement the changes required in the delivery of basic science teaching in the new curriculum have been a challenge for many medical schools. If they are to be of benefit, however, a control system is required to monitor and refine their role. A model taken from physiology (see Fig. 21.1) shows a control loop consisting of these elements, generally referred to as the integrating centre with its set level of controlled variable, sensors with afferent input, efferent output to effectors, and the control loop closed with negative

Fig. 21.1   Control loop

feedback. Demonstrating a transferable skill, it is possible to re-present, rename and restructure Figure 21.1 as a model for use in curricular development, management and 'control' (see Fig. 21.2). Figure 21.2 can be thought to operate at many levels of the hierarchy, whether the set level of variable be the curriculum outcomes, the objectives in a systems block of teaching or a single learning objective in a lecture. Points of note within this figure therefore relate not only to the integration of basic sciences but to the curriculum as a whole. Contemplation of Figure 21.2 should emphasise the importance of and need for:

- a set level of clearly defined variables
- communication both between and within elements
- feedback to close the loop.

A developing viewpoint in relation to defined variables may be found in curricular outcomes (Association of American Medical Colleges 1998). For these to succeed there is a paramount requirement to communicate between educationalists and educators, between groupings of teachers delivering either one section of the course or different sections of the curriculum, and between all teachers and all students. Good-quality communication can lead to commitment and is a key to success – as is good-quality intelligence feedback. Note in Figure 21.2 the additional lines of communication which emphasise this point.

Conceptually Figure 21.2 can be overviewed under different headings (see Fig. 21.3):

- theory
- practice
- reality.

It is in the reality, the students' learning experience, that there is most reservation. The weakness of most first-year students is an immaturity which prevents them from organising their own learning effectively. They set out either consciously or subconsciously to learn less than 100% of the core material. When students were overloaded a 70% learning of overload probably

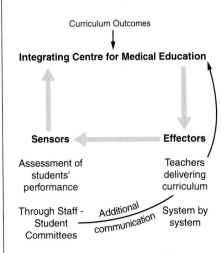

Fig. 21.2 Restructured for use in curriculum development

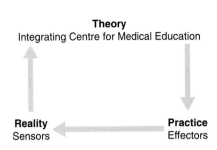

Fig. 21.3 Overview

"You will have to learn many tedious things, . . . which you will forget the moment you have passed your final examination, but in anatomy it is better to have learned and lost than never to have learned at all"

W. Somerset Maugham
1874–1965

"My students are dismayed when I say to them, 'Half of what you are taught as medical students will in ten years be shown to be wrong, and the trouble is, none of your teachers knows which half'"

C. Sidney Burwell 1893–1967

"Create something, perfect it and it will be yours forever"

Pliny the Younger c.61–c.112

prepared them to take a good knowledge of their basic sciences onwards. A 70% knowledge of a core basic sciences curriculum may in time prove to be less than adequate. Hence the ever-present need clearly to define, communicate and provide feedback on the integration of basic sciences into the medical curriculum.

Summary

Individual medical schools in the UK have been tasked by the GMC to set their own experimental conditions within which the recommended changes must evolve to reduce factual overload and didacticism. Set out specifically in this chapter are a number of facets for consideration when contemplating the task of integrating the basic sciences into a 'core curriculum'; these are identification and integration, delivery and assessment. No doubt in evolving curricular changes in undergraduate education medical schools will have their successes and failures. It is too soon in this experiment to know which approaches will be the mutant disappointments that need discarding and which approaches will see the survival of the fittest in achieving the desired goals.

References and further reading

Association of American Medical Colleges 1998 Report 1: Learning objectives for medical student education; guidelines for medical schools. AAMC, Washington, DC

Drake R L 1998 Anatomy education in a changing medical curriculum. Anatomical Record 253:28–31

Ellis J 1987–8 Integration of basic sciences and clinical teaching. Clio Medica 21:153–160

General Medical Council 1993 Tomorrow's doctors: recommendations on undergraduate medical education. GMC, London

Ginzberg E 1993 The reform of medical education: an outsider's reflections. Academic Medicine 68:518–521

Harden R M, Davis M H, Crosby J R, 1997 The new Dundee medical curriculum: a whole that is greater than the sum of the parts. Medical Education 31:264–271

Schmid R 1989 Medical schools in the year 2000 and beyond. Mayo Clinical Proceeding 64:1180–1184

Chapter 22
Communication skills

D. Snadden   J. S. Ker

Introduction

The evidence that doctors are not all good communicators and that communication skills can be taught is well established (Simpson et al 1991). There is now growing evidence that good communication has a positive effect on patient outcomes; thus effective communication teaching at all levels of medical education is imperative.

What are communication skills?

Until recently communicating with patients and traditional history-taking were often seen as the same thing. This is no longer so, history-taking now being seen as something that doctors do to patients as a way of extracting information from them, while communication is about how doctors and patients talk with each other in a search for mutual understanding and shared solutions to problems. This does not exclude history-taking, but rather includes it as part of an overall communication strategy to be used when appropriate.

Communication skills can be extended beyond the doctor–patient encounter to include communication between colleagues and other professionals and also written communications. As the doctor–patient interaction lies at the heart of medicine we will concentrate on that in this chapter and make some comments on team working.

"Communication skills are not an optional extra; without appropriate communication skills our knowledge and intellectual efforts are easily wasted"

Silverman, Kurtz & Draper 1998

"To do good and to communicate forget not"

Hebrews ch 13, v 16

Communication models

A number of communication models now exist, and each of these is well described in the literature with appropriate instruction on how to teach the model (Neighbour 1992, Pendleton et al 1984, Stewart et al 1995). They all emphasise the importance of understanding not only the patient's disease process but also their thoughts, beliefs, feelings and expectations in helping determine the best course of action for each person. In addition the models share similar understandings in terms of defining the basic elements of a successful consultation. These basic skills were described by Silverman, Kurtz & Draper as:

- initiating the session
- gathering information
- building the relationship
- explanation and planning
- closing the session.

More advanced skills consist of subjects such as breaking bad news, dealing with anger and dealing with addiction.

Rather than thinking about which is the best model, it is better to think about which one suits the purpose of your particular setting, whether it is a small teaching unit or a whole medical school. What is important for learners is that they are exposed to similar advice in different settings, particularly at medical school. This means that the types of communication training they receive in different hospital wards, clinics and primary care settings need to complement each other.

How to teach communication skills

As communication skills are something that doctors need in practice, teaching will be more effective if it contains practical experience and feedback. The latter means giving direct constructive feedback to a learner in a supporting environment. This could be in a one-to-one or small-group setting. Before giving feedback ground rules need to be established. These may include:

Concentrate on core skills before special skills. The core skills are:

- initiating the session
- gathering information
- building the relationship
- explanation and planning
- closing the session.

Giving feedback on communication is important, but the feedback needs to value the opinion and feelings of learners, as well as being constructive in helping them to improve. One way to do this is to ask:

- the learners what they were trying to achieve in the communication session
- the learners what they think went well
- the observers what they think went well
- the learners what didn't go so well or what they would do differently next time
- the observers what didn't go so well or what could be done differently next time.

- how the feedback will be given
- confidentiality
- what will happen to any material collected during the teaching session.

Learners need to be given examples of the core skills of communication, some background reading and models and then an opportunity to try out these skills with constructive feedback. Practice and feedback are the most effective ways to improve skills.

Resources
Various methods can be used to teach communication skills as they also provide opportunities for analysis and discussion. Whichever teaching method is to be used certain issues need to be resolved:

- If real patients are to be used fully informed consent needs to be gained. This is extremely important if video or audio tapes will be used.
- If a tape is used, how will it be discussed and how will constructive feedback be given? It is important that a climate is set in which it is safe for individuals to discuss difficulties openly and receive feedback on how to tackle them. This can only be done in one-to-one or small-group settings.

Demonstrations
Demonstrations can be created on video tape, on audio tape or as role-plays to show students examples of good and poor communication, or to give them practice at understanding or analysing various models. Taped consultations can be real or simulated. These can illustrate many medical settings from the hospital ward and the outpatient department to a primary care setting.

Simulations
Simulated consultations can be created using members of the teaching team, volunteer patients or professional actors. They have the advantages of not requiring informed consent, of being able to use the same people in different situations and of being able to be used in special situations, such as learning to break bad news.

Be prepared to lead by example and hold demonstrations of your own consultations for your students to criticise constructively.

In videoing real consultations informed consent is essential:

- Give a written information sheet and a consent form to sign prior to the consultation starting.
- The information sheet must say what the tape could be used for, who might see it and how long it will be kept.
- Patients must be allowed to say no.
- When the consultation is finished then patients should sign once more to show that they still consent to the tape being used for teaching purposes.

"Having the opportunity to take histories from simulated patients and get feedback on how you've done, gave me more confidence to go on to the wards and speak to real patients"

Medical student

"The thought of being videoed was scary, but once you got into the consultation you forgot the camera was there"

Medical student

The disadvantages are that all simulators need good training, expensive equipment is needed if video tapes are to be made, and professional actors are very expensive.

Simulations can be particularly powerful when the student meets the simulated patient in a one-to-one encounter and receives feedback on performance, either at once or later if the consultation is video- or audio-taped.

Observation

Observation of students can take place in any setting where they meet patients. The important thing is that feedback is constructive and specific, and relates to the communication model that students have learned about.

Video-audio-taping

Students can make video- or audio-taped consultations of their meetings with real or simulated patients. They can then bring them to meetings with a tutor or a learning group. This is particularly useful in postgraduate teaching.

Role play

Role play can also be used in consultation situations when students take on the roles of patient and doctor and carry out a simulated consultation.

Here is an example of the type of script which can be used either for role playing or for simulation.

Example 1 Simulated patient instructions
The student seeing you will have a limited time to speak to you. Please spend some time thinking yourself into the role. The student has been asked to explore your reasons for visiting the doctor today.

You are a 26-year-old male/female named Jones. You are at university in the second year of a PhD in biochemistry. For the last 6 months you have been getting a cough at night. When the student asks you why you have come say that you have 'been getting a cough at night' and wait and see what he or she asks you next.

It is likely you will be asked more about your cough. This wakes you up sometimes and you have been feeling a bit tired because of lost sleep. The problem has gradually worsened.

Give the following information if you are asked directly or if the student encourages you to talk with open-ended questions.

You are in the university swimming team and train regularly. Training nights are Tuesdays and Fridays. Your times have not been so good recently and during training you are feeling unduly short of breath and develop a sensation of tightness across your chest. Last Tuesday this got pretty bad and scared you – that is why you are here – your chest was making funny wheezy noises. This settled eventually but you had a really bad night with coughing.

You have no personal or social problems. You are happy as a student. Your only past history of note was eczema as a child. Your brother has hay fever; otherwise there is no relevant family history. Your parents are alive and well.

You think it is asthma because the swimming coach told you. A quick suck on one of your team's inhaler (Salbutamol) sorted you out; you will only admit to this if asked what you think is happening to you, what you think is wrong with you or some similar question.

If you are asked anything else make it up!

Notes for the student: This patient is consulting you as a doctor for the first time. Elicit his or her story. The patient is Mr/Mrs Jones. They are 26 years old – despite how old he or she may look!
You will be given feedback on the types of question you ask, your listening skills and how you acquire information.

Games – communication in teams
Learning to communicate with other health workers is increasingly important. Students can be shown examples of well-performing teams; intensive care units and

surgical teams are often good examples. Role play and games can be fun and very instructive; they do not tell students how to communicate but rather help them to experience the difficulties and problems of communicating between individuals and to learn from these.

Example 2 'Communicate'

One example of a game is 'communicate' (Crosby & Eastaugh 1994). This is a simple game for a minimum of four players. Each assumes a role and has a number of skills. The skills are as follows:

- Player 1 is fully mobile, but cannot see or talk.
- Player 2 can see and write, but cannot talk or walk.
- Player 3 can read and talk, but cannot move and cannot see the game area.
- Player 4 organises and observes.

The players are then positioned with players 2 and 3 sitting beside each other but facing different ways. Player 3 faces away from the game area and can only see to read. Player 2 can see the game area and has a clip board, paper and pen. Player 1 is blindfolded. The idea is that players 2 and 3 work together to give appropriate instructions to player 1 to complete a task.

Also needed are four balloons of different colours and a waste bin. The balloons are on the floor about 10 metres from the bin. The task is written on a flip chart at the start of the game: 'put the red (or whichever colour is available) balloon in the bin.' The team is given 10 minutes to accomplish the task.

It is better not to give teams too much preparation time, and more than one team can be used to introduce an element of competition.

At the end of the task de-role the participants as the game can provoke strong feelings. De-roling allows players to confirm that the game is finished and to explore what happened, what they felt and what the experience meant. Exploring the experience is where the learning comes from and where any other observers can make comments.

Feedback

It is difficult to see how students can improve their communication skills without practising them in safe settings and receiving feedback on their performance. Effective feedback is one of the cornerstones of effective communication teaching and needs to be:

- **C**lear. If you are vague you will not be understood. 'Well, I don't know if this matters or not, it might not be relevant, but the patient seemed a bit more upset after seeing you.'
- **O**wned. The feedback you give is your own perception, but comments such as 'I think the way you handled that situation was very clever' can be positively helpful.
- **R**egular. Feedback will be more useful if it happens regularly and is given close to events and in a way that an individual student can use to make changes. 'You say that your consultations tend to be too long. I've noticed that you seem to have a bit of difficulty stopping consultations. Do you want to think about this and try out some ways of stopping effectively and we'll discuss it next time?'
- **B**alanced. Feedback can be perceived as always being negative but constructive feedback is about discussing strengths as well as weaknesses.
- **S**pecific. Generalised feedback can be hard to learn from. 'You can be frustrating' may be less useful than 'I get frustrated if you are not talking about problems that occur around prescribing.'

Special situations

Once students have mastered basic communication skills there are a number of special situations which merit further study:

- breaking bad news (Buckman 1994)
- dealing with distressed patients who are angry or upset
- dealing with ethical dilemmas.

Teaching special situations requires preparation, patience and tact. It is difficult to arrange for students to experience these in the course of their clinical exposure. If they do meet these situations they are usually only able to observe experienced doctors handling them. As we have said before, real learning often comes from trying things out yourself so simulations and role play are often the best methods. These particular situations can provoke a lot of emotion in those involved in acting out the scenario. For this reason scripts need to be carefully created, everyone involved has to be well briefed, and there must be plenty of time for discussion and debriefing afterwards. Well-trained simulated patients are very helpful in this situation as, if things are not going well, the consultation can be stopped, the problem discussed and the student can try again. Particularly in these situations teachers need good skills in facilitation and counselling. The sessions can be most effective in small-group or one-to-one situations. Effective communication skill teaching requires time and preparation and is labour-intensive.

Assessing communication skills

Formative assessment

Feedback on a student's performance can be given using observation or audio or video tapes. Particularly in communication skills it is not what the student knows that is important; it is what the student does in practice. Therefore formative assessment is best carried out as close to the real clinical situation as possible.

Such formative assessment consists of feedback on the student's performance; if this is to be effective in supporting the student's learning it must use a constructive feedback model. It may be helpful for students or teachers to keep records of teaching sessions and formative feedback comments as these can give an indication of progress over time. It is, however, important that formative assessments are used to support learning – if they count towards formal assessments they can reduce experimentation and real exploration of weaknesses and inhibit learning.

Summative assessment

Communication assessments can be built into examinations such as the objective structured clinical examination where simulated patients can be used for standardised consultations. Standardised instruments for assessing communication skills now exist and can either be used as they are or further refined in different settings (Stewart et al 1995; Campbell, Howie & Murray 1995). More complex assessments have been developed using simulated surgeries (Rashid et al 1994). The latter are costly in terms of time and resources and may be more applicable in the postgraduate setting. In the undergraduate setting, however, it is imperative that robust assessments of student performances are devised so that students only qualify after they have mastered and demonstrated certain core communication competencies.

"Basic interviewing skills can be learned at undergraduate and postgraduate level, providing effective methods are used. These include demonstration of key skills, practice under controlled conditions, and audiotape or videotape feedback of performance by a tutor within small groups. More complex skills can also be learned but may not be used or maintained without ongoing training and supervision"

Maguire 1990

Summary

Effective communication skills can be taught at undergraduate and postgraduate level. Knowledge alone is insufficient to make an effective doctor as doctors have to be able to communicate genuinely with patients, colleagues and staff. Basic communication skills are most effectively taught using a recognised communication model in small groups or one-to-one situations. Role play, simulated patients and real patients are effective teaching methods, with video or audio recording or direct observation being well used to support constructive feedback to the student.

Good communication skills are at the core of the doctor–patient interaction. They are not an addition or an option but central to the effective practice of medicine.

Acknowledgements

We are grateful to Mary Thomas for help with the CORBS feedback model.

References and further reading

Buckman R 1994. How to break bad news. Papermac, London

Campbell L M, Howie J G R, Murray T S. 1995. Use of videotaped consultations in summative assessment of trainees in general practice. British Journal of General Practice 45(392):137–141

Crosby J, Eastaugh A 1994 A game exploring teamwork. Education for General Practice 5:269–273

Maguire P 1990 Can communication skills be taught? British Journal of Hospital Medicine March 43(3):215–216

Neighbour R 1992 The inner consultation 3. Kluwer Academic, London, pp. 3–296

Pendleton D, Schofield T, Tate P, Havelock P 1984 The consultation: an approach to learning and teaching. Oxford University Press, Oxford

Rashid A, Allen J, Thew R, Aram G 1994 Performance based assessment using simulated patients. Education for General Practice 5:151–156

Silverman J D, Kurtz S M, Draper J 1998 Skills for communicating with patients. Radcliffe, Oxford

Simpson M, Buckman R, Stewart M, Maguire P, Lipkin M, Novack D, Till J 1991 Doctor patient communication: the Toronto consensus statement. British Medical Journal 303:1385–1387

Stewart M, Brown J B, Weston W W, McWhinney I, McWilliam C L, Freeman T R 1995 Patient-centered medicine transforming the clinical method. Sage, London, pp. 1–238

Chapter 23
Ethics and attitudes

M. G. Brennan

Introduction

To be a doctor is literally to be a teacher. One of the most valuable lessons doctors can impart to their students is how to be a 'good' doctor, an ethical practitioner. Like all areas of medicine, this is a complex lesson, best learnt by hard work, application, reflection and experience. For the lesson to be successful it needs to be relevant, credible and well delivered; prior planning and preparation need to take place. For the teachers of ethics to be successful they also need to be credible, to be able to 'walk the talk', and to know how to plan, prepare and deliver the teaching.

This chapter provides a practical introduction to the teaching of medical ethics and attitudes. It uses a case study to illustrate recent innovations in the teaching of medical ethics, and focuses on some of the factors which have precipitated such developments. Above all, it is intended to show how ethics can be taught in a way that is enjoyable and effective for the life-long learner in medicine.

How it has been

Sir Lancelot Spratt lives on in medical education. He first appeared as an eminent consultant surgeon in *Doctor in the House* (Rank 1954), the film inspired by Richard Gordon's books. Sir Lancelot's attitude towards medical ethics was best displayed in the classic ward round scene. In this, he drew a long incision line across a patient's abdomen and then said 'Don't worry, my good man, this has got absolutely nothing to do with you,'

"Students should acquire a knowledge and understanding of 'ethical and legal issues relevant to the practice of medicine' and an 'ability to understand and analyse ethical problems so as to enable patients, their families, society and the doctor to have proper regard to such problems in reaching decisions' "

General Medical Council 1993

having first told him that 'you won't understand our medical talk.' Since then, he has made his mark in numerous hospitals and medical schools worldwide. Medical ethics for Sir Lancelot and some of his generation could be summed up as not seducing your patients, avoiding too much alcohol on duty, and not advertising your services.

Fortunately, times are changing. Most doctors and medical students have high ideals and aspirations, and want to practise medicine in an ethical way. At the very least, they are keen to avoid complaints by their patients and colleagues, or being sued for malpractice; this might be described as the default position. Medical litigation has increased exponentially over the past few years and seems set to continue its rapid growth.

With this background, it is actually not very difficult to capitalise on the willingness of doctors and medical students to practise medicine in an ethical way. New curricula have recently appeared in medical schools across the world; in many of them, the study of medical ethics has taken its rightful place at the centre of the curriculum. At a postgraduate level, there are very few medical training schemes or specialties prepared to neglect medical ethics in their provision of education, training, discussion and debate.

Moving forward

The dictionary defines ethics as 'moral principles or codes', and ethical as 'conforming to a recognised standard'. But medical ethics involves more than these definitions might suggest, encompassing the way a doctor lives his or her life and practises the art of medicine. It used to be assumed that, if one was taught by 'good' doctors, one would become a good doctor oneself – ethics would be acquired almost by a process of osmosis. Of course, this ignored the fact that there might be considerable variability in how good the teacher actually was at imparting the skills, qualities and precepts that enable a doctor to engage with medical ethics. In the past, medical ethics teaching might have

"With purity and holiness I will live my life and practise my art. Into whatever houses I go, I will enter them for the benefit of the sick, and will abstain from every voluntary act of mischief and corruption. Whatsoever I see or hear in the life of men which ought not to be spoken of abroad, I will not divulge, as reckoning that all such should be kept secret"

Hippocratic Oath 460–377 BC

amounted to a 1-hour lecture over 5 years of teaching. There was no structure, little coordination and very little relevance to everyday practice.

Medical ethics teaching in UK medical schools has been in a state of flux since the Pond Report in 1987. The recommendations of the General Medical Council on undergraduate medical education (GMC 1993) provided additional impetus for an increase in the teaching of medical ethics as part of the core curriculum to be implemented in every UK medical school. A survey in the *Journal of Medical Ethics* (Fulford, Yates & Hope 1997) reported that although the majority of schools in the UK were able to provide ethics teaching in one form or other, there was a wide variation in the quality and quantity available across the country. The report identified a number of key problems including a lack of teachers, teaching materials and library resources.

In 1998, the *Journal of Medical Ethics* and the *British Medical Journal* published a consensus statement, agreed by a number of British teachers of medical ethics. This provided a minimal 'core curriculum' in ethics and law which it was hoped medical schools would be prepared to incorporate in their undergraduate curricula (Gillon & Doyle 1998).

Organising medical ethics teaching – a case study

At an undergraduate level, ethics has often been taught in a variety of places in the curriculum by a wide range of teachers. This variety, though good in its way, has sometimes lacked coordination and lost educational impact as a result. The following describes the development of medical ethics in one medical school, where coordination and collaboration were critical factors in achieving a successful contribution to the curriculum.

The Bristol approach
At Bristol medical school the development of ethics teaching was given considerable impetus by the establishment in 1997 of a Centre for Ethics in Medicine.

Teaching ethics in small groups:

- use cases and vignettes.
- create a safe environment.
- use students' names.
- set out ground rules.
- encourage discussion.
- allow experiences to be shared.
- aim to develop:
  — tolerance
  — the ability to cope with ambiguity
  — the ability to appreciate different views.

Teaching ethics to large groups:

- Keep the session interactive.
- Use video clips and other media.
- Set up an ethics debate.
- Divide the students into 'buzz' groups.
- Team-teach with others.
- Vary the style and pace.

"As part of its full integration into the curriculum, teaching in ethics and law should feature in the students' clinical experience, consistently forging links with good medical and surgical practice. Each clinical discipline should address ethical and legal issues of particular relevance to it and its students should be subject to assessment as they would be for any other teaching in that specialty. Students should be encouraged to present problems which they have personally encountered in their course"

Consensus statement on the teaching of medical ethics 1998

Key points of the Bristol approach:

- student-centred teaching
- patient-centred ethics
- structured and incremental
- case-based
- grounded in theory but applied to clinical practice
- inclusive and humanistic approach
- team-teaching wherever appropriate
- interactive and non-didactic
- opportunity for discussion within a safe environment
- positive critique employed throughout.

This led to the introduction of a structured and incremental approach to the teaching of ethics in Bristol. Medical ethics became a vertical theme running all the way through the curriculum, which required considerable collaboration with preclinical and clinical colleagues. A core group of ethics teachers was formed (several of whom were from outside the university), whose role in contributing to the overall curriculum came to be described as either sole, joint or advisory. This group comprised specialists in medical ethics as well as clinical and preclinical teachers who had a long-established interest in the subject.

A nodal expansion of ethics throughout the curriculum was planned, which would allow the students to develop their understanding of ethics as their scientific and clinical grasp of medicine increased. Three major teaching nodes were built into the 5 years of the curriculum, with additional teaching taking place in clinical and specialist attachments. The teaching comprises core teaching, special study modules and an optional intercalated BSc in bioethics.

The ethics teaching in Bristol starts in the first week of the first year of the medical course. A session on the doctor–patient relationship is followed by a session jointly taught with anatomy teachers and the university chaplain. This takes place before the students enter the dissection room to begin their study of anatomy, and aims to provide a gentle introduction to what can be a somewhat traumatic experience for some. Both of these early sessions rely on accessing the students' views, opinions, fears and aspirations at the point of entry to the medical profession. An exercise is conducted in which the new students devise a list of core ethical values with which they identify as doctors-to-be.

In the second term of year one, the students undergo several afternoon sessions of ethics teaching spread over consecutive weeks. This core teaching forms part of the human basis of medicine unit. Considerable reference is made to their visits to general practice in their first term as medical students. Topics covered include:

- the patient's values
- the patient's narrative
- going into hospital
- professional obligations
- the individual and society
- justice and health care.

The afternoons take the form of a plenary presentation followed by small group tutorials. Tutors are drawn from a range of disciplines and include nurses, hospital doctors and general practitioners. Assessment is by the submission of an essay at the end of the course, and an integrated examination paper at the end of the first year.

In year three, an ethics symposium is held when the students return from their first clinical attachment in secondary care. This day comprises small group tutorials and large group discussion of the ethical issues encountered by the students in hospitals, followed by plenary sessions on a range of ethical dilemmas.

Joint teaching also takes place in a number of clinical attachments, including obstetrics and gynecology, where the use of ethical cases and dilemmas is tailored to the relevant clinical situation.

In year five, further ethics teaching is provided enabling the students to enter the pre-registration year with a renewed sense of confidence. This teaching will focus on the demands and realities of the house year, and provide further opportunity for the students to discuss their fears, concerns and experiences within a safe setting.

The development of appropriate attitudes is implicit in the teaching of medical ethics. Some of this occurs during small group teaching. However, attitudes are developed in a number of ways, and the example set by doctors, health professionals and senior medical students is an especially powerful form of teaching.

The most commonly used visual aid in clinical teaching is the patient. Frequently patients are used as the subject of a clinical teaching session without being asked for their consent, without them being involved in

How Bristol was able to develop ethics teaching:

- a clearly visible senior academic leader
- dedicated academic and support staff
- a physical focus for ethics teaching in the form of the new centre
- policy documents which strongly emphasised the requirement for medical ethics teaching
- synchronicity of a major process of medical curriculum change across the UK
- a remit to coordinate and improve ethics teaching across the curriculum
- the enthusiasm of fellow teachers and students to embrace the teaching of medical ethics.

the discussion or being referred to at all except in an off-hand way. This is obviously unacceptable, and the GMC have made it clear in *Duties of a Doctor* (GMC 1998), that doctors must:

- make the care of the patient their first concern
- treat every patient politely and considerately
- respect patients' dignity and privacy
- listen to patients and respect their views (Consensus Statement Journal of Medical Ethics 1998).

Walking the talk

Many medical students and doctors will be aware of teaching situations – primarily in hospitals – where these rules have not been observed and where they have often felt acutely embarrassed to be present. Medical teachers have a duty to act as appropriate role models to junior colleagues in medicine and to other health professionals.

Just as bullying of students and juniors is still part of medical education, so the humiliation of patients is present too – and it is up to all of us to change it! Nowhere is it more important that doctors display appropriate attitudes and ethical behaviour than in clinical teaching. This might be called 'walking the talk'.

Giving praise and developing collegiality

Medical teachers need to remember always that people respond much better to praise and constructive criticism than to criticism that is merely negative and destructive. Some medical teachers – principally in hospital and academic medicine – seem to believe that humiliation and constant negative criticism are acceptable and even successful teaching approaches. This is not so, and a change in this aspect of medical culture is needed. Positive critique in which the emphasis is on what has gone well and what can be improved can have significant effects on the learner's self-esteem and confidence.

The development of collegiality in medical education – treating student doctors with the respect, kindness and consideration with which one would treat any other professional colleague – is vital. One occasionally comes across doctors whose bedside persona is exemplary, yet whose behaviour – once offstage, as it were – towards their colleagues, juniors and students is, frankly, appalling. Ethics teaching should include this aspect of professionalism in its remit.

Sources of reference

Teaching materials for medical ethics abound. Perhaps the first resource of which to make use is the experience of fellow medical teachers, students and patients. Students rate very highly ethics teaching which is directly applied to clinical situations. Discussions and video clips can help to draw out these experiences, and videos are freely available which can assist this process. New books on medical ethics are published regularly. The *Journal of Medical Ethics* and *Bioethics* are perhaps the best-known journals, containing topical articles and academic papers. The main medical journals invariably contain papers or correspondence on ethical issues.

In the UK, the General Medical Council publish a number of pamphlets that are made freely available to doctors and medical students. Among these is the set of pamphlets, *Duties of a Doctor*, which includes 'Good medical practice'. Medical regulatory bodies in other countries will usually have their own set of guidelines for incorporation into the ethics curriculum where appropriate. The *Oxford Practice Skills Course Manual* (Hope, Fulford & Yates 1996) is a good source of materials for ethics teaching, containing as it does cases, vignettes and handouts. The Medical Defence Union (MDU) has provided each medical school in the UK with a teaching pack, *The MDU Introduction to Medical Ethics*, which contains materials and student handouts on consent and confidentiality. International and postgraduate versions of this pack are in preparation. As with the other defence organisations, the MDU also provides members with publications containing advice on ethical practice.

An obvious (but sometimes under-used) resource is the non-medical media, the output of which can help immeasurably to keep teachers and students informed about medical ethics in practice. TV and radio, newspapers and magazines often present medical stories from the patients' or public's perspective; medical students and doctors need to appreciate this perspective. Every day there is a news report or media discussion of an ethical dilemma in medicine and health care. This coverage – wherever it is found – often provides the perfect material for discussion of ethical issues.

Summary

A good understanding of medical ethics is central to the practice of good medicine. The study of ethics can act as the cement that binds the medical curriculum together, allowing the integration of preclinical and clinical teaching. Ethics teaching is able to benefit from the synthesis of many approaches from the arts, humanities and law, science, technology and medicine.

All medical teachers have the responsibility to develop knowledge, skills and attitudes in 'tomorrow's doctors'. We who teach medical ethics have the additional responsibility to help them develop their humanity. There can be no better reward or stronger incentive for a medical teacher.

Acknowledgements

I should like to thank all those who have taught me about ethics, especially my family; Professors Alastair Campbell, Ranaan Gillon and Ian Kennedy; Dr Richard Ashcroft and all my colleagues at the Centre for Ethics in Medicine at Bristol University. Most of all, I thank the students, doctors, health professionals and others with whom I have been privileged to work over the years. To all of you, I owe a great debt and express my deep appreciation.

Sources of information

Centre for Ethics in Medicine, University of Bristol, 73 St Michael's Hill, Bristol
  BS2 8HW, UK
Tel: 0117 928 9843

"Patients must be able to trust doctors with their lives and wellbeing. To justify that trust, we as a profession have a duty to maintain a good standard of practice and care and to show respect for human life"

General Medical Council 1998

General Medical Council, 178 Great Portland Street, London W1N 6JE, UK
Tel: 0171 580 7642 Fax: 0171 915 3641

Medical Defence Union, 3 Devonshire Place, London W1N 2EA, UK
Tel: 0171 486 6181 Fax: 0171 935 5503

References and further reading

Brennan M G, Schutte P 1997 The MDU introduction to medical ethics. Medical Defence Union London

Consensus statement on the teaching of medical ethics 1998. Journal of Medical Ethics, June

Fulford K W M, Yates A, Hope T 1997 Ethics and the GMC core curriculum: a survey of resources in UK medical schools. Journal of Medical Ethics 23: 82–87

General Medical Council 1993 Tomorrow's doctors. Recommendations on undergraduate medical education. GMC, London

General Medical Council 1998 Duties of a doctor. GMC, London

Gillon R, Doyle L 1998 Medical ethics and law as a core subject in medical education. British Medical Journal 316:1623–1624

Hope T, Fulford K W M, Yates A 1996 The Oxford practice skills course manual. Oxford University Press, Oxford

Pond D. 1987 Report of a working party on the teaching of medical ethics. Institute of Medical Ethics, London

Chapter 24
Preparing for practice

M. E. T. McMurdo

"Medical education is not completed at medical school: it is only begun"

William H Welch 1850–1934

"I embarked on my career as a doctor brim-full of textbook learning and realised by lunchtime of the first day that I was as useful as a chocolate tea-pot. I knew all the sub-types of glomerulonephritis, but did not know how to organise an urgent CT scan, or how to tell a young wife that her husband had died"

A junior doctor

"I was a keen medical student among the top dozen in my year, but it still took me four or five weeks in post as a junior doctor to learn the ropes. With hindsight, I am sure that my medical school could have done more to have me better prepared"

A junior doctor

Introduction

The student–doctor transition

The purpose of undergraduate medical training is to produce newly qualified doctors who are well prepared for the responsibilities of their first year of practice. Medical curricula have been justifiably criticised in the past for having produced inadequately prepared graduates.

Problems with conventional undergraduate teaching

Too often in the past, medical graduates have stepped on to the wards on their first day as a doctor only to discover themselves ill equipped for the task in hand. This disconcerting experience can be a shattering one for the young doctor, but also means that the quality of clinical care delivered falls short of the high standard to which all physicians aspire. There is a need to ensure that students qualify having demonstrated competence in key skills and arrive armed with sufficient insight and prior experience of life as a junior doctor to function as a productive member of the clinical team from day one. The concept of the 'steep learning curve' for the new graduate is undoubtedly true, but our students (and their patients) will be better served by some progress along that curve prior to qualification.

What areas may be lacking?

Undergraduates must be trained to recognise that, although in their early student years it may take 1 hour to derive a history and examine a patient, this process has to be refined through experience to be rapid, efficient and thorough. It is at the point of graduation that newly qualified doctors must learn to trust their own clinical skills and become adept at distinguishing the sick from the well. Good communication with colleagues, focused evaluations, knowing what elements of assessment can be deferred, and knowing when to seek senior help are all essential to the survival of any junior doctor.

Several areas may require further practice or experience before they are attained:

- Streamlined and efficient history and examination. Most students can take a history and examine a patient, but the art of doing this rapidly under pressure of time and with frequent interruptions is a key skill for junior doctors.
- Requesting investigations and obtaining results. This is one of the main functions of junior doctors and requires good time management, familiarity with the role of other professionals, and a sound grasp of diplomacy.
- Management of common medical and surgical emergencies. All junior doctors should be confident in the management of patients with chest pain, breathlessness, overdose, an acute abdomen and cardiac arrest.
- Competence in core practical skills. By the time they reach their first job students should feel they have had sufficient supervised practice at common procedures such as venepuncture and bladder catheterisation.
- Time management skills and an ability to prioritise tasks. One of the surprises of life as a junior doctor is how frequently your bleep sounds while you are in the middle of one task, which you may then have to leave to deal with a more pressing clinical problem. A clear mind, good note-taking and an ability to rank tasks in order of clinical need are essential. An ability to anticipate problems is the hallmark of a good junior doctor.
- Effective written and oral communication with patients, relatives and colleagues. Good

"it is the embracing of responsibility and accountability that matters the clinician"

Smith 1996

documentation is an essential part of good clinical care and can provide an effective response to clinical complaints. Knowing what to write and what not to write, and meticulously recording discussions with relatives are important skills. The effective exchange of information between all members of the multidisciplinary team is based on an understanding of each others' roles and respect for the contribution of non-doctors to patient care.

Opportunities to rectify these problems

Reorientation of the undergraduate curriculum
Some recent recommendations on changes to the undergraduate curriculum have been made specifically to prepare young doctors better for clinical practice. Opportunities exist in revising medical courses to identify the elements of core clinical knowledge which all graduates should possess, and generic skills in which graduates should be proficient. Good problem-solving and clinical reasoning skills are the foundation for learning effectively. An emphasis on teaching students how to acquire and evaluate information, and on self-directed learning will also prepare graduates for life-long learning.

Job shadowing
As an integral part of their training medical students should spend some time shadowing a junior doctor. Ideally this experience should be in the hospital in which they will undertake their first post after qualifying. This offers considerable potential benefits:

- familiarisation with the day-to-day working of the unit
- familiarisation with laboratory services and request systems
- meeting future nursing, medical and paramedical colleagues
- spending time shadowing the individual whose job they will be doing
- the senior staff having a vested interest in ensuring that the students:

— have a positive experience
— demonstrate appropriate clinical judgement
— participate in the work of the unit
— identify and rectify any deficiencies in skills or behaviour.

Job shadowing should involve defined responsibilities for both daytime and night-time duties, acute receiving, clerking, ward rounds, scrubbing up and assisting in theatre, as well as gaining an insight into the role of other members of the multidisciplinary team.

In conjunction with the unit consultant, students should draw up and agree a timetable for each week which should include targeting known areas of weakness. Progress towards these targets should be reviewed midway through the attachment and activities redirected as necessary. Performance during job shadowing attachments may usefully be assessed jointly by both senior nursing and medical staff. Nursing staff often have considerably more day-to-day contact than consultants with both students and junior doctors, making their perspective invaluable. Part of the assessment process should include review of a logbook of cases, procedures witnessed or performed, and other experiences. These should be countersigned by the member of staff who supervised it.

Induction days and handovers

Formal induction days are recommended for all junior doctors when arriving for their first medical post. Induction 'fairs' have been used successfully in some hospitals when information on key aspects of the young doctor's work can be presented to the entire cohort of new doctors.

Programmes should include:

- opportunities for discussion with key medical and nursing staff
- consultant and junior doctor views of the role of the new doctor
- teamworking with nursing staff
- time for a formal handover with the outgoing doctor
- duties of the doctor

- management of the dying patient
- pain relief
- cardiac arrest code and team
- medico-legal issues of consent, certification, reports to coroner
- dealing with complaints.

This introductory day should ensure the rapid integration of the new doctor into the working environment. It is, however, simply the beginning of what should be an ongoing process of education and information provided for junior doctors during their first year in practice.

Handbooks

For reference purposes, junior doctor handbooks can be very helpful. They should contain key information including topics such as:

- a list of useful contact phone numbers for laboratories, local doctors, accident and emergency
- practical procedures for arranging investigations within and outside normal working hours
- arrangements for resuscitation training
- the educational programme for the hospital
- local guidelines on the management of common presentations
- local drug formularies
- domestic arrangements such as accommodation, catering, security
- how to request annual and study leave
- on-call rotas.

Preparation courses

An alternative approach is to dedicate a portion of the final year of the undergraduate course to preparation for practice. Logically this should be timetabled near the end of final year when the impending realities of life as a junior doctor serve to concentrate the mind wonderfully. Such a course should not be seen as a 'stand-alone' item, but rather as an opportunity to polish those clinical and practical skills acquired throughout the curriculum which are necessary to function as a junior doctor. This

"The education of the doctor which goes on after he has his degree is, after all, the most important part of his education"

John Shaw Billings 1838–1913

Try to include only essential information in the junior doctor handbook. The longer you make it, the less likely it is to be read. Keep it short.

provides an opening for interactive sessions derived from the students' own experiences on:

- medical ethics – informed consent and refusal of treatment, confidentiality, death pronouncement and certification, dying and palliation, transplantation
- teamworking and relationships with other colleagues
- defusing complaints
- personal skills – time management and dealing with stress.

Presentations by junior doctors in post are greatly valued, and there is no doubt that this front-line troop perspective is appreciated by students. Likely topics include:

- prioritising
- when to ask for senior help
- relationships with nursing staff
- incident and accident forms
- arranging admissions
- discharge arrangements
- the function of the junior doctor on the ward round
- what to write (and what not to write) in case notes
- night-time rounds
- on-call rotas.

There is scope at this point for students to discover the role of their professional bodies in their future lives: for example, the medical defence unions, medical associations, and registration authorities such as the General Medical Council.

Most students will also appreciate a brief overview from personnel services on:

- contracts
- hours of work
- pay and conditions
- annual leave entitlement
- grievance procedures
- counselling services.

Students may be helped to organise their knowledge in preparation for practice by working through examples of common 'nurse calls'. None of the material should be

"It was only when the coroner telephoned me two hours before the cremation that I realised I should have reported that the patient's death was the result of a road traffic accident"

A junior doctor

Junior doctor preparation should give priority to life-threatening mistakes and avoidance of illegalities.

When considering the content of a preparation course, ask your own junior doctors what they wish they had known and what additional skills they wish they had possessed when they started.

"I vividly remember starting work as a junior doctor being asked to prescribe a laxative. I thought, hold on, I know four different types of dopamine receptor, but for the life of me, I couldn't come up with the name of a laxative. The staff nurse eventually told me what to write up"

A junior doctor

new; for example, all students will have covered the subject of 'pyrexia' during their course. Consideration of this material in the context of a clinical scenario with which they are certain to be faced in practice – 'Doctor, your patient has a temperature' – requires a subtle but crucially important change in thinking.

A session on practical therapeutics may be appropriate, and should certainly cover prescribing for common conditions and the use of analgesics, laxatives and hypnotics. It should include:

- the need for clear and unambiguous prescribing
- the use of generic names
- nurse prescribing
- warfarin/insulin/steroid/fluid charts
- prescription review and discharge prescriptions
- the legal implications of failure to comply with good prescribing.

Part of the time of a junior doctor is spent undertaking practical procedures. Medical students should qualify with confidence in their ability to complete these tasks. Ideally competence should be demonstrated in a group of core practical procedures prior to graduation. This may involve devising a practical procedures checklist carried by the students through their clinical years, specifying which tasks are required, how frequently each should be performed and what level of competence is required. The signature of a clinician is necessary to confirm that the task has been performed to the expected standard. Examples of such practical procedures include:

- venepuncture
- giving an intravenous injection
- peripheral cannulation
- running through a drip
- setting up a syringe driver
- arterial blood sampling
- suturing
- recording an ECG
- basic cardiopulmonary resuscitation
- bladder catheterisation (male and female).

For students who have failed to achieve these target skills or for others who simply wish to improve their technique, simulations involving models and manikins are now widely available. The ideal environment in which to practise and master such basics without the distraction of a patient is the clinical skills centre (see Chapter 8).

Continuing professional development

During the first year of medical practice new doctors will gain respect and learn from the knowledge and skills of their senior colleagues. Wise new doctors will be acutely aware that they do not 'know it all', and nor are they expected to. They will know when to ask for senior advice. The rapid rate of expansion of medical knowledge means that a commitment to continuing professional development is vital. Ample opportunity for attendance at block release training courses and educational meetings should be an integral part of each junior doctor's post. In addition, the emerging role of senior colleagues who act as educational supervisors and mentors for junior doctors is welcomed.

Summary

There has been much debate in recent years about appropriate curricula for undergraduate medical education with a specific concern being that the essential skills required by the graduate at the beginning of the junior doctor year are lacking. A variety of programmes and resources may be used to ensure that medical graduates 'hit the ground running'. Probably the most effective of these is job shadowing, undertaken ideally in the hospital in which the student will work during his or her first post after qualification. This usually works well as senior medical and nursing staff also profit from ensuring that the student develops appropriate skills and attitudes during the attachment.

Induction days and handovers are recommended for all junior doctors arriving for their first medical post. This should include time for a handover with the outgoing doctor, and ensure the rapid integration of the new doctor into the working environment.

Handbooks can be helpful reference guides, but should be kept concise. A dedicated preparation course is the alternative. It should incorporate interactive sessions on medico-legal topics and interpersonal skills, and should provide opportunities to practise key practical procedures. Where possible junior doctors should be involved in delivering the course as their front-line perspective is highly regarded by medical students. The course should not be seen as a 'stand-alone' item, but rather as the opportunity to hone the clinical and practical skills acquired throughout the entire curriculum. The first year in practice is a challenging period of rapid learning and professional growth but a variety of educational opportunities are available to ease the transition between medical student and junior doctor, and to ensure that medical graduates are better prepared for life in practice.

References and further reading

Consensus Group of Teachers of Medical Ethics and Law in UK Medical Schools 1998 Teaching medical ethics and law within medical education: a model for the UK core curriculum. Journal of Medical Ethics 24:188–192

English W A, Nguyen-Van-Tam J S, Pearson J C G, Madeley R J 1995 Deficiencies in undergraduate and pre-registration medical training in prescribing for pain control. Medical Teacher 17:215–218

Frain J P, Frain A E, Carr P H 1996 Experience of medical senior house officers in preparing discharge summaries. British Medical Journal 312:350–351

General Medical Council 1993 Tomorrow's doctors. GMC, London

General Medical Council 1997 The new doctor. GMC, London

Smith L G 1996 First year of practice: a year of rapid learning. Academic Medicine 71:580–581

Chapter 25
Informatics

F. Sullivan

Introduction

In the midst of the information revolution it may seem obvious that undergraduate education should be more firmly supported by informatics skills and evidence-based practice. Our students certainly believe so and the challenge for us as teachers is to meet and exceed their expectations. Encouraging students to identify and use information from a larger range of resources than their lecture notes and single textbooks demands more effort on their part to integrate information and it is more likely to result in deep learning.

It is apparent that the physician of the near future will be faced with patients who have already acquired, processed and used medical evidence from a variety of sources such as television screen Internet providers (see Fig. 25.1). Such patients will expect their physicians to be aware of everything that they know, and to be able to add further insights based on their own understanding of the issue from much more diverse sources. Patients may also begin to demand more computer use from their physicians as they realise that supported decisions are often better decisions (Coiera 1998).

Of course, informatics and evidence-based practice are not new concepts; an ability to interpret data, apply logic and manage uncertainty was taught by Hippocrates. However, the implications of the digital age are so profound that they have become important themes, which ought to run throughout the undergraduate curriculum. The conference of heads of medical schools in the UK recently published a report identifying four areas of informatics derived from 'Duties of a doctor',

"Informatics is the study of the acquisition, processing and use of knowledge"

Friedman & Wyatt 1997

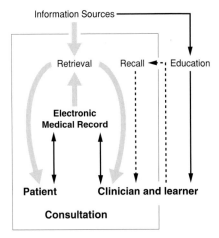

Fig. 25.1   Learning in an information age consultation

"It is astonishing with how little knowledge a doctor can practice medicine, but it is not astonishing how badly he may do it"

W. Osler, Aequanamitas, in Bryan 1906

'Tomorrow's Doctors' and 'New Doctor' (CHMS Joint Working Group 1998) These are:

- record-keeping
- ethical and legal imperatives
- professional communication
- education and research.

Various outcome attainments can be categorised in these areas.

Four areas of informatics

Record-keeping

The duty to keep accurate and contemporaneous patient records may be emphasised by clinical skills courses. Taking a careful history and expertly eliciting physical signs may be negated by a poor record of the encounter.

The use of simulated patients presenting the same challenges to several students allows learners to perform comparisons with their colleagues. Tutors who ask to see the written records which students keep about *every* patient seen will encourage good record-keeping. Paper or electronic formats to emphasise the structure of a patient record may be helpful, especially in the early phases of the clinical apprenticeship.

Ethical and legal imperatives

Briefing and debriefing of students may be used to direct attention to issues of security, confidentiality and the legal implications of what is recorded and stored about patients. Universities with a traditional forensic medicine 'course' need to supplement this with a 'right thing to do' theme as implemented in Glasgow; this runs throughout the curriculum and involves ethicists, moral philosophers, lawyers and medical defence union staff. Specialist contributors may be used to teach directly and to prepare teachers for the issues which arise in almost every encounter.

Professional communication

Keeping colleagues and others informed about issues which are relevant to patient care needs to be

"The medical record is the link to accountability to the outside world"

Conference of Heads of Medical Schools 1998

addressed in several ways. Writing referral letters and discharge summaries is one method often used. Role play, with medical undergraduates adopting the role of other professionals, may be useful in prompting a deeper understanding from an alternative perspective. In other situations shared learning may be appropriate, e.g. learning resuscitation with nurses (see Chapter 16). Comparisons between medical and nursing records on ward rounds or in practice may be useful, as may attendance at multiprofessional case conferences. Asking students to record what they told the patients emphasises the importance of this skill.

Education and research

In Oxford, David Sackett integrates education and research by asking learners on ward rounds to summarise 20 things about the patient in less than 2 minutes, including something they don't know about the patient but need to know. This forms the basis for critical appraisal of the relevant evidence, which can be stored as a critically appraised topic (CAT). Software to facilitate this process may be found at http://cebm.jr2.ox.ac.uk. Encounters with individual patients and communities could be used to build on this method more widely.

The 'virtual clinical campus': an ideal scenario

In an ideal situation undergraduate students would be provided with educational challenges in the optimal sequence and at the most appropriate rate for their learning needs (Friedman 1996). They would have easy access to patients, patient data, laboratories, libraries and teachers wherever they were. Their assessment processes would emphasise the importance of applying the best evidence to meet the needs of their future patients. This is technologically feasible and increasingly likely due to economic pressures, maturing technology and better infrastructure within the community. One of the key issues for educators will be to ensure that our students are able to appraise what they find critically (Jadad & Gagliardi 1998).

Why does complete curricular integration of this theme not occur universally already? Several studies have identified financial, practical and educational issues which impede progress, but there are reports of innovative teaching methods which teachers can use to overcome the barriers.

Practical methods of overcoming the barriers

Staff development

Although few medical teachers have had the benefit of IT training, most of us use a wide range of information sources in our scientific and/or clinical activities. This provides us with a sound basis for effective teaching in the four areas of informatics. However, some teachers have a narrower range of skills than others and their students might wish. The inevitable expansion in electronic educational resources means that we will all have to enhance our existing knowledge and skills in order to benefit our students. Responsibility for upgrading our capabilities should not only rest with individual teachers and occasional journal articles. Until the technology becomes easier to use, staff development needs to be provided by the medical school or university centrally.

Basic skills for students

Undergraduates describe themselves as nerds, norms and phobes. Nerds, self-evidently, need no training at all and may be useful resources for other students (and teachers). Norms need only an introduction to the facilities available. They may need some encouragement and support. Phobes may never have touched a computer and may not wish to do so. Gentle but firm reassurance that they will be able to cope may be required as well as extensive introductions to the facilities. Some medical schools have gone further by insisting that all new students buy a computer and a few such as Cambridge have supplied the students with a palmtop PC (Oswald & Alderson 1998).

Develop the teachers.

Provide basic skills (and equipment) for those students who require it.

Vertical integration

Skilled teachers who wish to facilitate deep learning will direct students to a wide variety of computer-assisted learning resources based on compact disc, digital video disc and Internet technologies. Many schools link these resources throughout the campus and some such as Stanford, California, link the learning resources for undergraduates and postgraduates via a simple search of high-quality, integrated knowledge resources and paper versions following electronic information. The University of Sydney has structured its graduate programme around Web-based multimedia. Internet-supplemented ward rounds, outpatient clinics and general practitioner surgeries could enhance the experience of the early years in medical school. Problem-based learning, (PBL) is a method of learning which is particularly suited to informatics integration within curricula. Students in PBL curricula will expect to go beyond the material presented by patients and teachers to retrieve more information and bring it into subsequent teaching sessions. Some useful websites for teaching have been identified and can be found in the Appendix.

Good use of new resources

New forms of IT are constantly being introduced into professional practice world-wide. In the UK, the NHS Information Management and Technology strategy states that *'information should be person based; systems should be integrated; management information should be derived from operational clinical systems; data should be secure and confidential; and data should be shared across the NHS'* (Leaning 1993). This policy can only serve to enhance educational opportunities. Rapid access to electronic laboratory data as well as in-patient, ambulatory and community records is becoming possible. Subject to the security concerns being addressed it is likely that the technology employed by current, innovative sites which permit this in health maintenance organisations (HMOs) in the USA will become generally available.

Ensure vertical integration of informatics as a theme.

"On the internet no-one need know you're a dog"
Cartoon in New Yorker 1997

"In 2021 computers will collect histories . . . together with the results of physical examination and special investigations. They will suggest diagnoses and therapy, taking into account previous experience and existing state of the art"

McManus 1991

Make good use of resources – existing+new.

Assess Informatics skills e.g. by emphasising project work.

Assessment in informatics

Any curriculum theme which is not examined will remain undervalued by a majority of students. A wide variety of assignments could be sent via e-mail to tutors or discussed more widely by all students in electronic discussion groups. Objective structured clinical examination (OSCE) stations could require students to review a patient record and decide whether a particular drug may be used safely. The Medical Independent Learning Examination (MILE) and the triple jump are methods of presenting students with a challenge which requires an initial review of a patient problem to be followed by critical appraisal of the literature and a second phase of examination based on the increased knowledge derived from the search (Smith 1993).

Essential skills

Ten essential clinical informatics skills have been identified by the University of Sydney Medical School:

- understand the dynamic and uncertain nature of medical knowledge and be able to keep personal knowledge and skills up to date
- know how to search for and assess knowledge according to the statistical basis of scientific evidence
- understand some of the logical and statistical models of the diagnostic process
- interpret uncertain clinical data and deal with artefact and error
- structure and analyse clinical decisions in terms of risks and benefits
- apply and adapt clinical knowledge to the individual circumstances of the patients
- access, assess, select and apply a treatment guideline, adapt it to local circumstances, and communicate and record variations in treatment plan and outcome
- structure and record clinical data in a form appropriate for the immediate clinical task, for communication with colleagues, or for epidemiological purposes

- select and operate the most appropriate communication method for a given task (e.g., face-to-face conversation, telephone, e-mail, video, voice-mail, letter)
- structure and communicate messages in a manner most suited to the recipient, task and chosen communication medium.

One method of assessing students' informatics skills is to require them to conduct project work such as an audit (see Fig. 25.2) (Morrison & Sullivan 1997). This has the added advantage of encouraging students to work at the higher levels of Bloom's cognitive taxonomy to integrate information from multiple sources (Bloom, Hastings & Madaus 1971). One example involves students on a 4-week general practice attachment being briefed about an evidence-based audit project and supported in the different phases of the project by departmental staff and tutors trained in evidence-based practice skills. The topic to be studied may be chosen on the basis of a critical incident during the early days of an attachment, a personal interest or a practice concern. Students need evidence based resources to decide which criteria should be studied in that topic, what level of performance denotes high-quality care, and what changes need to occur. The type of evidence used in projects by final year undergraduate students may include published studies, guidelines, policy statements and local protocols. This approach integrates many of the above practical methods of ensuring that informatics skills are employed to encourage evidence-based practice. Moreover, students and teachers seem to enjoy it.

Summary

Medical teachers need to obtain and transmit informatics skills and rely upon evidence to a greater extent than ever before. As the technology to sustain this change becomes more widespread, the task will become more straightforward. We should embrace the opportunities to integrate informatics and evidence-based practice

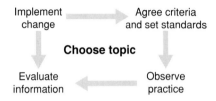

Fig. 25.2   **The audit cycle**

Implement change → Agree criteria and set standards

Choose topic

Evaluate information ← Observe practice

"A worthwhile exercise in information gathering and communication with the primary health-care team"
"It is very satisfying to be involved in something that the GP's could make use of"

Students commenting on an evidence-based audit project

throughout the curriculum to improve the quality of teaching and make it even more enjoyable.

References and further reading

Bryan C S 1906 Osler: inspirations from a great physician. Oxford University Press, Oxford

Bloom B S, Hastings J T, Madaus G F 1971 Condensed version of the taxonomy of educational objectives. In: Appendix. Handbook on formative and summative evaluation of student learning. McGraw-Hill, London

Coiera E 1998 Medical informatics meets medical education. Medical Journal of Australia 168:319–320

Conference of Heads of Medical Schools Joint Working Group 1998 Informatics in medical and dental undergraduate curricula. National Health Service Executive, London

Friedman C P 1996 The virtual clinical campus. Academic Medicine. 71(6):647–651

Friedman C P, Wyatt J C 1997 Evaluation methods in medical informatics. Springer, New York

Jadad A R, Gagliardi A 1998 Rating health information on the Internet: navigating to knowledge or to Babel? Journal of the American Medical Association Feb 25 279(8):611–614

Leaning M S 1993 The new information management and technology strategy of the NHS. British Medical Journal 307:217

McManus I 1991 How will medical education change? Lancet 337:1519–1521

Morrison J M, Sullivan F M 1997 Audit in general practice: educating medical students. Medical Education 31:128–131

Oswald N, Alderson T 1998 Basic medical education in primary care. The report and evaluation of the Cambridge community based clinical course 1993–8. GP Education Group, School of Medicine, University of Cambridge

Smith R M 1993 The triple jump examination as an assessment tool in the problem-based medical curriculum at Hawaii University. Academic Medicine 68:366–372

Chapter 26
Evidence-based medicine

S. Rennie

Introduction

Doctors are constantly faced with a rapidly changing body of relevant medical evidence and are expected to use this to maximum advantage in the delivery of quality patient care. To keep abreast of these advances in scientific information and technology doctors need to acquire new knowledge and learn new skills. Undergraduate medical education, therefore, should prepare students for life-long learning rather than simply enable them to master current information and techniques. Evidence-based medicine is an approach to clinical decision-making or problem-solving that involves applying external sources of information.

The aim for the future of medicine is that patient care should be evidence-based. Practising evidence-based medicine requires skills such as efficient and effective literature searching, critical appraisal and the application of these findings to the clinical problem. Shin, Haynes & Johnston (1993) showed that knowledge of appropriate clinical practice in graduates from traditional medical schools progressively declines. In contrast graduates from medical schools teaching life-long, self-directed, evidence-based medicine were found to be up to date as long as 15 years after graduation.

Teaching basic skills of evidence-based medicine

Five basic skills of evidence-based medicine have been identified:

- generating clinical questions

"Evidence-based medicine is the conscientious, explicit and judicious use of the best current evidence in making decisions about the care of individual patients"

Sackett et al 1996

"The dream of medicine for the new millennium is that the care of patients will be evidence based, supported by carefully designed randomised controlled trials and validated by focused outcome studies"

Felch 1997

- finding the evidence to answer the questions
- critically appraising the evidence
- applying the evidence to specific patients
- evaluating one's own performance.

Generating clinical questions

The challenge for the teacher is to formulate questions that are both patient-based and learner-centred. The questions may be grouped into categories such as diagnosis, management, prognosis or prevention. It is important to encourage students to formulate focused clinical questions that are directly relevant to the patient's problem. A well-constructed clinical question helps to direct the search for evidence and for precise answers.

A good clinical question has been defined by Sackett (Sackett et al 1999) as having four elements:

- the patient or problem
- the intervention (cause, prognostic factor, treatment)
- comparison intervention (if necessary)
- outcomes.

For example: 'In patients with acute otitis media does antibiotic therapy lead to faster resolution of symptoms compared with no intervention?'

It is important for the teacher to look for potential questions in the types of case that their students are exposed to and to select the best question to focus on. They should guide the student to construct the question well and assess their ability to design effective clinical questions.

Finding the evidence to answer the questions

Students must be aware of the hierarchy of evidence that forms an important principle in evidence-based medicine. In descending order, starting from the gold standard source, these are:

- carefully designed, randomised, controlled trials
- systematic reviews of studies
- large case series
- expert opinion
- personal experience.

"Good questions are the backbone of both practising and teaching EBM, and patients serve as the starting point for both"

Sackett et al 1997

Advances in technology have resulted in the development of databases such as Medline and the Cochrane Library. Students should be aware of the sources of information that are available and be taught how to use the questions they have developed to direct their literature search. They must have access to databases and be instructed in how they are organised, what search terms to use and how to operate the search software. Medical informatics teaching should begin early in the undergraduate curriculum as it is essential to ensure that students can perform computerised literature searches and to expose students to the strengths and limitations of other existing information sources, such as textbooks, personal experience and expert opinion.

Critically appraising the evidence

Once the best evidence has been found, the next step is to encourage students to appraise it critically for its validity and usefulness. Students need a fundamental knowledge of research methodology as a basis for critical appraisal of the literature. Guidelines to appraise critically and apply evidence are available, and teaching critical appraisal involves instructing students to ask key questions about the strength of the evidence. Software to help construct critical appraisals is available; the 'CAT-maker' can be found at the website of the Centre for Evidence-based Medicine (see Appendix). Once the students are comfortable with the principles of critical appraisal they should be encouraged to present the important points in the articles and their strength and weaknesses to their colleagues.

Applying the evidence to specific patients

The next step is to apply the answers that have been found from the critical appraisal of literature to the patient's problem. Students must be reminded that evidence-based medicine also involves applying the traditional skills of medical training. A good understanding of pathophysiology is essential in interpreting and applying the results of clinical research

"While present medical trainees may be gaining some familiarity with the basic uses of literature-searching programs such as Medline, we suspect that many trainees still lack the higher level skills required to develop efficient search strategies tailored to specific types of clinical questions"

Ghali, Lesky & Hershman 1998

"Medical students carrying out critical appraisals not only learn evidence based medicine for themselves but contribute their appraisals to teams and update their colleagues"

Rosenburg & Donald 1995

to their patient and they must also be sensitive to the emotional needs of the patient.

Evaluating one's own performance

Evaluating one's own performance is the final step in evidence-based practice and is essential in encouraging students to develop life-long learning skills. Students should be encouraged to assess their performance in a non-threatening environment, either in a one-to-one setting with the teacher or in small groups.

Teaching strategies for evidence-based medicine

A good teacher of evidence-based medicine needs general qualities such as good listening skills, enthusiasm and a willingness to help learners develop. No matter what teaching strategies are employed it is important to keep the sessions relevant and meaningful to the students. Adult learning theory stresses the importance of having a specific context in which to acquire new knowledge. It is also essential to keep students active and involved in the process of discovering and appraising the information and in applying it to the patient. Students should be assessed on their achievements in the skills of evidence-based medicine and provided with adequate feedback. A variety of educational strategies can be employed to teach evidence-based medicine, all resting on the fundamental principle of asking 'What's the evidence?'

Role model

All teachers must be effective role models for the practice of evidence-based medicine. In most undergraduate medical curricula there is an implicit apprenticeship learning model in which students observe what the teachers do and then emulate their clinical strategies without scrutinising their true value. Teachers who practise evidence-based medicine are excellent role models for training. An effective role model is one who forms good clinical questions in front of the students,

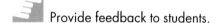 Keep sessions relevant and meaningful to learners.

Provide feedback to students.

identifies and admits knowledge gaps and specifies the strength of evidence that supports the clinical decisions.

Small group sessions

Small group sessions are a good approach to self-directed, problem-based learning which can incorporate the principles of evidence-based medicine. These sessions must keep the students' interest and will benefit from starting with a patient problem using either real or simulated patients. The website of the Centre for Evidence-based Medicine contains examples of clinical scenarios that can be used to teach evidence-based medicine. Students can be encouraged to discuss the case and identify specific learning issues. The students can work in groups or individually to formulate questions, and to find and appraise the evidence. The groups can then apply this evidence to the patient that they have discussed. Repeated cycles of problem-based learning enable students to gain a greater appreciation of their knowledge gaps and improve their ability to ask focused questions to direct their literature searches.

Journal clubs

Journal clubs provide a forum for learning how to appraise articles critically with a focus on study design and methods. Teachers need to recognise that medical students tend to be most interested in clinical material and should select articles that are of clinical interest. The articles should also be reviewed in the context of specific questions arising from real clinical encounters.

Discussion can be built around the clinical case, and two or more articles relating to the problem can be presented. The discussion can be guided by the teacher to encourage students to demonstrate both their knowledge of the hierarchy of research designs and the strengths and weaknesses of each design.

Educational prescriptions

Educational prescriptions were developed by Sackett (Sackett et al 1999) at McMaster University to enable students and teachers to keep track of questions that are formulated in encounters on the wards or in clinics. The

Be open about your own limitations and the things you don't know.

"Evidence based medicine can be practised in any situation when there is doubt about an aspect of clinical diagnosis, prognosis or management"

Rosenburg & Donald 1995

educational prescription specifies the clinical problem that generated the question, states the question and those responsible for answering it and gives a deadline for when the answer should be completed. It also contains a reminder of the steps of evidence-based medicine:

- searching
- critically appraising
- relating the answer back to the patient.

Special forms can be generated for the educational prescription or found at the website of the Centre for Evidence-based Medicine.

Computer-aided learning

Computer-aided learning packages are excellent for providing a grounding in the basics of epidemiology and the principles of research methodology. Evidence-based medicine packages can also be developed that use clinical scenarios to encourage students to generate questions and use critical appraisal software to guide students through their analysis of the literature.

Lectures

Lectures can also provide a setting for teaching the principles of epidemiology and research methods. Interactive lectures provide a strategy for introducing evidence-based medicine. A case can be presented to be analysed by the students. Their thoughts on the diagnosis and treatment are then discussed, and a clinical trial is presented to indicate that this evidence might then influence their initial thoughts.

What is needed to teach evidence-based medicine?

A barrier to the implementation of an evidence-based curriculum is frequently the limited number of faculty available who are capable of teaching and modelling the five steps of evidence-based medicine. The role modelling, practice and teaching of evidence-based medicine require skills that are not traditionally part of medical training, so staff development is an essential requirement for the introduction of a curriculum that integrates evidence-based medicine. It is also important to provide teachers with feedback on their performance as role models and teachers of evidence-based medicine and to provide them with appropriate peer support. Doctors who practise evidence-based medicine should be recruited into these teaching roles.

Another barrier to the teaching and practice of evidence-based medicine is a lack of the necessary infrastructure. The technology to find evidence and to review it must be available and, in an ideal world, it should be available where patients are being treated, on wards and in clinics. Computer equipment and support in these locations is vital.

Summary

Medicine is constantly changing and doctors are expected to keep abreast of new developments. Undergraduate medical education should promote life-long learning and teach students how to apply external sources of information to clinical decision-making. Through an evidence-based curriculum, educators have the opportunity to influence the learning style of students and create a new generation of evidence-based doctors.

The principal steps of evidence-based medicine are to formulate focused clinical questions related to a patient or problem, to perform an efficient literature search, to appraise the evidence critically and to apply it to the patient. A variety of educational strategies can be employed to teach students these key steps such as small groups, and ward and clinic teaching. Fundamental to these strategies is the teacher as an effective role model for evidence-based medicine.

"An immediate attraction of evidence based medicine is that it integrates medical education with clinical practice"

Rosenburg & Donald 1995

References and further reading

Batstone G 1997 Practising by the evidence: the role of pathology. Journal of Clinical Pathology 50:447–448
Bigby M 1998 Evidence-based medicine in a nutshell. A guide to finding and using the best evidence in caring for patients. Archives of Dermatology 134:1609–1618

Chessare J B 1998 Teaching clinical decision-making to pediatric residents in an era of managed care. Pediatrics 101:762–766

Felch W C 1997 Bridging the gap between research and practice. The role of continuing medical education. Journal of the American Medical Association 277:155–156

Ghali W A, Lesky L G, Hershman W Y 1998 The missing curriculum. Academic Medicine 73:734–736

Rosenburg W, Donald A 1995 Evidence based medicine: an approach to clinical problem solving. British Medical Journal 310:1122–1126

Sackett D L, Richardson W S, Rosenburg W, Haynes R B 1999 Evidence-based medicine. How to practise and teach EBM. Churchill Livingstone, Edinburgh

Sackett D L, Rosenburg W M, Gray J A, Haynes R B, Richardson W S 1996 Evidence based medicine: what it is and what it isn't. British Medical Journal 312:71–72

Shin J H, Haynes B, Johnston M E 1993 Effect of problem-based, self-directed undergraduate education on life-long learning. Journal of the Canadian Medical Association 148:969–976

SECTION 6
ASSESSMENT

SECTION 8
ASSESSMENT

Chapter 27
Formative and summative assessment

S. McAleer

Introduction

This chapter describes the different ways in which assessment can be used.

Summative assessment

In the quotation opposite Peter Cook seems to be complaining about the difficulty encountered when faced with summative assessment. This is usually undertaken at the end of a training programme or teaching course and determines whether the instructional objectives have been successfully achieved. With summative assessment the student usually receives a grade or a mark. It indicates what has been learnt.

Good summative assessment should involve the analysis of evidence from as many sources as possible. For example, summative assessment used by the Joint Committee on Postgraduate Training for General Practice (JCPTGP) in the vocational training of general practitioners ensures that doctors have the knowledge, consultation skills and clinical competence for their role. They are assessed in various ways:

- multiple choice questions
- video-taped assessment of consultation skills
- structured report of performance in practice
- trainer's report.

In any form of summative assessment it is important that every aspect of the curriculum which is considered essential, or which had significant teaching time

"Yes, I could have been a judge but I never had the Latin, never had the Latin for the judging, I just never had sufficient of it to get through the rigorous judging exams. They're noted for their rigour. People come staggering out saying, 'My God, what a rigorous exam' – and so I became a miner instead"

Peter Cook, *Beyond the Fringe* (1961 revue)

"The introduction of summative assessment of vocational training for general practice is one of the biggest innovations in medical education in recent years. It introduces a new competence-based approach to assessment in the largest branch of the medical profession"

Pereira Gray et al 1997

designated to it must be assessed to ensure that a valid report on a student's ability results.

The reasons behind summative assessment may include the following:

- a statement of achievement, e.g. obtaining a university degree
- a guide as to the wisdom of continuing with further programmes of study
- an entrance requirement to an educational institution
- a certification of competence
- a determinant of programme effectiveness.

A key issue pertaining to this type of assessment revolves around the feedback given to students. The 'event' assessed has taken place and feedback in many cases will be of a generalised nature. However, with some thoughtful planning the tutor can invariably provide quality information on individual performances. This is an area that is often overlooked because many teachers ignore the opportunity to supply feedback on summative assessment as they feel the benefits are negligible.

Formative assessment

Formative assessment should emanate from a wish to foster learning and understanding. Students should know what is required of them and the learning environment should promote opportunities that permit the application of their knowledge, skills and attitudes. For this reason the tutor–tutee relationship is of paramount importance. All too often what appears to be an effective formative assessment in theory stumbles on the lack of dialogue between teacher and student. Formative assessment must be properly introduced into teaching. It must be built into the coursework in a relevant and non-threatening fashion. It may be appropriate for students to self-assess and then discuss the outcome with the teacher. Laurillard (1993) commented that one of the greatest dissatisfactions with student performance was that students did not appear to understand what was required of them. He stressed, 'the

"Formative assessment is used to monitor students' progress through a course or period of training. It 'involves using assessment information to feed back into the teaching/learning process'"

Gipps, 1994

greatest service teachers can do for themselves and for their students is to take time to clarify assessment requirements, check that they are understood, and if not, take steps to make them understood better. It is not unreasonable to maintain a continuing dialogue about this, so important is it for the success of any teaching method'. The same could equally well be said of summative assessment.

Understanding what is happening and why it is happening are key ingredients for student learning. In relation to formative assessment, there is evidence which demonstrates that considerable benefits to students do take place (Black 1993). Why then is it not a prerequisite for any teaching? One of the main reasons, suggested by Black (1997), is that summative assessments often dominate teaching because of the importance given to the results. Entry to colleges, universities and professions is primarily determined by end-of-course examinations. In contrast formative assessment must be carefully planned and must not be added on as an afterthought. Black argues that it 'has to be built into the scheme, if only because its use to guide pupils' learning according to their different needs can only happen if the teaching plans allow the extensive time for planning and organisation that such use requires'.

The assessment can be used in:

- observing practical work
- gauging clinical abilities
- appraising projects
- evaluating small group discussions.

For formative assessment to act as an effective means of improving competencies students must have a clear idea of what they should be able to achieve. The tutor must have a similar view. Comparisons with a standard can be made and remedial action taken if necessary. The quality of the feedback is critical. There is no point in the tutor telling students that they did well and giving a B⁺. Such information will not help in indicating strengths and weaknesses in performance. Feedback used in summative assessment can, with some time and effort, be used in a formative capacity.

For example, the objective structured clinical examination (OSCE) station checklist below, used as part of a summative assessment, could easily be adopted as part of the training process.

Example: Angina Patient

The patient is a 50-year-old man who has recently moved house and joined your list. This is the first time that you have seen him and his records have not arrived. He has angina. Please take a history with a view to future management.

Symptoms
- Characteristics of pain
- Frequency
- Radiation
- Precipitating factors
- Distance walked on flat ground
- Meals
- Cold
- Stress/Excitement
- Alleviating factors

Background
- Job
- Family history
- Smoking
- Dependent family

Medication
- Current medication
- Past medication
- Response to medication

- Previous investigations
- Serum cholesterol
- ECG stress test
- Angiography
- Ever seen a cardiologist?

Technique
- Correct phrasing of questions
- Answers followed up appropriately
- Systematic approach

Attitude to patient
- Introduces self
- Greets patient warmly
- Attempts to establish rapport
- Considers patient's feelings
- Establishes eye contact

The above checklist could be used to give valuable feedback to students at various stages of their training. Each item could be checked to see if it was:

(a) carried out satisfactorily
(b) carried out unsatisfactorily
(c) not attempted.

It could be a focus for group discussion and lead to decisions over the relative importance of the various items. The allocation of a pass/fail grade need never be an issue. Students could also use the checklist as a method of self-assessment or to assess their peers. In addition the trainer could use the results to assess the quality of the teaching.

The importance of feedback

Feedback informs students about how they are performing in relation to the learning situation. It can come in various forms, e.g. end-of-term grades, a verbal reprimand, a prize for an essay, or an informal discussion between trainer and trainee over a cup of coffee. Feedback should concentrate on both the good aspects of a performance and the not so good. It can come from within the student (intrinsic) or it can emanate from another person, e.g. teacher or trainer. Intrinsic feedback is gained from being aware of the strengths and weaknesses of one's own performance. It involves a degree of insight linked to the skill of effective self-assessment.

Feedback from the teacher should concentrate on improving learning and students should experience a gain in motivation and in information if it is carried out effectively.

Characteristics of effective feedback
To be of value to students feedback should be:

- Timely. Feedback is best given immediately after the response to learning, if possible. However, there are times when it is more appropriate to wait for a period, as the environment that the student is working in may not be conducive to a prompt reaction, e.g. to give feedback in the middle of a patient examination may do nothing for the student's confidence, not to mention the probable embarrassment to both student and patient.
- Specific. It is more beneficial to give specific feedback rather than a more general response. This will ensure

 Effective feedback should be:

- timely
- specific
- accurate
- not embarrassing
- sufficient
- constructive
- relevant.

that the student knows exactly what was appropriate/inappropriate about his/her actions.

- Accurate. Good feedback necessitates accurate appraisal of the student in the learning situation. If you are incorrect in what you are saying the result will be demotivation among the learners and the role of the teacher will be severely undermined.
- Not embarrassing. Try to avoid personalising the feedback. Focus on specific behaviour rather than on the individual responsible. This is particularly important when pointing out weaknesses. Neither should the student feel embarrassed (through effusive praise) or diminished (through scathing criticism).
- Sufficient. Always consider the individual student's needs. There are those who will be confident learners and they will respond to a minimum of feedback. Others may need more frequent and regular input.
- Constructive. Feedback should be constructive and not destructive. Ensure that the student sees it as something positive and beneficial. Strike a balance between what was carried out well and those areas in need of further work.
- Relevant. Provide the student with relevant information on how to improve on performance. Quality feedback revolves around a healthy dialogue between trainer and trainee. If this is fostered it will encourage a situation where feedback is actively sought.

Self-assessment

Self-assessment is a key way of developing in students an appreciation of what 'quality in performance' signifies. It encourages a responsibility for each stage in the learning process and fosters skills in making judgements as to whether work is of an acceptable standard. In essence it improves performance.

For successful self-assessment both teacher and student need to have a commitment to the process. Certain requirements are integral:

- Enhancing learning should be the central motive.

"Arguably, the most important skill medical educators need to cultivate in nascent physicians is the ability to accurately evaluate personal strengths and weaknesses"

Wooliscroft et al 1993

- Students should be directly involved in establishing the criteria.
- Students must understand why they are doing it.
- It should not be imposed.
- Quality feedback is essential.
- It should not be viewed as a replacement for other forms of assessment.
- It should actively engage students in the learning process.
- A good rapport should exist between staff and students.

Self-assessment for the student means monitoring progress and deepening the learning process, for the teacher a recognition of responsibility and a sharing in the control over assessment, and for the medical school a firm commitment to improved teaching.

Self-assessment techniques

Most forms of assessment can be adapted to a self-assessment format. For example, multiple choice questions, modified essay questions, objective structured clinical examinations (OSCEs) and rating scales can all be used by students to gauge their progress. Whatever the technique, the student must be aware of the standards required for a competent performance. Although the student should have responsibility for his/her own assessment, the climate should be such that staff–student dialogue fits easily into the process. Figure 27.1 gives an example of the type of rating scale which could be used.

Peer assessment

With peer assessment students are required to assess not only themselves but also their colleagues. It is important that they are able to fully justify the marks they award. This task can be particularly rewarding, as the reasons for grading can be catalysts for high-quality discussions. In addition, important skills such as the ability to work with others and professional insight are honed.

Rate your ability to do the following:

	Little Ability			High Ability
Establish rapport with patient	1	2	3	4	5
Provide patient education	1	2	3	4	5
Interact with consultants	1	2	3	4	5

Fig. 27.1 Trainee self-assessment rating form

Norm-referenced and criterion-referenced assessment

Norm referencing is where the assessor describes a student's performance in terms of his or her position in the class. Individuals are judged by comparison with the marks of their colleagues. It does not give:

- an accurate representation of what a student can or cannot do
- useful feedback in terms of specific strengths and weaknesses
- an encouragement for group learning; rather it is more likely to promote individual competition.

One example of norm referencing is an examination where the top 25% of students are deemed successful. In this case students are ranked and the top quadrant receives a pass. A second example is where an individual mark is compared to the average mark obtained by the class.

Criterion referencing is used to determine whether a student has achieved mastery in a particular skill or knowledge component. In the majority of cases it is used as a formative assessment as it highlights areas that are causing problems and it is not concerned with who came first or second. In carrying out criterion referencing it is important to establish clear behavioural objectives:

- a clear definition what the student should know or be able to do
- the context in which the learning outcomes should take place
- a standard which indicates an acceptable level of performance.

The assessor sets the level of performance which is required of the student. This can range from complete mastery of a task to the minimal acceptable level. This will be influenced by the subject content and the experience of the individuals being assessed.

The purpose of the assessment should determine whether one uses criterion or norm referenced testing.

"As the principal objective of medical education is to produce a competent physician, then, unquestionably, the raison d'être for the evaluation process is to assess the competency and not the rank order of students. To this end, criterion-referenced testing is necessary and must become the principal method of evaluation within medical education"

Turnball 1989

Standard setting

The setting of a standard will be dependent on the reason why you are assessing in the first place. Standards may be norm-referenced, i.e. the student mark is compared against the rest of the class, or they may be criterion-referenced, i.e. the mark is compared to a specific level. Defining an accepted standard is something that remains unresolved. Over the years a variety of methods have been developed mainly in the area of knowledge-based assessment. The Angoff method, the Hofstee method and the Ebel method are a few of the attempts to arrive at a satisfactory method of standard setting. It is clear that assessment within the field of medical education must be based on performance criteria that have been carefully established. The use of criterion referencing for performance-based tasks makes the issue of standard setting of paramount importance. Subjective elements in the process must be removed as far as it is possible.

In the United Kingdom, the General Medical Council has advocated a move towards a core curriculum with additional special study modules (SSMs). It is essential that any assessment establish that the students have achieved the standard for the core before continuing to the SSMs. Students, of course, learn at different rates and subsequently will vary in the time they take to reach the core standards. Assessment at a fixed time may penalise the slower learners. If the time is extended then the faster students may become demotivated and bored. An alternative is to assess all students after the minimum time for the course. Those who pass move on to new learning. Those who fail continue to study and are reassessed at a later date; if they pass they continue with the next course (see Fig. 27.2).

Computerised adaptive testing (CAT)

Adaptive testing is a method whereby candidates are presented with a minimum number of questions via the computer. Candidates can work at their own pace. The questions will vary as they are based on responses to

"The resulting standard, however, must be defensible in that it must identify practising physicians who provide an acceptable level of patient care"

Cusimano 1996

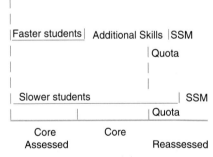

Fig. 27.2   Assessment after minimum time

prior test questions. Each question gives maximum information about the candidate, based on the skill level indicated by the previous answers. Once the computer has reached a decision about a candidate's competence, the examination is terminated.

CAT can provide an accurate measure of performance. Results may be given immediately and candidates may retake the test at agreed dates. Questions asked in successive tests will vary, which counteracts any practice effects.

Summary

Although we need to be rigorous in the application of assessment and to integrate it into professional training so that it becomes accepted as the norm, it is also wise to remember that discovering the perfect assessment is akin to finding the Holy Grail.

Involvement with the assessment process does, however, mean a continual search for 'getting it better' next time. It is this type of philosophy which goes a long way to ensuring all-round quality.

"There is no such thing as a process of assessment that is without critics. Whatever efforts are made to improve assessment someone is bound to be unhappy with the process"

Hager, Gonczi & Athanasou 1994

References and further reading

Black P J 1993 Formative and summative assessment by teachers. Studies in Science Education 21:49–97

Black P J 1997 Evaluation and assessment. In: Tiberghien A, Jossem E L, Barojas J (eds) Connecting research in physics education with teacher education. International Commission on Physics Education

Boud D 1995 Enhancing learning through self-assessment. Kogan Page, London and Philadelphia

Cusimano M D 1996 Standard setting in medical education. Academic Medicine 71(10):S112–S120

Gipps C 1994 Quality in teacher assessment. In: Harlen W (ed.) Enhancing quality in assessment. Chapman, London

Hager P, Gonczi A, Athanasou J 1994 General issues about the assessment of competence. Assessment and Evaluation in Higher Education 19:3–16

Laurillard D 1993 Rethinking university teaching. Routledge, London and New York

Pereira Gray D, Murray S, Hasler J, Percy D, Allen J, Freeth M, Hayden J 1997 The summative assessment package: an alternative view. Education for General Practice 8:8–15

Turnball J M 1989 What is . . . Normative versus criterion-referenced assessment. Medical Teacher 11(2):145–150

Wooliscroft J O, TenHaken J, Smith J, Calhoun J G 1993 Medical students' clinical self-assessments: comparisons with external measures of performance and the students' self-assessments of overall performance and effort. Academic Medicine 68(4):285–294

Chapter 28
Choosing assessment instruments

S. McAleer

Introduction

When it comes down to deciding on the best instrument for assessment the choices on offer are not as depressing as those suggested by Woody Allen. Nevertheless getting it right or wrong can have long-term effects for the students involved in the process. Therefore in selecting appropriate assessment instruments it is essential to understand the key principles involved. Assessment is a measure of performance, which can be used as a feedback mechanism for three important aspects of the learning situation. It can provide:

- a measure of the level of student performance
- an indication of the effectiveness of the teaching situation
- a measure of the appropriateness of the content input.

There are a number of important questions which must be asked before making a choice of assessment method:

- What should be assessed?
- Why assess?

When an assessment instrument is being considered it must be asked:

- Is it valid?
- Is it reliable?
- Is it feasible?

In answering these questions the basic principles of assessment will be brought into play. What is assessed

"More than at any other time in history, mankind faces a crossroads. One path leads to despair and utter hopelessness. The other, to total extinction. Let us pray we have the wisdom to choose correctly"

Woody Allen: Side Effects (1980)

"Examinations are formidable even to the best prepared, for the greatest fool may ask more than the wisest man can answer"

Charles Caleb Colton, 1780–1832

and which methods are used will play a significant part in what is learnt. Decisions on what students should learn and the reasons for making those decisions must be established first. Afterwards the type of assessment can be determined. For example, if you want your students to read a textbook then tell them there will be a series of multiple choice questions (MCQs) on each chapter in their end-of-term examination. If you want your students to show competence in minor surgical techniques then inform them that there will be a practical examination in these skills.

At this stage it is probably useful to make the distinction between assessment method and assessment instrument. For example, the method of assessment selected may be self-assessment and the instruments used could be MCQs or perhaps an objective structured clinical examination (OSCE). Table 28.1 illustrates the difference by comparing assessment to travel and instruments to types of conveyance. Of course, different assessment instruments may be used within a particular method.

Table 28.1   Difference between methods and instruments

Method of travel	Conveyance	Method of assessment	Instrument
By land By sea By air	Train/Bus/Car Ferry/Speedboat/Liner Helicopter/Glider/Jet	Performance Written	Checklist/Simulators Essay/MCQs

Try to use more than one assessment instrument, and more than one assessor especially if you are looking at skills and attitudes. Gather as much data on the candidate as is feasible.

There is currently a wide range of assessment instruments available and in order to make an informed choice it is necessary to be familiar with what is on offer:

- essays
- patient management problems
- modified essay questions
- checklists
- objective structured clinical examinations
- projects
- constructed response questions
- objective tests
- critical reading papers
- rating scales

- tutor reports
- portfolios
- short case assessments
- long case assessments

What should be assessed?

Harden (1979) suggested that many teachers failed to address this question with sufficient thought. This claim is still worthy of consideration as it stresses the importance of educational objectives defined by Mager (1984) as the performance to be exhibited by a learner before being considered competent 'An educational objective is therefore an intended result of instruction, rather than the process itself.'

Useful objectives relate to:

- the task the student is to perform
- the conditions under which the performance should be exhibited
- the level of performance that will be considered acceptable.

Clear objectives are important in the planning of authentic assessment. These objectives should not only be worth measuring but they should also be measurable. The more specific the objective, the more useful it is likely to be in indicating the assessable behaviours expected of students. Specific objectives are also extremely useful as a springboard for developing a suitable assessment programme. Morgan & Irby (1978) emphasise the importance of the precise wording of objectives so that student, teacher and assessor are all exactly clear about what must be performed to show competence. For example, rather than saying that a medical technologist should '*know* the characteristic appearance of different types of blood cell', the objective should state that 'the medical technologist will *identify* and *interpret* blood cells on a blood smear.'

Writing objectives that are well defined and precise can be difficult and can be influenced by the subject being taught. Objectives are always output measures and in determining what they are, the assessment writer has

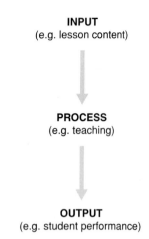

INPUT
(e.g. lesson content)

PROCESS
(e.g. teaching)

OUTPUT
(e.g. student performance)

Fig. 28.1   **Assessment process**

to start at the end of the process illustrated in Figure 28.1. The teacher usually thinks about the content first and then develops the assessment instruments second. Focusing on the output measures, although educationally sound, goes against the natural instincts of many teachers.

Output measures should contain:

• a knowledge component
• a skill component
• an attitudinal component.

The knowledge component domain relates to the learners' ability to remember and understand. The skill component encompasses those psychomotor tasks which are deemed prerequisite for professional competence. The attitudinal component includes the key personal qualities thought necessary of a professional. Before choosing an assessment instrument it is vital to define clearly what exactly is to be assessed. What may be appropriate for testing knowledge is unlikely to be useful for assessing psychomotor skills. A number of taxonomies are available which can help by providing lists of the competencies available and in setting an appropriate level of performance: for example, Bloom (1956), Harrow (1972), Krathwohl, Bloom & Masia (1964).

Why assess?

Assessment is an important part of the curriculum for the following reasons:

• It is an integral part of the learning process in which students are informed of any weaknesses and of how to improve on the quality of their performance.
• It illustrates progress and ensures a proper standard has been achieved before progressing to a higher level of training.
• It provides certification relating to a standard of performance, e.g. the award of a degree.
• It indicates to students the areas of a course which are considered important.

- It acts as a promotion technique.
- It acts as a means of selection for a career or as an entrance requirement for a course.
- It motivates students in their studies.
- It measures the effectiveness of training and identifies curriculum weaknesses.

Validity

Whatever assessment instrument is used it must be valid for the task it is to do. In other words the answer to the question 'Am I measuring what I am supposed to be measuring?' must be positive. A particular examination might be valid for one purpose but invalid for another. For example, a series of MCQs which test factual recall may be a valid measure of whether a student has read a textbook on diabetes but invalid as the indicator of whether that same student can actually manage a patient suffering from diabetes.

The measure of validity is not a straightforward process as a variety of types of validity are described and 'degrees of validity' are recognised. Building up a dossier to support a claim of validity can involve looking at five major types:

- content validity
- concurrent validity
- predictive validity
- construct validity
- face validity.

It is important to be familiar with all of these but the emphasis attributed to each is dependent on the reasons for assessing.

Content validity
This refers to the extent to which a test or examination actually measures the intended content area. For an examination to have content validity it must have 'item validity' and 'sampling validity'. These terms are best explained in the following example. If a test is designed to measure knowledge of the human anatomy then good item validity is present if all the questions deal with facts

pertaining to the human body. However, poor sampling validity will be apparent if all the questions focus on the lower limbs.

The issue of content should be seen in relation to:

- the subject matter you are teaching
- the students who are being taught.

How to establish content validity

- Define the subject matter being assessed.
- Identify the cognitive/behavioural/attitudinal process involved.
- Establish the outcomes expected.
- Draw up a specifications grid (see Table 28.2).

Table 28.2   Table of specifications for an MCQ in physiological psychology

Content	Knowledge	Comprehension	Application	Higher processing	Total
Neurones/ Gross anatomy	6	4	2	1	13 (26%)
Motor mechanisms	4	3	2	1	10 (20%)
Sensory systems	3	2	2	1	8 (16%)
Alerting mechanisms	3	2	2	1	8 (16%)
Motivation/ Emotion	2	2	1	1	6 (12%)
Memory/ Learning	2	2	1	—	5 (10%)
Total	20 (40%)	15 (30%)	10 (20%)	5 (10%)	50 (100%)

This type of grid should:

- identify the content areas (n=6)
- specify learning outcomes (n=4)
- determine the number of items for each content area and learning objective
- ensure that the number of items in each cell is in proportion to the time spent in teaching and learning.

Content validity is based on expert judgement and the assessor should compare what is taught with what is measured by the examination. If you are testing for achievement you must ensure content validity.

Concurrent validity

This refers to the degree to which scores on a test correlate with the scores on an established test administered at the same time. The procedure is to:

- Administer the new test.
- Administer the established test.
- Correlate the two sets of scores.
- The greater the positive correlation, the greater the validity.

Predictive validity

Predictive validity relates to the certainty with which a test can predict future performance. It is particularly important if you are using your assessment for selection purposes. No test will have perfect predictability so it is wise to base any decision on more than one predictor. The procedure is to:

- Administer your test.
- Collect measures of the new behaviour.
- Correlate the two results.
- The magnitude of the correlation coefficient will determine the predictive validity.

Construct validity

Construct validity is the extent to which a test measures a hypothetical construct (e.g. empathy, intelligence) or a trait that explains behaviour but is not easily observed. For example, if a theory of schizophrenia hypothesised that high scorers on a test will take longer to problem-solve than low scorers, then if high scorers do indeed take longer it would provide evidence for construct validity. It can be difficult to determine and all forms of validity should be used as evidence for its presence.

Face validity

Face validity is concerned with appearance; i.e. does the exam *seem* to measure what it is supposed to measure? If candidates feel that the assessment is fair and relevant then they will be better motivated. The teaching and learning environment will also benefit. Face validity is determined by feedback received from all those involved in the assessment.

Factors influencing validity

There are a variety of factors which may influence the validity of an assessment instrument. Check for the following:

- vague or misleading instructions to candidates
- inappropriate vocabulary or overcomplicated wording
- too few test items causing poor sampling validity
- problems of time – insufficient time for answers turns the test into one based on speed
- items inappropriate for the outcomes being measured
- item difficulty – items that are too easy/difficult will fail to discriminate.

Reliability

It is important to be able to trust any assessment instrument used. Reliability is the degree to which a test consistently measures whatever it is supposed to measure. The more reliable the examination, the greater the confidence that the result would be the same if the examination were re-administered. For example, if a student scored 60% in an MCQ examination and in two subsequent sittings shortly afterwards scored 30% and 90% then you would assume the test lacked reliability. As with validity a number of different kinds of reliability are described, as outlined below.

Test-retest reliability

Test-retest reliability measures the consistency of an examination over time. It is calculated by correlating the scores on a test with scores produced by a repeat administration to the same group. A high positive correlation indicates good reliability. One problem is deciding on the appropriate time period between the two administrations. If it is too short then the students are likely to remember their previous answers. If there is too lengthy a gap then students may have benefited from further learning. This type of reliability is important for tests used as predictors.

Equivalent forms reliability

This type of reliability refers to the consistency of scores across two different formats of the same test. The tests are identical in terms of number of questions, structure and the level of difficulty. The only difference is in the wording of the specific items but both tests measure the same objectives. To calculate reliability the scores on format 1 of the test are correlated with the scores from format 2. Not surprisingly a major difficulty is constructing two versions of the same examination that are essentially equivalent. The main use for this form of examination is in studies which require a pre-test and a post-test to be given.

Split half reliability

The internal consistency of an examination is measured by this method. With split half reliability the examination is divided into two parts, e.g. all the odd numbered questions and all the even numbered questions. The scores for both halves are correlated and the degree of correlation reflects the internal consistency of the instrument. Only one administration of the test is necessary and the method is particularly suitable for tests with many items. The more questions in an examination, the greater the likelihood of high reliability. There are various statistical techniques for discovering the internal consistency of a test. The KR20 and Cronbach's Alpha are two of the most common.

Scorer/rater reliability

If you are using an instrument where the scoring involves a certain amount of subjectivity it is important to check for both inter-rater reliability and intra-rater reliability. The first type refers to the reliability of two or more independent markers to give the same marks to each student. The second kind relates to the scoring of assessors: will a marker give the same score to a student if the work is remarked at a later date? The reliability for both versions is calculated by correlational statistics.

Factors influencing reliability

- Test length. The more items included in an examination, the greater the reliability.
- Objectivity in scoring. Lack of objectivity, for example, will reduce reliability use of long essay questions.
- Environmental errors. Performance may be poor in candidates who are required to sit an examination at the end of a long day.
- Processing errors. Mistakes may be made in calculating candidates' marks.
- Classification errors. A marker may interpret what may really be a candidate's anxiety as rudeness.
- Generalisation errors. The examiner may generalise from a specific answer.
- Bias errors. Some examiners may place too great an emphasis on a particular trait. Others may be prejudiced against certain students. The previous overall impression of a student can sometimes influence the mark given to a student. Certain examiners may be 'easy' markers while others may be 'hard' markers.

Feasibility

When selecting an assessment instrument it is paramount to check that it will be feasible to use it. This will involve calculating the cost of the assessment, both in terms of resources and time. The following questions should be asked:

- How long will it take to construct the instrument?
- How much time will be involved with the marking process?
- Will it be relatively easy to interpret the scores and produce the results?
- Is it practical in terms of organisation?
- Can quality feedback result from the instrument?
- Will the instrument indicate to the students the important elements within the course?
- Will the assessment have a beneficial effect in terms of student motivation, good study habits and positive career aspirations?

Always look at the way you assess and ask 'How will this benefit my students?'

Summary

In selecting an assessment instrument it is necessary to know exactly what it is that is to be measured. This should reflect the course outcomes, i.e. what it is you want your students to be able to do. Different learning outcomes necessitate the use of different instruments. It is inappropriate to assess a performance skill with an MCQ. It is essential to use an instrument that is valid, reliable and feasible. An instrument may be perfectly reliable but totally invalid. For example, an MCQ examination may show high reliability but is it really a valid measure of whether students are competent in resuscitation skills? Finally, no assessment instrument is of any value if it is unfeasible to use it. If a full variety of instruments are used then there will be more confidence that the results obtained are a true reflection of the students' performance.

References and further reading

Bloom B S (ed.) 1956 Taxonomy of educational objectives. Handbook I: Cognitive domain. David McKay, New York

Harden R M 1979 How to assess students: an overview. Medical Teacher 1(2):65–70

Harrow A J A 1972 A taxonomy of the psychomotor domain: a guide for developing behavioural objectives. David McKay, New York

Krathwohl D R, Bloom B S, Masia B B 1964 Taxonomy of educational objectives. Handbook II: Affective domain. David McKay, New York

Mager R F 1984 Preparing instructional objectives. Pitman Learning, California

Morgan M K, Irby D M (eds) 1978 Evaluating clinical competence in the health professions. C. V. Mosby, Saint Louis

Thomson B, Daniel L G 1996 Seminal readings on reliability and validity: a 'hit parade' bibliography. Educational and Psychological Measurement 56(5):741–745

Chapter 29
Objective testing

S. McAleer

Before starting to set a question ask yourself what it is you want to find out.

Introduction

The use of objective tests in assessing the knowledge base of students is now commonplace in most medical schools throughout the world. Speed, in both marking and examination time, allied to high reliability are major advantages. There are a variety of types available and it is important to be familiar with what is on offer in order to arrive at an assessment instrument which truly provides you with relevant information. What exactly do you want to find out about your students in terms of knowledge? Is it simple factual recall you are interested in? Or do you want to look at higher-level components such as understanding relationships and identifying principles?

Types of objective test

There are four major types of objective test and each one has a variety of formats:

- short answer items
  — question format
  — completion format
  — association format
- true/false items
  — true/false format
  — correction format
  — multiple true/false format
- matching exercises
  — simple matching exercises
  — multiple matching type
  — extended matching items

- multiple choice questions
  — correct answer format
  — best answer format
  — multiple response format
  — rearrangement format.

Each type will be described here in turn and illustrated with examples. Advice on how to construct such questions and their advantages and disadvantages will follow. By doing this, it is hoped to provide you with practical guidelines for developing objective tests which are appropriate for your own specific assessment needs.

The short answer item
In this type of test the student answers with a word or a phrase.

Question format
A specific question is presented and a direct answer requested. For example:

- What is the largest organ in the human body?_____

    This is a good example because there is one and only one answer.

- What is the main cause of mortality in babies under 3 months?_____

    This is a poor question because the answer is dependent on which part of the world you consider.

Completion format
The student must supply the missing word. For example:

- The largest organ in the human body is the_____

Association format

The student has to supply the appropriate letter or number that is linked to a particular word or phrase. For example:

- Write the symbol for each of the following elements
  Mercury_____

"*Learning to write good items is important if the test is to be of value to students and teacher. Not only do teachers need to understand the subject matter they teach, but they also need to determine how well such knowledge has been taught to their students*"

Sax 1989

Silver_____
Radium_____

Advantages and disadvantages of short answer items
All the formats are quite easy to construct and can be objectively scored. The marker need not be an expert but should have a general background in the area being assessed. It is essential to have a clear set of answers. The probability for guessing correctly is quite low and the test is primarily used as a way of measuring information recall.

The main disadvantage relates to what it is you wish to assess. The test is not ideal in the assessment of complex learning outcomes: for instance, where the ability to synthesise and analyse information is required.

Constructing short answer items
There are a number of rules which should be adhered to when developing a bank of short answer questions:

- Ensure the question is brief and has only one correct answer.
- Avoid any possible ambiguities relating to the phrasing.
- Avoid if possible using wording taken directly from textbooks as the context may not be appropriate.
- A direct question is preferable to an incomplete statement. For example: 'In what year did Sir Alexander Fleming discover penicillin?' is better than 'Sir Alexander Fleming discovered penicillin in _____'
- If you are asking for an answer which has a numerical value always stipulate the unit of value.
- Blank spaces should be of a standard length in order that candidates are not given a clue to the answer.

True/false items
In recent years there has been a move away from this type of objective test. Why do you think that is? A closer examination of the format may give you an

indication. The true/false item consists of a statement, which the candidate must indicate as being either true or false.

True/false format

A simple choice is required. The respondent is asked to circle the correct answer. For example:

The patella is located in the knee T F

Correction format

This is somewhat more complicated. Here a student is asked to circle the T if a statement is true. If it is false the F must be circled and the underlined word changed so that the statement is true. The new word must be written in the allocated space. For example:

- Autonomic nerves carry sensory fibres from the receptors in the *viscera*
  T   F_____

- The tenth cranial nerve is known as the *trochlea*
  T   F   *vagus*

This type of true/false question can be difficult to mark and it requires very clear instructions.

Multiple true/false format

This is composed of a stem with a number of items which may be either true or false. For example:

- Lesions in the ventromedial nucleus of the hypothalamus cause:

Hyperphagia	T	F
Blindness	T	F
Obesity	T	F

Advantages and disadvantages of true/false items

One advantage often cited relates to the ability of true/false items to cover a wide range of topics within a subject. This is not always the case, as many topics do not lend themselves to such absolute judgements.

Shades of grey are not catered for. Undoubtedly the statements are easy to construct. The difficulty arises in attempting to write unambiguous questions that measure complex learning outcomes. They are of course easily marked, except for the correction variety. Their main use is in the simple identification of facts or definitions and a key criticism is their encouragement of basic rote learning. Richardson (1992) has suggested that by changing the way in which they are used they could measure concept mastery. Another major disadvantage is the high probability of guessing the correct answer – a one in two chance. Employing negative marking where students are penalised by deducting marks for an incorrect answer may discourage guessing. Perhaps the biggest downside to true/false questions is their inability to discover if the student who correctly identifies a statement as false actually knows the correct answer.

Constructing true/false items
- Avoid general statements.
- Be careful not to use unnecessarily specific statements. For example: 'The stethoscope was first used in July 1971'.
- Double negatives can be confusing.
- Avoid unwieldy and lengthy statements.
- The actual length should be about the same for both true and false statements.
- The number of true statements should be approximate to the number of false statements.
- Ensure that each statement is definitely true or definitely false.
- Keep the wording as simple as possible.

Matching exercises

Simple matching exercises
Respondents are asked to match pairs of items from a list of premises and a list of responses. It is important that clear instructions are given to avoid any inconsistencies or ambiguities relating to the nature of the task. For example:

- Below are two lists. Column A contains the three major golf tournaments and Column B international golfers. Choose the letter from Column B that fits the premises in Column A.

Column A
Winner of the 1998 US Open
The winner of the 1998 Open
The winner of the 1998 US Masters

Column B
A Mark O'Meara
B Tom Kite
C Tiger Woods
D Jack Nicklaus
E Cory Pavin
F Ernie Els
G Lee Janzen

Multiple matching type

The candidate has to make the right 'connections' from two (or more) lists. For example:

- For each of the novel titles (Column A) identify the author (Column B) and his/her nationality (Column C). Write your choice of name and country in the blanks spaces provided.

A	Author	Nationality	B	C
1984	———	———	Joyce	British
			Pasternak	French
The Great Gatsby	———	———	Tolstoy	American
			Hugo	Irish
War and Peace	———	———	Orwell	German
			Fitzgerald	Russian

Advantages and disadvantages of matching exercises

Matching exercises are relatively easy to construct and particularly appropriate for measuring associations. Guessing the correct match is not so simple as the list(s) of responses should contain more items than the list of premises. You can also cover a number of associations with one exercise. However, there is a tendency to focus on basic factual information. In addition matching exercises are open to the presence of irrelevant clues.

Constructing matching exercises

- Use only premises and responses which have a similar theme.
- Include more response options than premises.
- Avoid a lengthy list of premises.
- List the responses in a logical order (when appropriate).
- Always ensure that the basis for matching is made clear.
- Keep all the items on the same page.

Extended matching items (EMIs)

This is a variation of the above technique. It consists of a topic, a list of possible responses, the basis for the matching and a number of scenarios.

For example:

Topic: Investigations

Response options:
A Plain X-ray
B Isotope scan
C CT scan
D MRI scan
E Ultrasound scan
F PET scan
G Intravenous pyelogram
H Myelogram
I Cholecystogram
J Lateral chest X-ray

Instructions: For the patients described below, which is likely to be the *single* most helpful investigation? Place the letter corresponding to the investigation in the space provided.

Scenarios:

1. Ten days after a knock on the head during rugby a 19-year-old complains to you that he has been unable to concentrate on lectures because of drowsiness and headaches. General neurological examination is unremarkable.

   C

2. A 16-week pregnant 24-year-old complains of loin pain and tenderness from the previous day.

   E

3. A 66-year-old man with a history of partial pneumonectomy for bronchogenic carcinoma has

presented acutely with a transverse fracture of the femur. The injury happened as he got up from a chair. Plain X-ray shows a fracture through a secondary deposit.

B

(By kind permission of Dr C Walker, Ninewells Hospital, Dundee)

Advantages and disadvantages of extended matching items
This type of format allows for the assessment of the application of knowledge. Obviously, EMIs are difficult to construct, as there are a number of different components involved and relevant scenarios need to be well crafted.

Constructing extended matching items
- Identify the outcomes you wish to assess and the context in which they occur.
- It is usually best to write the response options first and then build the appropriate scenario for each one.
- Keep the options concise (one or two words).
- Ensure the reasons for matching are clear.
- The scenarios should not be overly complex and should contain only relevant information.

Case & Swanson (1993) provide useful information on the writing of extended matching items. The same authors have written a manual which gives guidance on the writing of test questions for the basic and clinical sciences (1996).

Multiple choice questions
Multiple choice questions (MCQs) consist of a stem followed by a number of options, usually four or five.

Correct answer format
A specific question is asked and the candidate is required to select the correct response from the list of options. For example:

- What is the only sensory nerve that goes directly to the telencephalon without synapsing in the thalamus?

In EMIs each of the ten distractors must appear to be plausible answers for each of the scenarios described.

A Cranial nerve
B Optic nerve
C Olfactory nerve
D Facial nerve
E Auditory nerve

There may be areas you wish to assess which are rather imprecise in that answers are not easily categorised into a simple yes or no. A particular response will be more appropriate than the other options on offer. Therefore the good candidate should hopefully select the best answer.

Best answer format
This assesses understanding coupled with application. Therefore it is essential that there is a consensus among the question setters as to what is the best answer. For example:

- What is the most likely cause of gout in a 50-year-old overweight businessman?
  A Heavy smoking
  B High-fat diet
  C Lack of physical exercise
  D Stress at work

Multiple response format
This requires the candidate to select more than one of the designated options. For example:

- What are the main types of visual receptor in the vertebrate eye?
  A Rods
  B Curves
  C Cones
  D Indicators
  E Photospins

Rearrangement format
This requires the candidate to place the options in the correct sequence. For example:

- Circle the letter corresponding to the correct sequence in terms of length, moving from the smallest to the largest.

1 Inch
2 Yard
3 Foot
A 1 2 3
B 3 2 1
C 1 3 2
D 2 1 3

Advantages of multiple choice questions

MCQs can readily sample a wide range of learning outcomes in a short period of time. It is relatively easy to ensure that the questions are free from any ambiguity. The probability for guessing the correct answer is quite low, e.g. a one in five chance with a question providing five possible answers. There is also the opportunity to use such questions to provide a diagnostic profile relating to a candidate's strengths and weaknesses across a particular subject. With a little extra effort it is possible to construct high-quality items that test the ability to process and interpret facts. In such instances the information provided by the stem has to be written as a problem-solving exercise.

On the negative side fixed choices do not allow the candidate any opportunity to provide pertinent additional material. This is common to all objective tests, i.e. that is what ensures objectivity. On occasion it may be difficult to construct plausible distractors. Distractors are those choices which are incorrect but which should appear to the candidate as a valid answer. There is also a tendency to build items around a relatively trivial fact in order to fulfil the question quota.

Constructing multiple choice questions

- Ensure that the stem is meaningful and presents a clear problem.
- Do not include irrelevant material in the stem.
- Distracters should be plausible. Avoid using any options which are blatantly incorrect or just plain silly.
- Try to avoid the use of negatives in the stem. There is no need to confuse the candidate unnecessarily.
- The choices must fit grammatically with the stem.

- Avoid the use of words like generally, occasionally and sometimes in the stem.

Uses of multiple choice questions

- To discover if there is an understanding of important terminology. This can be ascertained by asking the candidate to select the correct definition of a particular word (or phrase) from a number of options.
- To assess knowledge of specific facts. Questions of the who, what, when and where type are the standard offerings.
- To discover if there is a knowledge of principles. Here you are wishing to find out if the candidate can explain how a certain principle works. For example:

  The principle of hydrostatics is used in
  - **A** Fashion design
  - **B** Shipbuilding
  - **C** Electronics
  - **D** Aviation
  - **E** Astrometry
- The justification of procedures or processes.

  For example:

  Why do nurses regularly change hospital bed-linen?
  - **A** To prevent wound infection
  - **B** To prevent bed sores
  - **C** To ensure the patient feels comfortable
  - **D** To maintain a high standard of ward hygiene

Constructing plausible distractors

- Look at previous examinations and use candidates' most frequent errors.
- Ensure that the option is relevant to the stem.
- Use phrases that appear as if they come from an authoritative source.
- Use incorrect answers that are likely to result from a candidate's carelessness, e.g. misinterpreting metres for yards.
- Distractors are not there in order to create a trick question.

Summary

The objective test item, in whatever format it presents itself, is a hardy annual in assessment terms throughout medical schools the world over. It is efficient, reliable and economic and provides diagnostic information about both the student and the course. However, when using such tests it is essential to take a hard look at what it is you wish to assess. Too often they are pressed into service without due consideration. Good questions take time and careful thought. Look at the intended learning outcomes and then match them with the format that is most appropriate.

"In examinations those who do not wish to know ask questions of those who cannot tell"

Raliegh 1923

References and further reading

Case S M, Swanson D B 1993 Extended-matching items: a practical alternative to free-response questions. Teaching and Learning in Medicine 5(2):107–115

Case S M, Swanson D B 1996 Constructing written test questions for the basic and clinical sciences. National Board of Examiners, Philadelphia

Joorabachi B 1981 How to construct problem-solving MCQs. Medical Teacher 3(1):9–13

Raliegh W 1995 Some thoughts on examinations. Laughter from a cloud. In: Shettin N (ed.) The Oxford Dictionary of Humorous Quotations. Oxford University Press, Oxford

Richardson R 1992 The multiple choice true/false question: what does it measure and what could it measure? Medical Teacher 14(2/3):201–204

Roid G H, Haladyna T M 1982 A technology for test-item writing. Academic Press, New York

Sax G 1989 Principles of educational and psychological measurement and evaluation. Wadsworth, CA

Chapter 30
Constructed response questions

M. H. Davis

Introduction

What are constructed response questions (CRQs)?

A CRQ is any question requiring the candidate to generate an answer rather than select from a small set of options (Bennet & Ward 1993). The question may be asked in a variety of formats and generating the answer involves the student in carrying out an intellectual and/or physical task.

A CRQ may be posed as:

- a written question
- a statement, journal article or report
- a problem scenario: clinical, basic science or community
- photographic or other visual material
- a test result or other investigative data.

The response generated by the student may be:

- a very short answer – one or several words
- a short answer – notes or lists
- a long answer – essay, dissertation, referral letter or report
- a physical task – a project or other complex performance such as cardiopulmonary resuscitation or conducting an investigation.

Responses such as essays, dissertations, projects and complex performance will be considered in other chapters. In this chapter we deal with responses made in writing by the student.

Some advantages of CRQs

There has been increasing interest in this type of assessment as carefully constructed CRQs may be employed to assess important curriculum outcomes and to drive the learning approaches of students. CRQs can be designed to assess not just the candidate's knowledge base, but also the application of that knowledge to interpretation of data, clinical reasoning and problem-solving which are important outcomes of medical education.

The higher-order thinking involved in applying knowledge to answer the question requires a deeper approach to learning on the part of the student than the simple recall of factual information.

Another advantage is that simulations of important or common clinical situations are possible with this type of question and increase the reality. The approach is free from the cueing effects which are a potential drawback with multiple choice formats.

The CRQs described in this chapter can be

- used summatively, to assess candidates in both undergraduate and postgraduate examinations
- used formatively, for self-assessment.

Some disadvantages of CRQs

Although preparation of CRQs is relatively easy, some expertise is required to avoid ambiguity. A content expert is required to mark the paper. An optical mark reader cannot be used to mark the students' responses. For some formats, double marking is necessary to achieve the required level of reliability. This tends to slow down the marking process and the presentation of results. A large number of questions is needed to reduce sampling errors and this tends to make CRQ examinations rather long and time-consuming.

Posing the question

The curriculum outcome being assessed and the context in which it is to be assessed must first be identified; for example, health promotion in the cardiovascular system

"CRQs are more relevant than having essays in exams. They relate to the patient problems that we will have to deal with as doctors"

Medical student

or problem-solving in surgery. Then the most appropriate method of presenting the question to students can be selected from a range of formats.

A statement, journal article or report

A statement or other documentary material such as a journal article may be presented to candidates giving them the opportunity to comment, analyse or make notes on the information presented.

An article by Ebrahim et al (1997) was distributed to students 2 weeks before an examination which included assessment of critical thinking and the ability to assess evidence in medicine in relation to a course on ageing and health. The article reported the results of a randomised controlled trial to evaluate the effects of brisk walking on bone mineral density in women who had suffered an upper limb fracture. Students were told they would be asked questions relating to the design of the trial, the conclusions reached by the authors of the study and the implications for health promotion advice to patients.

A clinical problem

In a clinical or patient-management problem (Harden 1983) information about the patient is presented to set the scene and provide sufficient information for the candidate to come to some informed decision about the patient. This information should include:

- patient details
- a description of the patient's problem
- duration of the presenting complaint
- how the patient presents to the doctor
- further details including past history or family history
- a description of the medical care setting
- physical findings.

Diagnostic test results, initial treatment and subsequent findings may also be included where relevant.

Clinical problems can be used to test application of knowledge in patient care situations. In selecting the clinical problem for use in assessment, Case & Swanson (1996) recommend:

- selection of common or potentially catastrophic problem scenarios and avoidance of rare or esoteric situations
- involving the types of clinical decision that successful candidates will soon be expected to take in their professional situation
- avoidance of clinical situations that would be handled by a sub-specialist.

Example clinical problem designed to assess basic science and clinical and therapeutics knowledge in relation to the nervous system

A 72-year-old, right-handed man presents with a 6-month history of increasing tremor of his right hand that causes him severe embarrassment, such that he avoids going out. On examination, the tremor is most marked at rest and decreases on maintaining a posture and during movement. There is no intention tremor.

Example questions
- the name of this type of tremor
- the anatomical site of the pathological lesion
- drugs causing this phenomenon as a side-effect
- additional signs to look for on physical examination
- how to treat the condition.

A basic science problem

'Laboratory vignettes' can be useful in preparing constructed response questions that test the application of basic science knowledge (Case & Swanson 1996). Laboratory experiments are presented and candidates are required to use their understanding of basic science principles to predict or explain the results. Candidates are required to apply their knowledge, make a prediction or select a course of action based on the information presented.

The use of such problems to assess the application of knowledge has several advantages:

- The face validity of the examination is enhanced.
- Important information rather than trivia is emphasised.

"Such questions effectively shift the focus of assessment from knowledge of isolated facts to use of basic science principles to solve problems"

Case & Swanson 1996

- It identifies candidates who have memorised a substantial body of factual information but are unable to utilise it.

A community problem
Items appearing in newspapers may provide sources for community problems.

Example community problem
A photograph is presented along with an accompanying newspaper story describing the concern felt by a middle-aged, overweight taxi driver. His request for renewal of his taxi driver's licence had been withheld pending medical examination. Candidates were asked why the licensing authorities had requested a medical report; if they were his general practitioner, what advice they would give the taxi driver; and, if they discovered his blood pressure was 184/105, what initial advice/treatment they would provide for him.

The question was designed to assess candidates' knowledge of cardiovascular risk factors and their attitudes to health promotion in the context of cardiovascular disease.

Photographic or other visual material
Where a written description may provide candidates with clues or prompts, it is often useful to present the candidate with a photographic illustration or other visual material such as a 35 mm slide.

A written description of a wound or of a skin rash may provide the candidate with prompts to the diagnosis, which could not have been made from the appearance alone. Candidates may be asked to identify the cause of the lesion and describe its management.

Test results or other investigative data
The question may be put to candidates in the form of test results when diagnostic skills or data interpretation are being assessed.

Example
Test result question
The two abnormal forced expiratory volume-time curves from breathless patients shown in Figures 30.1 and 30.2 were presented to candidates along with the patients' predicted normal FEV_1 values for age and height.

Candidates were asked to calculate, for each patient, the FEV_1, the FEV_1 as a percentage of predicted normal, the forced vital capacity in litres and the forced expiratory ratio as a percentage. They were also asked to identify, for each patient, the pattern of abnormality: i.e., whether obstructive or restrictive.

The question was designed to test candidates' numeric skills and data interpretation in the context of the respiratory system.

Responses generated by the students

As already stated, the response generated by the student may be:

- a very short answer – one or several words
- a short answer – notes or lists
- a long answer – referral letter or report.

Example
Necropsy photograph of haemopericardium
Question 1   What is the condition called?
Answer   Haemopericardium
Question 2   State three causes which can lead to this condition.
Answers i   Myomalacia cordis following a myocardial infarct
    ii   Dissecting aortic aneurysm
    iii   Penetrating chest injury

The first question requires a very short answer and the second a short answer in the form of a list. Both questions were testing the candidates' knowledge.

Example of a long answer question
Students are presented with the following information:

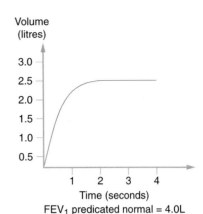

Fig. 30.1   Patient A

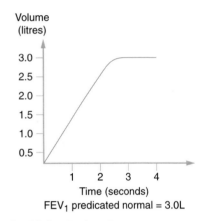

Fig. 30.2   Patient B

Mrs Jones is a 40-year-old lady who consults you because she hasn't had a period for 2 months. She usually has irregular periods and was therefore not initially concerned, but has never been so late before. She has been using condoms for contraception. Examination reveals a 12-week-size palpable uterus. You perform a pregnancy test that is positive. After discussion with her husband they decide to continue the pregnancy. She is concerned about the chance that the baby will have Down's syndrome. She has two teenage children. Both of these pregnancies and deliveries were uncomplicated. She has no significant past medical history.

Students are then asked to write a referral letter for Mrs Jones to attend the hospital for antenatal care, including all the points they consider relevant.

This question is designed to test applied knowledge and report writing in the context of the reproductive system.

Media available for the presentation of CRQs

A range of different media is available for presentation of the CRQ:

- print
- video tape
- audio tape
- 35 mm slides
- computer
- overhead projector

Print

Print is the most commonly used medium for the presentation of CRQs. It has the advantage of being relatively inexpensive and may be produced economically using readily available equipment. Illustrations, such as graphs and diagrams, and test results may be included in the printed text. Photographs and laboratory reports may be included in examination books or attached to question papers.

Video tape

Video tape may be used to present the question particularly within OSCE stations or in computerised

Resolution problems create difficulties in the successful reproduction of printed radiographic material and producing multiple copies of original radiographs is prohibitively expensive. Assessment of interpretation of radiographs is more easily and effectively carried out within the objective structured clinical examination (OSCE), with viewing boxes provided at OSCE stations.

examinations, when the question topic involves movement such as epileptic seizures or abnormalities of gait, or interactions such as consultations between doctor and patient. Clinical material which is difficult to provide for examinations on a predictable basis such as abdominal wound dehiscence can be successfully presented on video tape.

Audio tape

Audio tape may be used to present questions when recognition of voice quality is important or when conversations or interactions between individuals as in consultations or other communication skills are being assessed.

35 mm slides

A back projection system for the presentation of slides can be viewed by candidates in OSCEs without darkening the examination room.

Computers

Computers are increasingly used to present questions to candidates. Advantages include the ability to integrate multimedia material in the questions and so enrich the simulation. Computing skills can be assessed as a component of an examination where the acquisition of information technology skills is an important curriculum outcome.

Marking CRQs

Even when marking keys are used, random double marking of individual questions reveals significant variation between markers. It is good practice to double mark all CRQ examinations. The marks allocated by the two markers are compared. If there is good agreement between the markers (i.e. if the variation is no greater than 3%), the mean mark is used. When the variation between markers is greater than 3% in individual questions, the markers are asked to review the candidate's answer together, identify the reasons for the variation and agree a mark.

An answer key must be supplied to guide the markers of CRQs.

There can be wide variation in terminology used in candidates' answers even in questions requiring single word answers. Content experts are thus required rather than lay markers for all CRQ examinations.

The allocation of marks for each question in the examination is made known to students prior to the examination and again at the time of the examination in written instructions. The allocation of marks for each CRQ is decided on the basis of the importance of the curriculum outcome being assessed. Within each question, marks are allocated on the significance or importance of each component within the core curriculum. The candidate who correctly answers the core parts of the question has demonstrated mastery of core and should achieve the pass mark.

Examination design

Examinations should be designed to assess the individual candidate's ability to meet the course objectives or curriculum outcomes, and should cover the main content areas of the course. While examiners might wish to include the entire course content in the examination, in practice it is rarely possible to be so comprehensive; some degree of sampling is usually essential to provide an examination which is practicable.

A grid can be constructed to ensure that the parts of the CRQ test an even sample of curriculum outcomes and topics from the material presented during the course (see Table 30.1).

Summary

The CRQ examination provides a flexible framework for assessing a range of curriculum outcomes. CRQs can be posed as a written question, a statement, a journal article or report, as a clinical, basic science or community problem or as photographic or investigative material.

Student responses can be requested in a variety of formats including very short answers, short answers or a long answer which may take the form of a referral letter or report.

An examination can be constructed to sample widely among curriculum outcomes and topics presented in the course but a disadvantage is that content experts are required to mark the candidates' papers.

Acknowledgements

The author gratefully acknowledges the contribution of examination questions by Dr R Roberts, Professor B Lipworth, Dr A Evans and Dr G Mires of the University of Dundee Medical School.

References and further reading

Bennett R E, Ward W C 1993 Constructed versus choice in cognitive measurement. Lawrence Erlbaum, Hillsdale, NJ

Case S M, Swanson D B 1996 Constructing written test questions for the basic and clinical sciences. National Board of Medical Examiners, Philadelphia

Ebrahim S, Thompson P S, Baskaran V, Evans K 1997 Randomised placebo-controlled trial of brisk walking in the prevention of postmenopausal osteoporosis. Age and Ageing 26:253–260

Harden R M 1983 Preparation and presentation of patient-management problems. Medical Education 17(4):256–276

Table 30.1   Year 2 Constructed response paper

	Professionalism and role of doctor	Knowledge	Clinical skills	Communication skills	Clinical reasoning and data interpretation	Attitudes/ethics	Health promotion	Patient management	Investigations	Info handling	Transferable skills
CV risk factors		✓				✓	✓	✓			
Angina and peripheral vascular disease		✓						✓	✓		
Myocardial infarction		✓			✓			✓	✓		
Cardiac failure		✓			✓			✓	✓		
Asthma/Chronic obstructive airways disease		✓			✓			✓	✓		
Lung cancer		✓			✓			✓	✓		
Ventilation/Perfusion problems		✓	✓		✓			✓	✓		
Anaemia		✓			✓				✓		
Bleeding haematological malignancy		✓			✓			✓	✓		
Blood/Systemic disease/Immunology		✓			✓						
Upper gastrointestinal problems		✓	✓				✓		✓		
Abdominal pain		✓			✓		✓	✓	✓		
Jaundice	✓	✓			✓		✓				
Nutrition/Gastroenteritis/Eating disorder		✓									
Lower gastrointestinal problems		✓						✓	✓		
Diabetes		✓		✓	✓			✓			✓
Thyroid			✓		✓			✓	✓		
Pituitary/Adrenals calcium metabolism	✓				✓			✓	✓		
Breast disorders	✓	✓			✓			✓	✓		

Chapter 31
Tutor reports

M. H. Davis

"In contrast with the unstructured descriptions of behaviour gathered in anecdotal records, rating scales provide a systematic procedure for reporting observers' judgements"

Gronlund & Linn 1990

It is also important to include in the report a written comment area where tutors can list the major strengths and weaknesses of the student and identify what specific feedback points have been given to the student.

Introduction

Clinicians may be asked to provide reports on students or trainees who are attached to their units for a period of time. These reports are best provided in a structured format, based on an assessment of the student's performance in specific areas during the attachment period. Reports have sometimes been provided in the form of letters containing the tutor's opinion of the student's performance. Such unstructured reports are subjective, their reliability is low and their use is not recommended.

Most structured tutor reports employ rating scales designed to rate the student's performance over a range of competencies or curriculum outcomes. These rating scales can be used to assess whether or not the student meets the required standard over the range of outcomes being assessed.

Some advantages of tutor reports

Tutor reports are particularly useful for assessing areas which are difficult to test by conventional methods, such as:

- personal attributes
- attitudes
- generic competencies
- professional values – for example, reliability and trustworthiness, ability to work with other members of the health-care team, time-keeping.

As assessment occurs over a period of time, sustained performance is assessed rather than the snapshot obtained during an examination; tutor reports are actual and ongoing. Well-designed tutor reports allow for assessment against an agreed standard and are useful for identifying the underperforming student and for providing feedback to students at the end of a clinical attachment.

They are one of the few assessment methods that assess performance within the working context and thus have high content validity.

Tutor reports are flexible, unobtrusive and can be employed at minimal cost. Often they are the basis on which references are provided for students who have left the medical school some time previously as they provide a clearer picture of the individual than do examination grades.

Some disadvantages of tutor reports

Disadvantages of tutor reports include:

- problems in the use of rating scales
- subjectivity
- low reliability
- potential for adverse influence on the relationship between tutor and student.

Problems in the use of rating scales

Guilford in 'Psychometric Methods' (1974) lists six common errors made by raters when using rating scales:

- Error of leniency. Difficulties may arise if the rater likes the candidate. Some raters may give the candidate a higher rating than is appropriate, while others may overcompensate and give a lower rating.

Raters should be made aware of this potential problem and trained to separate the candidate's performance from their feelings about the candidate.

- Error of central tendency. Many raters tend to ignore the extremes of the scales and concentrate on the rating points near the centre of the scale.

Instruct raters to make full use of the scale, and anchor points on the scale using descriptors.

Use several raters' opinions to minimise the positive and negative influences of attributes that are not being assessed.

The provision of clear descriptors distinguishing the competencies will help to avoid this tendency.

Place similar traits some distance apart on the rating form.

Point out this tendency during rater training sessions.

- Halo effect. The appearance of the student may influence the rater's judgement.

- Logical error. Where competencies appear to be logically related, e.g. empathy and verbal communication, the raters tend to give similar ratings.

- Proximity errors. Raters tend to give similar ratings to traits which are placed close together especially if they are not disparate traits.

- Contrast error. If raters think that they are exceptionally good at certain skills, they tend to rate candidates lower than most other raters.

Subjectivity

If only one person completes the report, even when well-designed rating scales are employed, there is a possibility that the assessment may be subjective and open to the influences of hawks and doves.

Low reliability

The reliability of the tutor report may be low when only one tutor's view is represented and when the contact time between student and tutor has been short.

Adverse influence on relationship between tutor and student

A potential risk is that the observation of the student necessary for continuous assessment may affect the relationship between the student and the tutor. Emphasis placed on a consistently high level of performance during the observation period in order to obtain the highest point on the scale may be unrealistic and students may be discouraged.

Improving the quality of tutor reports

Several measures can be employed to improve the quality of tutor reports.

Provide feedback to tutors on the quality of their reports

The quality of tutor reports can be variable and depends on the effort the individual tutor expends in ensuring high standards and in following best practice when completing the report. It is important to maintain pressure on tutors to ensure that the reports are taken seriously and that adequate attention is paid to their completion. Those who are consistently hawks or doves should be informed of their stance.

Provide training in the use of the report form

Training in the use of the structured form improves reliability. Training should be directed at ensuring that tutors understand the form and its various components, are given practice in the use of rating scales, understand the common errors listed above and can defend their views particularly to their superiors. Although a consensus view is needed, there may be a tendency for the views of the head of department to dominate. Raters need to be trained to defend their views on students and for heads of department to accept consensus opinions.

Use several raters

Increasing the number of people who contribute to the report and taking into consideration the views of several tutors and other members of the health-care team working with the student will increase its objectivity. The use of several raters who reach a consensus for one report is likely to improve both objectivity and reliability.

Recognise the limitations

The tutor report is not a good way of testing knowledge.

Anchor the rating scales

Where rating scales are employed it is important to anchor the scales: that is, to define areas concretely to compensate for doves and hawks and to improve reliability.

Compensate for a central tendency

Raters may be unwilling to rate students at either end of the rating scale. This may effectively reduce a five-point scale to one of three points, which may be insufficiently discriminating. This problem can be overcome by:

- anchoring the scale with clearly defined descriptors
- the use of seven or more points in the scale, so that raters still have the choice of a number of points; in practice it is wise to limit the number of points to below 10 as beyond this anchoring is difficult and the range of choice becomes confusing
- varying the number of points on the scale so that raters cannot run down a central point on all scales
- using even numbers of points so that raters must choose one or other side of the midline.

Ensure adequate contact time between rater and student

In practice, it is not likely to be worthwhile employing tutor reports where the clinical attachment is under 4 weeks.

The design of structured tutor report forms

Structured tutor report forms may appear complex and may deter the rater from using them. They must therefore be designed to facilitate ease of use. However, the design and testing of the report forms are time-consuming and it may be useful to pilot the forms in restricted situations before full implementation.

Competencies to be assessed

Designing a structured report form begins with identifying the competencies to be assessed. As stated earlier these will probably include a number of areas, some of which are difficult to assess by other means:

- relationship with patients
- attendance
- interest and motivation
- reliability
- clinical skills
- dress code/appearance.

"The specific learning outcomes specify the characteristics to be observed and the rating scale provides a convenient method of recording our judgements"

Gronlund & Linn 1990

Wording of descriptors

Rating scales are then developed for each competency with clearly defined descriptors. The following are examples from report forms used in phase 3 of the undergraduate medical programme in the University of Dundee.

Relationships with patients

1 Causes concern by being discourteous and/or not empathetic with patients. Puts personal convenience above patients' needs
2 Fair rapport. Occasionally discourteous if patient is hostile
3 Generally good rapport with patients but may be erratic
4 Widely recognised as being courteous and empathetic. Gives patient's needs priority even with hostile/unpleasant patients
– Not observed or applicable.

Attendance

1 Zero attendance
2 Sporadic attendance
3 Occasional unexplained absence. Does not always produce supportive documentation
4 Attends all sessions. If absent makes request known in advance or produces support documentation, e.g. medical certificate
– Not observed or applicable.

Interest and motivation

1 Poor self-motivation. Has to be prompted to participate in activities. Sometimes refuses to participate. Shows little interest.
2 Frequently needs prompting to participate. May lack confidence. Demonstrates variable level of interest.
3 Always participates. Asks spontaneous questions.
4 Highly self-motivated. Mature approach to activities. Makes specific requests.
– Not observed or applicable.

Reliability

1 Poor reliability. Work not well done or incomplete. Often absent/late for duties.
2 Occasionally forgetful.
3 Usually reliable. Work always done. Always present and prompt for clinical responsibilities.
4 Always reliable. Takes initiative for routine matters.
– Not observed or applicable.

Clinical skills

1 Unable to demonstrate basic procedures appropriate to stage in course.
2 Minimal level of basic skill. Needs work on procedures. Little progress.
3 Satisfactory basic skill appropriate to stage in course. Steady improvement.
4 Demonstrates superior mastery of basic skills. Performs in advance of clerkship level.
– Not observed or applicable.

Dress code/appearance

1 Appearance may cause offence to patients.
2 Dress/appearance may be inappropriate, unkempt or immodest.
3 Generally conforms to standard but may be untidy.
4 Appearance appropriate. Conforms with professional image.
– Not observed or applicable.

The development of accurate descriptors is a skilled process requiring knowledge of student behaviour at different ability levels in the range of competencies being assessed. Facility with language and an accurate description of the behaviours being described are also required. The descriptors should paint a picture of real and recognisable behaviour. The ability of the tutors to identify with the described behaviour is the key to the success of the structured tutor report. The descriptors minimise the effects of the presence of hawks and doves among raters and increase inter-rater reliability.

There should be space in the report for a written comment on the student and completion of this area should be enforced. The number of contact hours between student and tutor should be noted somewhere on the report.

Who should see the tutor report?

Tutor reports that are discussed with the student at the end of the attachment or better still at an intermediate point during the attachment are useful for providing feedback to students. Tutor reports can be included in the student portfolio and during subsequent portfolio assessment a number of reports from different tutors may form the basis of discussion between examiners and student.

Summary

Tutor reports provide the opportunity to assess students in areas which are difficult to test by other methods. They are useful in identifying students who are underperforming in the areas of personal attributes, attitudes, reliability or ability to work with other members of the health-care team. Some disadvantages however have been identified so guidelines should be followed if a tutor report is to be appropriately designed, used and evaluated. The construction of descriptors helps a tutor to grade student performance more accurately.

References and further reading

Das M, Mpofu D, Dunn E, Lanphear J H 1998 Self and tutor evaluations in problem-based learning tutorials: is there a relationship? Medical Education 32:411–418

Engel C E 1982 Clinical supervisor's report Medical Teacher 4:151–154

Gronlund N E, Linn R L 1990 Measurement and evaluation in teaching, 6th edn. Macmillan, New York

Guilford J P 1974 Psychometric methods, 2nd edn. McGraw-Hill, New York

Chapter 32
Portfolios, projects and dissertations

M. H. Davis

Introduction: what are portfolios?

A portfolio is literally 'a collection of papers'. Portfolios have been used to assess students – for example, in the fine arts – where material such as artwork produced by students during the course is just as important as written material.

Uses of portfolios

Interest in the use of portfolios for assessment in the health-care professions has developed as part of the move away from testing described in the quotation opposite, towards a broader use of assessment described as an assessment culture. This culture includes:

- closer links between assessment and learning
- the use of assessment to improve learning outcomes through the provision of feedback
- attempts to assess students in areas difficult to assess by traditional methods such attitudes and personal attributes.

The use of portfolios provides an opportunity to assess:

- Student course work and its documentation.
- Student attitudes through selection of material for inclusion in their portfolio. What students include in their portfolio highlights what they consider to be important. The portfolio contents are, therefore, a statement of what the student values.
- Student learning and progression of learning during the course. Through the use of commentaries on students' learning experiences during the course and

annotations of submitted work, teachers can explore the learning that has taken place.

Portfolios used for assessment purposes in undergraduate medical education may include:

- case reports
- a checklist of practical procedures undertaken
- video tapes of consultations
- descriptions of learning experiences
- commentaries on books or journals
- research project reports
- published work
- other achievements: for example, work undertaken on behalf of the student body or on the organisation of meetings or conferences.

Portfolios used formatively in postgraduate general practice training by Snadden & Thomas (1998) included:

- critical incidents of trainees' experiences with patients
- reflections on their difficulties and successes during the training period.

Many teachers in the health-care professions now assemble a teaching portfolio for job-seeking purposes. They identify the following ideas underlying the use of professional teaching portfolios. Portfolios:

- are reflective compendiums of self-selected artefacts
- are representations of teaching credentials and competencies
- offer holistic views of teachers
- provide documentation for strengthening interviews.

In this section, we deal with the use of portfolios in the undergraduate medical curriculum.

Construction of the portfolio

To construct the portfolio students may be given guidance in general terms about what contents to include, but they should make the selection. In preparing material for inclusion in the portfolio the student:

- takes part in a planned learning experience
- identifies how the experience relates to course

"These professional teaching portfolios provide teachers with vivid visual representations of themselves – self-portraits – as they apply for teaching positions"

Hurst, Wilson & Kramer 1998

objectives and outcomes
- identifies what has been learned
- identifies what further learning is required
- undertakes the further learning
- describes the further learning achieved.

If, for example, the learning experience is clerking a patient with thyrotoxicosis, the student identifies the course objectives to which this experience relates, such as patient examination, clinical diagnosis and initial patient management. The student is asked to reflect on what has been learned – perhaps that he or she has palpated a goitre and auscultated a bruit or that thyroid disease can be a serious problem but can be treated. The student may then identify that further learning needs to take place: for example, in relation to the familial incidence of the condition, the action of drugs or the reason for the choice of treatment. A description of the further learning undertaken is provided, possibly citing a chapter in a book or in a journal. The student then describes what further learning has been achieved in relation to the patient, such as the indications for surgery and for radio-iodine treatment.

The material below is from the portfolio of a fourth-year medical student at the University of Dundee Medical School. This phase of the curriculum employs a task-based learning educational strategy where student learning is focused around 100 tasks or core presentations (Harden et al 2000). This material related to a patient with a sore throat, one of the core presentations.

Description of patient

A 13-year-old girl with a long history of recurrent sore throats which tended to make her systemically unwell (fever, malaise, dysphagia) was seen as an in-patient in the ENT wards. Five years ago she had been seen by an ENT specialist as she was suffering from persistently discharging ears, enlarged adenoids and tonsils and suspected obstructive sleep apnoea. Although grommets were fitted at this time, no operative intervention was advised for her tonsils and adenoid problems.

Commentary

She was seen in September 1997 having had many days off school because of recurrent episodes of acute tonsillitis. On examination her tonsils were markedly enlarged and jugulodigastric nodes palpable. No abnormalities were detected in her ears. An elective tonsillectomy was arranged.

In December 1997 she had the tonsillectomy performed, the only complication being quite severe nausea and vomiting post-operatively for which she was prescribed ondansetron.

Immediate lessons

Recurrent ear infections such as described above do not necessarily lead to problems in later life if adequately investigated and treated. Repeated attacks of tonsillitis resulting in repeated school/work absences are an indication for surgical intervention.

Further learning required

- More precise indications for tonsillectomy
- Hazards/risks of such operative intervention
- Complications of acute tonsillar infection
- Causative organisms
- Non-operative treatment of tonsillitis

Methods of further case study

- Discussed with ENT consultant
- Studied ENT colour atlas and text
- Read ABC of otolaryngology

Discoveries made

Tonsillectomy is usually indicated in children with recurrent sore throats with lymphadenitis, for recurrent acute suppurative otitis media, for obstructive sleep apnoea syndrome, in children with a history of systemic complications of haemolytic streptococcal infection and for the rare condition of chronic tonsillar infection.

Risks of tonsillectomy include inhalation of blood during the operation, respiratory obstruction due to laryngeal spasm immediately after the operation, post-operative haemorrhage, and accidental damage to structures adjacent to the operating site (e.g. palate, uvula, cervical vertebrae and internal carotid artery). In small children, risks associated with blood loss are far greater due to their small blood volume. Complications of acute tonsillar infection include various abscesses: acute retropharyngeal abscess, peritonsillar abscess (quinsy) and acute otitis media. In addition, systemic diseases may occur as immunological responses to streptococcal infections. These include rheumatic fever and acute glomerulonephritis.

Causative organisms may be viral (~ 50%), bacterial or fungal. Viruses involved are influenza, parainfluenza, adenoviruses, respiratory syncytial viruses and rhinoviruses. Causative bacteria are usually haemolytic streptococci, less often *S. pneumoniae* and *H. influenzae* and rarely diphtheria and gonococcal infection. Finally, monilia is the commonest fungal infection that occurs in debilitated patients.

Treatment of acute tonsillitis should be started after taking throat swabs if at all possible. Penicillin is the drug of choice. The first dose should be given intravenously and the course continued orally for 10 days. Erythromycin, co-trimoxazole or augmentin are alternatives.

Advantages of portfolios

Assess difficult-to-test areas

There has been increasing interest in the use of portfolio assessment in medicine to assess curriculum outcomes that are not easily assessed in written tests. These outcomes include independent learning and taking responsibility for continuing professional development, critical thinking and professionalism.

Portfolios can be used to assess components of these curriculum outcomes:

- record keeping and report writing
- analysis, critical thinking and other attributes of scientific behaviour found in the reflective practitioner
- application of theory to practice
- use made of resources for learning

- attitudes
- progress made by the individual student.

Attitudes can be assessed
The learning identified by the student in the extract on pages 346–348 relates to knowledge of the basic and clinical sciences, clinical judgement and patient management. If, throughout the portfolio, the student consistently identifies learning in these areas and ignores learning associated with other curriculum outcomes such as ethical approaches and awareness of health promotion issues, then an attitude on the part of the student is revealed.

Curriculum outcomes can be emphasised
During discussion of the portfolio the tutor can explore the reasons for ignoring some curriculum outcomes and emphasising others. Thus the importance of all curriculum outcomes can be emphasised.

More effective student learning
Student learning can be made more effective through the use of portfolios. Opportunities for feedback to the student are provided during discussion of the portfolio with the tutor/teacher. The importance of the learning experiences provided for students is emphasised.

Other advantages
- Reflect a student-centred approach to learning. Students identify their own further learning needs and differences between students are acknowledged.
- Partners in learning. Partnerships between students and teachers are encouraged through discussion of learning needs.
- Continuous assessment. Opportunities for continuous assessment are provided through regular review of the portfolio.
- Learning progress. Progression of student competence can be demonstrated.
- Extent of learning assessed. Both the breadth and depth of student learning can be assessed.

- Self-expression and creativity. Opportunities for self-expression and creativity through selection of material and its presentation are provided.

Portfolio assessment can be used in undergraduate and postgraduate medical education. Portfolios are used for formative assessment and work is ongoing to evaluate the use of portfolios in summative assessment.

Snadden & Thomas (1998) described portfolio learning with general practice vocational trainees and emphasised its usefulness for providing feedback. They found the portfolio was used in four ways:

- as a tool for reminding, planning, tracking and encouraging reflection
- as a route to exploring attitudes and values to stimulate feedback
- as encouragement not humiliation
- as a bridge from hospital practice to general practice.

Disadvantages of portfolios

There has been little work published on the reliability and validity of portfolios when used to assess outcomes of the undergraduate medical curriculum and their use in summative assessment is an area of research interest. Many medical teachers are unfamiliar with the use of portfolios and staff development is needed before they can be employed in the undergraduate curriculum.

Assessing portfolios

To increase reliability between two and four examiners should be used to assess each student portfolio. A formal meeting is arranged between the student and the examiners at which the student presents the portfolio and discusses the contents with the examiners. It is important that the examiners have the opportunity to review the contents of the portfolio beforehand to ensure familiarity with the material the student has selected. The portfolio contents and the student responses during the discussion are assessed by the examiners using criteria distributed to students in advance of the examination. Examples of some of the criteria we employ are identified in Table 32.1.

Table 32.1   Criteria used in portfolio assessment

Points awarded	Grade	Descriptor
Record Keeping: Presentation of content		
1	Fails to meet the standard	Chaotic, no emphasis, accessing items generally difficult
2	Borderline	Disorganised/muddled at times. Some difficulty accessing material. Little attempt at emphasis.
3	Meets the standard	Clear layout, organised material, easily accessed. Key points emphasised.
4	Exceptional	Shows flair in layout and organisation. Portfolio 'shines'
Discussion of the portfolio		
Students are asked to identify the important features of an individual patient.		
1	Fails to meet the standard	Failure to identify salient features
2	Borderline	Identifies clinical features only in relation to presenting complaint
3	Meets the standard	Correctly identifies key features and links them to patient's ideas, concerns and contexts
4	Exceptional	High level of empathy with patient's situation. Student appropriately identifies key features and links them to patient's ideas, concerns and contexts
Patient management		
1	Fails to meet the standard	No suggestions
2	Borderline	Is able to provide one option but is unable to supply reasons regarding its acceptability/suitability
3	Meets the standard	Provides at least one acceptable management option with reasons
4	Exceptional	Is able to provide a range of different management options with reasons for acceptability or lack of it
Task-based learning		
This scale is designed to assess the student's ability to link theory to practice.		
1	Fails to meet the standard	Inability to link relevant theory to the cases discussed
2	Borderline	Sometimes uses inappropriate linkage of theory to the case
3	Meets the standard	Demonstrates ability to link theoretical aspects of the course appropriately to the cases discussed
4	Exceptional	The case is instrumental in driving theory acquisition
Further learning		
This scale is designed to assess utilisation of educational resources.		
1	Fails to meet the standard	Doesn't know what educational resources are available. Doesn't ask others
2	Borderline	Unsure of educational resource availability. Leans heavily on referral to colleagues/other health-care professionals

Points awarded	Grade	Descriptor
3	Meets the standard	Makes a reasonable attempt to answer patient problems by accessing other health-care professionals plus more than one educational resource
4	Exceptional	Uses a wide range of learning resources including other health-care professionals and knows how to access them without support

Scientific behaviour

Is the student able to reflect on what has been learned from seeing the patient?

1	Fails to meet the standard	Only addresses the issues of what, when and where
2	Borderline	Analytical skills becoming evident but poorly constructed
3	Meets the standard	Demonstrates the ability to analyse the case critically. Adequately assesses the whys and hows
4	Exceptional	Demonstrates the ability to analyse the case critically and apply the analysis to his or her own potential future situation

Portfolios are important records of student achievements. A public display of portfolios provides useful information for various stakeholders in medical education: for example, members of faculty, other students and employing authorities.

Implementing portfolio-based learning and assessment

The introduction of portfolio-based learning and assessment needs careful planning if it is to succeed. The contents of the portfolio need to fit in with course objectives; for example, if a skills checklist is a component of the portfolio, the skills included in it must be part of the course objectives. Students need clear guidelines about the type of material to be included in the portfolio and deadlines for submission of material are helpful to enable students to pace their work. This information may be included in student study guides or in handbooks provided at the start of the course.

We have found interim feedback helpful to both students and staff and we provide this by identifying the rate of student progress in meeting deadlines for submission of portfolio material and by giving feedback

"Students need considerable guidance if they are not to use a 'supermarket trolley' approach to portfolio assembly ('just shove it all in')"

Brown 1999

to students on their portfolios as part of end-of-course objective structured clinical examinations (OSCEs).

The estimates of student and staff time involved in completion of portfolios must be realistic.

Portfolios are important documents and their significance needs to be emphasised to all involved when they are introduced.

Staff development is essential for the successful introduction of portfolios, for training assessors in providing feedback and in using the rating scales to assess student learning in relation to the portfolio.

Projects and dissertations

What are projects and dissertations?

A dissertation is a piece of written work based on personal research. The research may be either a literature review or a piece of original work or both. The research is usually supervised and the level of supervision needs to be identified before the research starts. Discussion between the student and the supervisor is required to identify the appropriate level of supervision.

The term 'project' is usually applied to a smaller piece of research that may be carried out either individually or by groups of students. Medical students may be asked to carry out projects as part of the undergraduate programme, often as one afternoon per week over a period of several weeks.

Projects may be:

- questionnaire surveys
  - staff: violence and abuse in teaching hospitals
  - students: student attitudes to assessment in the undergraduate curriculum
  - patients: a survey of patients in a city general practice who are prescribed H_2 antagonists
  - other groups: a look at parental stress and the provision and adequacy of services provided to families with autistic children
- interview surveys
  - staff: which drugs do GPs carry in their emergency bags and are they in date?
  - patients: antenatal care – what do women want?

"Portfolios take a lot of looking at!"

Race 1996

"Most tutors will at some stage have faced a pile of written projects which are derivative, tedious, full of unreferenced, photocopied, unacknowledged material, which represent a vast amount of student work but do not represent a vast amount of student learning"

Brown & Knight 1994

If the student is allowed to select the area of research, it is likely to be personally relevant and motivation may be increased.

The opinion of pregnant women in two areas of Scotland with regard to provision of antenatal care
— other groups: a comparative view of school carers' and patients' perceptions of feeding difficulties occurring in children with neurological problems
- library reviews
  — investigations into medicinal uses of maggots
- practical research
  — laboratory: does the activity of glutathione S transferase modulate the expression of multiple self-healing squamous epitheliomata?
  — clinical: the effects of local anaesthetic on intravenous cannulation
- audit projects
  — assessing the quality of dialysis using the quality of dialysis scoring system
- case note surveys
  — the outcome of diabetic pregnancies in the city.

The outcomes of the research may be presented by the individual student or by the group as a report, a poster, a video tape, an audio tape, a short computer program, an oral presentation or written material.

Projects and dissertations are used for assessment purposes at both undergraduate and postgraduate levels.

Advantages of projects and dissertations

Projects and dissertations can be used to assess a range of curriculum outcomes. They can provide evidence of creativity through the way that the students present their results. They promote knowledge of the literature in the area of the research topic and an understanding of the importance of carrying out literature searches.

Through project work students can acquire a range of competencies:

- knowledge of a specific topic
- improved communication skills through interview surveys
- competence in practical procedures such as laboratory techniques or investigative procedures

- heightened awareness of ethical stances through access to patients and their records
- accuracy in dealing with data
- ability to handle and retrieve information
- improved critical thinking
- problem-solving skills
- time management.

Because the research is carried out over a period of time, projects and dissertations provide the opportunity to assess continuous work. They overcome the problems inherent in the 'big-bang' examination when short-term illness or 'an off-day' may adversely influence performance.

The research work may produce publishable material for inclusion in the student's portfolio.

Projects prepared by students can be used to teach subsequent cohorts of students, capitalising on the saying that 'to teach is to learn twice.'

Disadvantages of projects and dissertations

Identification of a piece of research that is capable of completion within the available time is critical to the success of this type of assessment. Experienced supervisors are necessary to recognise over-ambitious projects. The research needs to be realistically costed in terms of staff time, resources and finance, and adequate funds to cover the cost of the work must be identified. The agreed level of supervision must be provided and a series of short-term goals are useful for monitoring progress. Fraud and plagiarism are potential problems with this type of assessment. The requirement of a signed statement stating that the work is original is one way of validating this work.

How to assess projects and dissertations

The dissertation requires the ability to handle large quantities of information and to criticise, analyse and evaluate the information. Deadlines need to be met. The work needs to be presented in a coherent, lucid and compelling way. The significance of the conclusions needs to be appreciated and made explicit.

Criteria for assessment of the project or dissertation should be based on the competencies being assessed and need to be identified before the work begins. Rating scales are useful for this purpose, particularly where a number of people are involved in assessing the projects/dissertations. Peer assessment of project work – for example, voting on the best poster presentation – adds excitement to the process and is motivating for students and supervisors alike.

Summary

A portfolio is an innovative method of assessing student abilities and attitudes in areas which are less suitably assessed by traditional examinations. Students not only choose the material which they wish to include in their portfolio but also are encouraged to reflect on their work to identify what has been learned and what is yet to be learned.

The advantages and disadvantages of this approach are discussed and a method of assessing portfolios is described.

The completion of a project or a dissertation usually takes several weeks of part-time study during a senior year of the undergraduate medical course. Whether a survey, practical work or an audit project is chosen, close supervision and guidance from a tutor are required. Innovative methods of assessment can be employed to add extra interest to this approach.

References and further reading

Brown S, Knight P 1994 Assessing learners in higher education. Kogan Page, London

Brown S 1999 Assessment matters in higher education. The Society for Research into Higher Education and Open University Press, Buckingham

Gipps C 1994 Beyond testing. Falmer, London

Harden R M, Crosby J R, Davis M H, Howie P W, Struthers A D 2000 Task-based learning; the answer to integration and problem-based learning in the clinical years. Medical Education 34:391–397

Hurst B, Wilson C, Cramer G 1998 Professional teaching portfolios: tools for reflection, growth and advancement. Phi Delta Kappan April: 578–582

Race P 1996 The art of assessing: 2. New Academic 5(1):3–6

Snadden D S, Thomas M L 1998 Portfolio learning in general practice vocational training – does it work? Medical Education 32: 401–406

Chapter 33
Objective clinical examinations

I. Hart

Introduction

The need for performance-based testing
The basic underpinnings of clinical competence are:

- knowledge
- skills
- attitudes

Competence in a clinical situation is the complex ability to apply these appropriately as needed. Performance is the translation of competence into action.

In simple terms the basics are 'do they know it' and 'do they know how'; competence is 'can they do it' and performance is 'do they show how'.

Although we have many methods for evaluating student and postgraduate trainees' knowledge and some for measuring skills, our ability to measure clinical performance reliably is quite limited.

Assessment methods must meet three criteria to be fair and credible to those being assessed. They must be:

- valid
- reliable
- feasible

In its simplest sense, validity is the concept that the test method is actually capable of measuring that which it purports to measure; for example, writing a brief essay on how to do a lumbar puncture in no way predicts someone's ability to carry out the procedure. Reliability, in its simplest form, is the reproducibility of the results for example, would the same candidate, given the same examination repeatedly score the same? Finally,

"When evaluation is judgmental, people will try to hide their ignorance. What we really want is for people to reveal their ignorance so that we can remedy it"

George Miller

"I believe that teaching without testing is like cooking without tasting"

Ian Lang, Scottish Education Secretary

The OSCE is now used routinely in over 50 countries worldwide. There is a national OSCE in Canada, taken by all medical school graduates before they are granted a licence to practise.

although rigorous repetitive testing might give answers closer to the truth, examination processes must be feasible within the constraints of the limited time and resources available in most clinical training settings.

Examinations of clinical competence have traditionally used the long and short case viva approach. Although this approach appears to have validity – the candidates are tested on real patients and asked clinical problem-solving questions – since candidates are tested on different cases, of different difficulty and judged by different standards by different examiners, reliability of the results may be somewhat suspect.

In order to overcome the poor reliability of clinical examinations, objective clinical examinations were developed in the 1970s and are gaining in use worldwide.

The prototype of these is the objective structured clinical examination (OSCE).

The objective structured clinical examination (OSCE)

In the OSCE, candidates rotate through a series of stations at which they are asked to carry out a (usually clinical) task. In most stations they are observed (by one or more examiners) and scored as they carry out the task; in others they may interpret clinical materials (e.g. laboratory data, X-rays), write notes or answer questions.

The major difference from other types of clinical examination is that over the course of the OSCE, all candidates are given the same clinical and other challenges and assessed by the same judges using the same preset standards.

In a way, the OSCE is not an examination method; rather it is an examination format or framework into which many different types of test method can be incorporated. There are certain basic ground rules:

- There are multiple stations, each testing different competencies.
- Each station has a time limit (usually the same).

- All candidates rotate through all the stations and thus are tested on the same material.
- All are judged by the same preset standards – usually using checklists or rating scales.

Providing these are followed, the OSCE can incorporate tests of:

- various skills – history-taking, physical examination, procedure (on models), communication, interpersonal skills
- knowledge and understanding
- data interpretation
- problem-solving
- attitudes.

A variety of test methods may be used, including

- short cases
- oral exams (vivas)
- interpretation of laboratory results and images
- computerised problem-solving.

In order to ensure that all candidates are tested on the same clinical material (patients), trained volunteers role-play as so-called standardised patients (SPs), particularly for history-taking but also for some physical examination stations. Real patients are sometimes used but should be coached on giving their history in a reliable fashion.

Trained SPs are widely used in North America for both teaching and assessment (including OSCEs). Most medical schools there have such programmes established as an integral part of their curriculum.

The original OSCE stations tended to be only 4–7 minutes in length. Although this suffices for some basic clinical skills or some very focused history-taking or examination, longer stations are required for more complex performance-based testing and many multiple-station examinations for senior students and postgraduate trainees are longer in duration – even up to 20 minutes.

Obviously since longer stations allow fewer candidates to be tested in the same length of time there has to be some kind of balance between the duration of the stations, the number of stations and the number of

"The great end in life is not knowledge, but action"

Thomas Huxley

The OSCE is all about measuring actions.

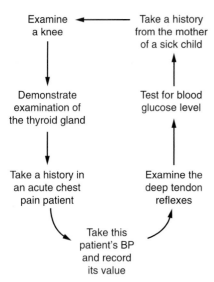

Fig. 33.1   Example of OSCE testing

"*The trouble with our evaluation system is that we use it as a drunk uses a lamppost, more for support than illumination*"

Steyn

Generalisability theory, a psychometric approach to the reliability of testing, indicates that you cannot generalise from affirmed competence in one area to assumed competence in all others. In other words, you cannot assume since someone performs well in depth in one long neurology case that that person is competent across the whole wide range of medicine.

candidates in order to meet the restraints of time and resources.

Figure 33.1 gives an example of what a small OSCE testing basic clinical skills might look like (5-minute stations).

The real power of multi-station objective clinical examinations

It may seem that such examinations simply improve the reliability of clinical examinations by segmenting and compartmentalising individual skills. OSCE-type examinations do, or can do, much more.

Advantages of multiple station examinations

- Since each station can test a totally different content area, the candidate's knowledge and skills over a whole range of topics can be tested. The psychometric evidence is good that testing in less depth over many topic areas gives a more reliable and valid indication of an individual's competence than testing in depth in one or two areas.
- As they test a wide variety of competencies – knowledge, skills or attitudes over a wide range of content areas, they force the use of different test methods – vivas, writtens, practicals, computer-based as appropriate.
- The breadth of content areas tested and the flexibility in test methods used allow testing to encompass not only knowledge and skills, but attitudes as well, e.g. a station may have a component that requires ethical decision-making.
- They allow the efficient use of limited resources, e.g. even though every patient sees the same 'Mrs Jones', the same computer and the same set of X-rays, so everyone sees them at different points in time, you need only one set of each.
- Since the items on the checklist and/or rating scale for each station are agreed upon by a group of experts before the examination and a scoring scheme is predetermined, the examination is more objective

than subjective (i.e. the judgement of only one person).

- Finally, this type of examination, with its formalised marking and scoring scheme, allows specific profiling of each component by performance. This allows each student's performance to be profiled precisely, e.g. station by station, component by component (history-taking, physical examination, data interpretation etc.) and by knowledge, skills and attitudes.

The real power of this type of examination lies in the ability of those responsible for teaching and testing to examine their trainees with imagination and forethought, in a reliable way, in areas seldom or never tested before.

With care and planning, most learning objectives for most courses can be tested using this technique. However, it is important to emphasise that the OSCE does not replace all other examination formats. Knowledge testing and writing skills are still more efficiently tested in written examinations (increasingly delivered electronically online).

Figure 33.2 gives an example of a higher-level (postgraduate surgical) OSCE using longer stations (12–15 minutes) and demonstrates the wide range of competencies that can be tested in this type of format. Most of the stations shown have actually been used; the others have been projected as possibilities for future inclusion.

Not only would such an examination cover a variety of content areas within surgery – from gastroenterology through orthopaedics and urology to trauma; it also uses a variety of test methods – written, practical, clinical, computer-assisted testing and simulations – to test the whole range of knowledge, psychomotor skills, attitudes and interpersonal skills.

Breaking down the elements of competence that such an OSCE would be testing demonstrates the range that can be covered in one examination meeting the generalisability test. Such a breakdown is outlined in Table 33.1.

The OSCE allows very specific feedback, not only to the candidates, but also to those who taught them and to those who set the examination.

If there is a set of explicit learning objectives for the course, these can be used along with imagination to develop a series of stations that can test them in as close to real-life situations as possible.

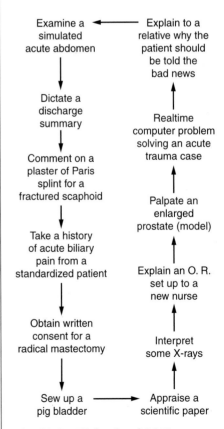

Fig. 33.2 Higher level OSCE

Table 33.1   Elements of competence tested in an OSCE

Task	Content area	Type	Cognitive	Psychomotor	Attitude
Abdominal examination	GI	SP encounter	+	+++	++
Discharge summary	General	Essay	+++		
PoP scaphoid	Orthopaedic	Practical	+	+++	+
Biliary history	GI	History	+++		++
Written consent	Oncology	Counsel	++		+++
Suturing	General	Practical		+++	
Scientific appraisal	Research	Essay	+++		
X-rays	General	Data interpretation	+++		
Explain O.R.	General	Oral	+++		+
Prostate examination	Urology	Clinical		+++	
Computer simulation	Trauma	Simulation	+++		
Interview relative	General	SP encounter	++		+++

Planning, preparing and running objective clinical examinations

Planning the outline

The first step in planning the outline of the overall examination is to review the course learning objectives. If, as is unfortunately still too often the case, no complete set of objectives is available (and there is not enough time to prepare one), those responsible should come to a consensus as to exactly what competencies they wish to test.

This whole process is made much easier if the planners already have a bank of OSCE stations that they have already used – or access to someone else's bank from which they can borrow and (with permission) possibly modify appropriate stations.

The rest of this outline for planning an OSCE assumes that the stations are being developed *de novo*.

The steps involved are as follows:

• Come to a consensus on the list of areas of competence that need to be tested.

For each – define the:

• content area to be addressed

"The devil is in the detail"

Planning an OSCE is much easier if the course being tested has a set of explicit learning objectives. Not having these, however, should not be an excuse not to run this type of examination. If it were, we would run no examinations at all! Develop them as you go.

- problem or challenge in the station that addresses it
- clearly state whether the station will attempt to measure knowledge, skills or attitudes
- Map out the plan of all of the stations indicating in a simple phrase the scenario being used – similar to the flow charts in Figures 33.1 and 33.2. This approach keeps the outline simple and easy to understand at a glance.

Planning the details of each station

For each station the following details must be addressed by the planning group:

- List the specific:
  - content area – organ system/problem/disease
  - domains – cognitive/affective/psychomotor
  - objectives – behavioural
- Write a scenario:
  - who/when/why/where/what
- Develop instructions to the candidate:
  - precise
  - concise
  - unambiguous
- Develop a checklist containing:
  - key features
  - a score for overall technique
  - if applicable – a score for attitude
- Draw up a scoring scheme which assigns a percentage of the station mark for:
  - the checklist
  - possibly a weight for each item or group
  - the score for overall technique
  - the attitude score
- Draw up a list of resources including:
  - space – i.e. the site to run the examination
  - people
  - equipment
  - materials
- Write instructions to the simulator and, if necessary, a script for role-playing.

Getting and training volunteers to act as standardised patients is not as difficult as you might think. Many medical schools have a group of these who assist not only in testing but also in teaching.

Devising a scoring scheme and setting the standard for pass/fail

Usually each station counts equally in the overall score of the examination, but this must be explicit.

Since each station has a scoring sheet which usually consists mainly of a checklist of each component of the skill being tested, decisions have to be made concerning the weighting given to each item on the checklist. Usually each is rated as '1' but sometimes decisions are made that certain items are weighted at more or less than '1'.

If the scoring sheet uses rating scales to rate overall technique and/or attitude, it must be predetermined how much each of these contributes to the station score.

If there are answers to be verbalised or written, how much each contributes to the overall station score must be decided.

Finally, how are decisions going to be made regarding who passes or who fails? The commonest approach is to add up the candidate's scores for all the stations and express them as a percentage of the potential total score. Sometimes, however, an approach is taken that assigns a pass/fail mark for each station and the overall pass/fail decision is based on the candidate passing a set number of stations.

The very complex issue of deciding on how and at what level to set pass/fail marks is beyond the scope of this chapter.

Running the objective clinical examination

When it comes to running the OSCE, the devil was really in the planning and preparation phases. If the preparations were complete and rigorous, the running of it should be simple. The one major factor that has not been addressed is the site for the examination.

The ideal place for this type of examination is a clinical skills unit of appropriate size. If this is not available, the second-best choice is an outpatient department on a day that it is not being used for patients. Failing those possibilities, an empty ward is probably the best alternative, though privacy can be an issue in such a setting.

Knowledge is information stored in learners' minds. Either they have it or they do not. In a way it is digital – yes/no.

Skills are actions (and reactions) which a person performs in a competent way in order to achieve a goal.

One may have no skill, some skill or complete skill. Acceptable mastery must be set appropriate to the level of the student's training: not yes/no, but analogue along a spectrum.

Because of the relatively small numbers of stations that it is practical to set up for any given examination (12–18 is common, though up to 30 have been used in some high-stakes examinations) and the not uncommon problem of large numbers of students to be tested (even within single institutions up to 200 or more) sometimes the set of stations has to be 'cloned' either in space or in time.

Where possible, this is done by setting up clones of the examination at several sites – e.g. wards – or even different hospitals – and running them simultaneously. Even then, sometimes it is necessary to run more than one iteration of the examination. If possible these should be run on the same day and, for credibility's sake, attempts should be made to prevent sharing of examination experiences between candidates from different streams.

Interestingly enough, it appears from a number of studies that, providing the confidentiality of the checklist contents and scoring schemes is kept intact, students sharing information about the general nature of the stations (e.g. those who took the exam one day those taking it later in the week) do not apparently influence student scores.

Obviously, conducting the OSCE at multiple sites or over different times or days increases the logistical complexity, but providing the responsibilities of the key organisers of the examination are clear and are taken seriously, this is not exponential. Similarly, running an OSCE for the first time may seem formidable, but each subsequent time for the same team is much easier.

A preparation timeline
Depending on the importance of the examination and the number of candidates and stations the timetable for planning and implementing an OSCE will vary. An example for a relatively small (e.g. end-of-attachment) examination follows.

Before the examination
- 8 weeks   Select date and appoint overall coordinator and site coordinator

An attitude is a feeling about an object, concept or idea which may be based on knowledge or experience, and which results in an action tendency (positive or negative) about that object, concept or idea. Attitudes have valence, i.e. they may be strongly or weakly positive or negative.

- 6 weeks — Decide on station tasks, book site and refreshments, make local arrangements Allocate individual station responsibilities to specific faculty members. Ensure they know what they have to do. Note requirements for SPs, recruit people and start training
- 3 weeks — Review all station details and have them approved by overall coordinator; revise where necessary
- 2 weeks — Have all station paperwork printed, signs made, equipment prepared; remind station examiners of the examination
- 24 hours — Walk through examination site with site coordinator. If possible, i.e. if site is now available, set up signs, equipment, furnishings etc.
- 2 hours — All coordinators on-site
- 1 hour — Final briefing of examiners and SPs
- 30 minutes — All examiners and SPs at stations Students' orientation/briefing

Examination

After the examination
- Immediate — Feedback from those involved
- 1 week — Results and feedback to students.

Summary

One of the major problems with traditional clinical examinations (e.g. long and short cases) is that they all too often test very limited content areas and seldom measure much beyond factual recall and a few basic skills. In addition, since all the candidates are tested on different cases, by different examiners and often using different standards, such examinations, though having face validity, lack reliability and fairness.

Objective clinical examinations consist of a circle of stations through which each student rotates while the

*"There is something much more scarce.
Something finer far.
Something rarer than ability.
It is the ability to recognize ability"*

E Hubbard

examiner(s) remain constant. At each station a different clinical task is performed, usually observed by the same examiner using checklists or rating scales. This ensures that each candidate is faced with the same tasks or cases and judged by the same preset standards.

This type of examination, if well planned, also ensures that candidates are tested over several content areas within the discipline being tested and allows a wide variety of attributes to be tested including interpersonal skills, knowledge and understanding, psychomotor skills (e.g. physical examination, procedures etc.), data interpretation and attitudes. The station format allows the use of test methods appropriate to the task being tested including the use of real patients, standardised (simulated) patients, written, short structured vivas, computers, simulators and others.

OSCEs provide an efficient use of resources (patients, SPs, computers, X-rays) since although candidates are tested on the same set, they all do it at a different point in time.

The scoring and marking infrastructure of this type of examination allows the profiling of student performance by station and by attribute, e.g. history-taking skills, interpersonal skills, data interpretation, problem-solving. This enables specific and useful feedback to be given to each candidate. It also provides the curriculum planners and teachers with useful feedback regarding learning deficiencies or gaps involving the group, thus enabling planning for remedial teaching for the current set of students, and fine-tuning of the curriculum of the course being tested.

This type of examination can be run for small groups of students or postgraduate trainees, but by cloning the set of OSCE stations, either at different sites or over a period of time, as many as several hundred candidates can be tested.

Though complex to set up and run at first, the development of a management team, an organisational plan, a timetable and ultimately a bank of reusable OSCE stations makes later examinations decreasingly demanding on those involved.

References and further reading

Brailovsky C A, Grand'Maison P, Lescop J 1992 A large-scale multi-centre objective clinical examination for licensure. Academic Medicine 67:S37–39

Harden R M 1990 Twelve tips for organising an objective structured clinical examination (OSCE). Medical Teacher 12:259–264

Harden R M, Gleeson F A 1979 Assessment of medical competence using an objective structured clinical examination. ASME Medical Education booklet no. 8

Hart I R 1986 The objective structured clinical examination. In: Lloyd J S, Langsley D G (eds) How to Evaluate Residents, American Board of Medical Specialties, Chicago, Il, pp. 13–146

Mann K V, MacDonald A C 1990 Reliability of objective structured clinical examinations: four years of experience in a surgical clerkship. Teaching and Learning in Medicine 2:219–224

Smee S M, Blackmore D E 1997 Preparing physician examiners for a high stakes, multi-site OSCE. In: Scherpbier A J J A, van der Vleuten C P M, Rethans J J van der Steeg A F W (eds) Advances in Medical Education (Proceedings of the Seventh Ottawa Conference on Medical Education, Maastricht). Kluwer Academic, Dordrecht, pp. 462–464

Van der Vleuten C P M, Swanson D B 1990 Assessment of clinical skills with standardized patients: state of the art. Teaching and Learning in Medicine 2:58–76

Chapter 34
External examiners

C. D. Forbes

Introduction

No matter what course of education is undertaken, it is critical for the candidate to be assessed or examined in some shape or form. In medicine, it has long been agreed that external examiners are required as assessors from outside the medical school to ensure that a common national standard is reached. This chapter will explore a variety of aspects of the role of external examiners and the problems associated with their use (Walters, Sivanesaratnam & Hamilton 1995). It is also clear that it is not just within countries that external examiners are required; they are needed to compare standards across Europe and internationally.

The alternative to having external examiners is to have external examinations and this has become the norm in the USA and Canada where various National Boards have been constituted. These include the national board of Medical Examiners (NBME), the Federal License Examinations (FLEX), the Educational Commission for Foreign Medical Graduates (ECFMG) and the Board Examinations in most specialties. These national examinations are an attempt to impose a standard at national level while allowing individual schools to develop their own curricula and to draw on their own strengths. By their very nature they consist of paper-based questions. To introduce a standardised objective structured clinical examination (OSCE) raises major logistical problems which still require to be overcome. The strength of such examinations is that they can act as a comparator, comparing the end results of a course in medical education delivered by a variety of means in

"we make the examination the end of education, not an accessory in its acquisition"

Osler 1913

"The concept of the external examiner appeals to notions of the universality of educational standards and justice for the individual student"

Walters, Sivanesaratnam & Hamilton 1995

"A major guarantee of quality and equality in higher education"

Piper 1985

" . . . would promote higher quality medical education across the Continent"

Nystrup & Mårtenson 1992

different schools. In addition a national examination would allow comparison of the achievements of the teaching process in different schools as part of the recent Teaching Quality Assessment (TQA) exercise seen in the United Kingdom.

What is an external examiner?

Most universities in the UK accept the Committee of Vice Chancellors and Principals' Code of Practice for external examining in universities at first degree and taught masters level (CVCP 1985). This has since been extensively modified but sets down the rules for the appointment of external examiners. They should be of high regard within their profession and should be acknowledged leaders academically, clinically and as teachers in their medical subjects. They have to be objective in their assessment of the school they are visiting and remain impartial and dedicated to the setting and maintenance of national medical standards. They must also understand that as well as a global role in the examination system they have a responsibility to ensure that individual students are also looked at objectively, especially if there have been previous problems of discipline or performance in any individual.

Appointment

External examiners are appointed by the university court on the recommendation of the appropriate department and the appointment is endorsed by the relevant dean. It is usual for the head of department to have already approached the potential external examiner to ensure that he or she is willing and able to undertake the duties which are set out below and therefore willing to serve as and when required for the appropriate duration. The usual duration of appointment is 3 years in the first instance and may be extended to 4 years. It is not usual for the external to be reappointed after that time for another period of office. It is also not usual for previous staff members to be appointed as external examiners to their previous department until a period of 3 years has elapsed.

An external examiner should not usually hold more than two other external examinerships for undergraduate courses. Care must be taken that the external examiner is not from a department in another institution in which a member of staff of the home department is currently serving as an external examiner. This is to avoid the possibility of a 'quid pro quo' situation. It is important that external examiners feel no pressure is brought to bear on them to provide a report other than a totally objective assessment of the quality of the course and it is usual that the report goes directly to the principal of the university and not directly to the department.

Duties of the external examiner

Duties of the external examiner will vary with the different phases of the curriculum. In the first year of the course, where the emphasis is on the scientific background of disease, it is difficult to find a single external examiner who is sufficiently knowledgeable in anatomy, biochemistry and physiology to cover all these requirements. It is therefore usual to have a panel of people with specialist knowledge. The middle years consist of mechanisms of disease and the start of the clinical curriculum. These are now totally integrated and a small panel of examiners overview the various subjects. By the last 2 years the curriculum is wholly clinical, covering the specialties of medicine, surgery, obstetrics, gynaecology, child health, psychiatry and general practice. Appropriate external examiners with the required clinical skills are appointed in each of these subjects, even though some of the examinations are now coordinated.

Special study modules present rather different problems because of their diverse nature and content and examiners for these must be chosen with special care (see Chapter 5).

Requirements for an external examiner

There is much more to being external examiners than just being present at the medical school on a few days per

"a visiting assessor of high academic standing and possessed of absolute integrity and objectivity"

Walters, Sivanesaratnam & Hamilton 1995

Choose a respected senior from another university:

- who has a reputation for ability in teaching/assessment and clinical care/research
- who can give the time commitment
- who has been involved in curriculum development
- who has a robust personality.

year. They must now expect to fulfil a contract with the other medical school which requires them to:

- have time to do the job
- have a broad range of knowledge
- be an established teacher
- be intimately aware of the curriculum to be examined before starting the examinations; prior briefing is required or better still a 'dry run' as an observer
- accept a firm brief or job description of the particular task
- be prepared to do the job for 3 years with the option of a further year
- be prepared to attend several times for the one examination which may be in different parts, and also to attend the meeting of the board of examiners and provide detailed discussion on students who fail to meet the standards.

It is important to say that external examiners are not to be appointed to rubber-stamp the processes of an individual school, subject or the internal examiner and preferably should not be appointed because they are old friends of the head of department.

They must have neutral attitudes to:

- gender
- race
- colour
- creed.

Approval of examination papers

All examination papers for a particular part of the course must be approved by the external examiners of the course. External examiners should contribute to the questions and ensure that their contribution is actually added to the examination paper. It would then be usual for an external examiner to be asked to mark that particular question, having provided an optimal outline answer. The external examiner should see the final format of the paper to check it for errors of omission or commission. There is now a requirement for papers to be marked by two examiners and to be marked anonymously. It is the duty of the external examiner to see that this is carried out. It is also usual for the external examiner to look at a range of approximately 10% of all the candidates' answers, once marked, to ensure that an appropriate standard is met. If there is to be an oral examination after the written examination, then this survey of the works should be done before the oral takes place. The external examiner should look at the better students in the year if there is a question of grading their marks as a 'merit' or 'distinction', as well as looking at all the borderline candidates. At the oral examination, external examiners should identify themselves to the candidate (wear a name badge) and clearly indicate that they are from outside that school and hence 'neutral'. In addition, external examiners should look at all other pieces of work which are part of the assessment system and in particular course work which may include essays, projects and posters. It is more difficult for externals to come regularly to a far-off university to look at presentations and attend seminars and so on, and probably this should not be required of them, but they should be in a position to make comments about the content of the course and the assessment system. The alternative is for course work to be sent in bulk to the external examiner.

Clinical examinations

External examiners should be prepared to give up enough time, often 2 or 3 days, to take part in the clinical examinations of a particular part of the course. This now tends to be done at the end of each teaching block so it may involve three or four visits to the school each year. Normally they would be paired with an internal examiner of equivalent seniority and, once again, they should see the top and bottom ends of the spectrum of students. The profile of marks in previous internal examinations of the same course should be made available to them. It is particularly important that external examiners be involved with students who are likely to be deficient and at risk of not passing the diet of

On appointment external examiners should be given:

- a detailed briefing on the curriculum with a focus on the part they are to examine
- a 'job description' of what is expected of them
- an agreement which they sign to indicate their willingness to attend as required over the period of the appointment.

examinations. They should make available sufficient time to attend the board of examiners when each of these candidates is discussed in detail, especially if there is compensation in terms of other marks which might allow a candidate's work to be upgraded. External examiners report directly to the principal of the university and not to the head of department, the dean or the faculty.

Their report should follow the recommendations of the Committee of Vice Chancellors and Principals' Code of Practice (1985). The following questions are based on the requirements of the Academic Standards Committee, University of Dundee (1996):

- Was the information supplied on the course structure, content and methods of assessment adequate?
- Was the administration of the external process satisfactory?
- Was the assessment process appropriate to the subject matter and to the students?
- Were the examinations sufficiently comprehensive with regard to the course examined?
- Were the facilities and material for practical and/or clinical examinations adequate?
- Was there adequate opportunity to see scripts of borderline candidates and also of students at the top end of the scale?
- Was there access to a sufficient number and range of papers to enable a view to be formed as to whether internal marking was appropriate and consistent?
- Was there sufficient access to course work to enable the exercise of effective external judgement?
- Were the procedures followed by the board of examiners impartial and equitable?
- Were course objectives sufficiently well defined and appropriate to the subject matter and to the students?
- Was the course structure and content appropriate to the level at which it was taught?
- Were the quality of teaching and the methods used, as revealed in examinations, effective and appropriate?
- Was the general quality of candidates' work satisfactory?

- Was the failure rate acceptable?
- Was the distribution of final honours, merit or distinction comparable with other institutions?
- Were the standards achieved by students consistent with standards elsewhere in UK universities?

It is to be noted that the payment of the external examiner's fee is only authorised under receipt of this report and that this ensures almost 100% compliance!

Examination exemption and curriculum development

External examiners should also be involved in exemption schemes and should be consulted by departmental boards if new courses are to be introduced or if there are substantial changes to existing courses. As a result of the General Medical Council's (GMC) drive to change the curriculum, it is also appropriate now to involve external examiners in curriculum development. The above information applies to the United Kingdom currently but in countries such as Canada, the United States and Australia there is movement towards a national curriculum with accreditation of medical schools and courses and centralisation of the examination system. The British system continues to be used in many former colonies and it is common for external examiners to be required for these medical schools. Indeed it is common for the GMC to employ experienced examiners in this role for their own purposes abroad and in the UK for the examination of the Professional and Linguistic Assessment Board (PLAB).

The cost of external examination

There is little doubt that universities will continue to want objective assessment of their courses and require external reviews despite the costs for travel and accommodation plus fees. Thus it is important that the system does not degenerate into a 'freebie' for academic chums. Care must be taken also to offer hospitality

" . . . against retention of the external examiner system is its high cost"

Walters, Sivanesaratnam & Hamilton 1995

during the stay which is commensurate with the job but which does not attract criticism as being too lavish or having any other motivation.

Summary

The role of the external examiner remains critical to universities to ensure the maintenance of educational standards both nationally and internationally. Careful selection of the individual examiner is necessary. As considerable abilities are required in the development of innovative curricula the external examiner is often involved with contributing to the oversight of the whole course and not just of the written papers, clinical examinations and vivas. It must be recognised that such a position brings kudos to the home university and consequently appropriate time and resources should be given to enable the role to be filled adequately.

References and further reading

Academic Standards Committee 1996 External examiners for undergraduate and postgraduate courses. University of Dundee, Dundee

Committee of Vice Chancellors and Principals 1985 The external examiner system for first degree and taught masters courses. Revised code of practice. CVCP, London

Nystrup J, Mårtenson D 1992 Reflections on possible virtues of European medical education. Medical Education 26:350–353

Osler W 1913 An introductory address on examinations, examiners and examinees. Lancet 11:1047–1050

Piper W D 1985 Enquiry into the role of the external examiners. Study on Higher Education 10:331–342

Walters W A, Sivanesaratnam V, Hamilton J D 1995 External Examiners. Lancet 345:1093–1095

SECTION 7
STUDENTS AND STAFF

Chapter 35
Student selection

I. C. McManus

Introduction

Selection seems deceptively easy; with more applicants than places, one simply selects the best applicants. In practice the process is much more complicated and may be:

- of dubious validity
- statistically unreliable
- a vulnerable process within the medical school
- open to legal challenge on grounds such as discrimination
- criticised by society at large
- under-resourced, particularly when compared with a medical school's implicit expectations of what it can do.

Why select?

A selection programme must clearly state the reasons for selection. If the only reason is reduction of numbers a lottery-type process would suffice. In reality selection is a complex process with several different stages.

Selection of students by the medical school

The straightforward reason is to choose the best students. Although seemingly simple, this contains many complexities.

Selection by applicants of medicine as a career

The pool of applicants for medical schools to choose from consists only of those who have selected medicine

"Selection is of key importance to medical education. What sort of students are recruited at the beginning is a major determination of what kind of doctors come out at the end"

Downie & Charlton 1992

"although there are reasons for being anxious about medical school selection, not all of the blame can be laid at the door of the selectors. Self-selection and preselection out of the applicant pool is extensive"

Johnson 1971

as a career. The majority of the population who did not apply cannot be selected, even if they might make excellent doctors.

Selection of the medical school by applicants

Applicants study *all* medical schools and then choose which to apply to. There is no point in running a good selection system if most good applicants have already applied elsewhere. An effective selection system must encourage the best students to apply to a school.

Explicit selection of medical schools by applicants

Applicants receiving offers from several medical schools make an explicit choice and select one from those on offer. McManus et al 1999 have shown that schools which interview are twice as likely to be preferred to schools which do not.

Selection for a particular course

Increasingly medical schools are developing courses with different emphases. A course, for example, with a large component of problem-based learning in small groups might choose to select students who can work together in a cooperative rather than a competitive fashion.

Selection by staff

If staff have been actively involved in the selection process and have met the students as applicants a relationship can develop which can enhance the educational process. Staff feel ownership of selection and students feel membership of the institution.

The limits of selection

There is a fundamental misconception that medical schools receive numerous applications. In practice the ratio in the UK is about two applicants for every place, although from the perspective of admissions officers it may seem much more than that, because each candidate makes multiple applications. The power of selection depends to a large extent on the 'selection ratio', the

"The aim is not to pick men and women for specific tasks but to train wise, bright, humane, multipotential individuals who will find their niche somewhere in medicine"

Richards & Stockill 1997

number of applicants for each place. As the ratio grows, so selection can be more effective.

The limits of selection can be shown in a straightforward mathematical model. For example, if selecting on a single criterion (such as intellectual ability), assuming that this ability has a normal distribution and that the selection ratio is two applicants for every place the optimal selection is as shown in Figure 35.1. Place the candidates in rank order and take those above the median.

The limits of selection appear when two or more criteria are introduced. For example, if selecting on two independent (orthogonal) criteria (intellectual ability and communication skills) there will now be a bivariate normal distribution (see Fig. 35.2) and the aim is to take the best 50% of candidates on the joint criteria. The dashed lines indicate the means of the distributions, which would be the threshold if there were only one characteristic.

There are several ways to select the best 50%, according to the extent to which high ability on one criterion can compensate for poorer performance on the other, though all have similar effects (McManus & Vincent 1993). If selected candidates have to be above a certain threshold on *both* criteria they must be in the top right-hand corner of the figure. The important thing is that the threshold on either criterion must be substantially below the median. In fact, with two independent criteria, candidates selected are only in the top 71% of the ability range, rather than the top 50%. Therefore they are less able on average on either criterion than if it had been the sole criterion.

So if one selects principally on just one attribute, and wishes to select also on a second attribute, it is necessary to reduce one's criterion on the first attribute. In the UK medical student selection is currently based predominantly on academic achievement. If it is felt desirable to take non-academic factors into account then current academic standards will have to be lowered.

Once medical schools have started considering non-academic attributes for selection then they rapidly

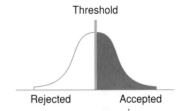

Threshold

Rejected   Accepted

Fig. 35.1   A simple model of selection when there is a single characteristic on which selection is taking place. Those above the threshold are accepted, those below are rejected

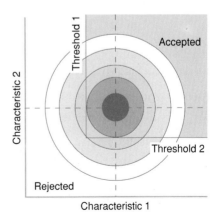

Fig. 35.2   Example showing joint criteria

Table 35.1   The effects of selection on multiple criteria (McManus & Vincent 1993)

Number of independent selection criteria	Proportion of applicants rejected on any single criterion
1	Bottom 50%
2	Bottom 29.3%
3	Bottom 20.6%
4	Bottom 15.9%
5	Bottom 12.9%
6	Bottom 10.9%
10	Bottom 6.7%
20	Bottom 3.4%
50	Bottom 1.4%
N*	Bottom $100.\left(1-N\sqrt{\tfrac{1}{r}}\right)$%

* N = number of criteria: r = selection ratio (i.e. 1/r is the proportion of applicants accepted).

develop a long list. Even if these are not all statistically independent, one rapidly ends up with a system with 5, 10, 20 or even 50 statistical dimensions. Extending the selection process (see Figure 35.2) to three, four or five criteria and so on shows how the limits of selection rapidly appear. In Table 35.1 the proportion of candidates eliminated on a single criterion (shown in the second column) becomes smaller as the number of criteria rise. The criteria are assumed to be independent, and the selection ratio to be two (i.e. 50% of candidates are selected). To summarise it pithily, 'if one selects on everything one selects on nothing.' Therefore:

- Selection should aim at a relatively small number of what we will call 'canonical traits'; the three or four characteristics which are likely to be predictive of future professional behaviour and can be assessed reliably at the time of application to medical school.
- Schools where selection is currently based almost entirely on academic ability will have to reduce those academic standards if they wish also to select effectively on non-academic criteria.
- Selection should be recognised as being very limited in its power. The really powerful implements for effecting change are education and training (McManus & Vincent 1993).

What are the canonical traits which should be selected for?

Four principal canonical traits for selection have been identified (McManus & Vincent 1993).

Intelligence

Doctors probably cannot be too intelligent. Meta-analyses of selection across a wide range of different occupations at all social levels show that the best predictor of both job performance and the ability to be trained is intelligence (Schmidt & Hunter 1998).

Learning style and motivation

University students in general are motivated to study for different reasons and adopt different study habits and learning styles which are consistent with that motivation. Table 35.2 summarises the typology of Biggs (Biggs 1987, Newble & Entwistle 1986). Deep and strategic learning (but not surface learning) are both compatible with a self-directed, self-motivated approach to learning, which is likely to result in the life-long learning necessary of modern practitioners.

Communicative ability

The majority of complaints about doctors involve problems in communication so it makes some sense to

"'A' levels tell us nothing about some of the most desirable attributes of the doctor. The four desiderata are technical competence, human sympathy, wisdom and experience"

McKeown 1986

Table 35.2   Summary of the differences in motivation and study process of the surface, deep and strategic approaches to study (based on the work of Biggs 1978, 1985, 1987, 1993)

Style	Motivation	Process
Surface	Completion of the course	Rote learning of facts and ideas Focusing on task components in isolation
	Fear of failure	Little real interest in content
Deep	Interest in the subject	Relation of ideas to evidence
	Vocational relevance	Integration of material across courses
	Personal understanding	Identication of general principles
Strategic	Achieving high grades	Use of techniques that achieve highest grades
	Competing with others Being successful	Level of understanding patchy and variable

include it in selection. Although communication skills should have been developing during life they can be further refined. However, individuals who are communicating poorly at age 17 are less likely to respond well to training. Assessment is not straightforward but questionnaires are available (McManus, Kidd & Aldous 1997).

Conscientiousness

The meta-analysis of Schmidt & Hunter (1998) showed clearly that the best predictor of job performance and trainability, after taking intellectual ability into account, was integrity or conscientiousness. Conscientiousness is one of the five personality dimensions assessed in the 'Big Five', which together account for the majority of important variations in personality (Matthews & Deary 1998), the other four being extroversion, neuroticism, agreeableness and open-mindedness. Conscientiousness probably gains a large part of its impact through the simple fact that highly conscientious people tend to work harder and be more efficient, and thereby gain more and better experience.

Surrogates for selection

Although intelligence, learning style and motivation, communicative ability and conscientiousness should probably form the basis of selection, it is sufficient to select on other measures which correlate highly with them. Selection on school-leaving examinations is one surrogate as high grades correlate to some extent with level of intelligence, appropriate learning styles and a conscientious approach to study. Of course a person of lower intellect may pass exams by prodigious rote learning, conscientiously carried out, but it is relatively unlikely. Playing in an orchestra or for a sports team can imply conscientiousness at practising, an ability to communicate well with other individuals when collaborating on an enterprise, and perhaps a certain interest in the deeper aspects of a skill (intrinsic motivation). Good selection processes should not use such surrogates uncritically, but should ask what underlying psychological traits this biographical data (biodata) is purporting to assess.

Methods and process of selection

The process of selection and the methods used to carry it out are entirely separate (Powis 1998). Medical schools should have a selection policy which clearly states how selection takes place, how appropriate information is collected, and how a decision will be made based on that information. Once the information has been acquired the selection policy can be implemented and a decision made. This decision-making should be an entirely administrative process. Although seemingly absurd at first sight, this ensures good practice and avoids suggestions of discrimination or unfairness, or apparent inconsistencies in selection. The academic and educational input to the system should be in deciding the protocol and, where necessary, making subtle judgements about the information (such as evaluating aspects of the application form or interviewing). A corollary of the principle is that the separate items of information should be assessed separately. If interviewers are asked to judge a candidate's knowledge of medicine as a career then that is what they should do; they do not need information about interviewees' GCSE or 'A' level results, hobbies or so on as this information can result in a halo effect on the judgement interviewers are required to make.

Assessing methods of selection

There are many methods of selection, each of which has its strengths and weaknesses. Each may be assessed in terms of:

- Validity. All assessments in selection are implicit predictions of the future behaviour of a candidate. If there is no correlation with those future behaviours then they are not useful, however much assessors may agree about them.
- Reliability. If selectors disagree about a characteristic, or re-assessment gives different answers, then the information is unlikely to be useful.

"A multitude of ad hoc policies implemented by miscellaneous admissions officers of various medical schools cannot be properly evaluated or criticized, and is open to considerable abuse. Selection itself is problematic enough, without trying to make it a panacea for the world's ills. If selectors are trying to do too much too well, they will end by failing to do anything properly"

Downie & Charlton 1992

- Feasibility. Assessments can usually be made more reliable and more valid by extending them. The result is greater cost, financially or in staff time, the gain from which may not be worth the resource expended.
- Acceptability. Candidates and their teachers, friends and relations must feel that selection methods are appropriate.

Different methods of selection

Administrative methods
A method typically used by office staff, processing information from application forms is relatively objective and is mostly used for rejecting candidates. It is usually reliable, cheap and acceptable but of uncertain validity.

Assessment of application forms
Application forms often contain unstructured personal statements and referees' reports, which must be assessed by a shortlister who attempts to determine a candidate's motivation and experience of medicine as a career. Like interviewing, it is subjective and often of moderate or even poor reliability and of uncertain validity. It is, however, cost-effective and acceptable to applicants. Reliability can undoubtedly be improved by training and the use of structured assessment protocols, clear criterion referencing and careful constructed descriptors of the various characteristics to be identified.

Biographical data (biodata)
This can be assessed either indirectly from an open-ended application form (e.g. the 'personal statement') or more reliably from a specially designed structured or semi-structured questionnaire. It derives its usefulness from the psychological principle that the best predictor of future behaviour is past behaviour. It is usually reliable, valid (Cook 1990), cost-effective and acceptable to applicants.

Referees' reports

These can be useful if they are totally honest, but referees often feel a loyalty to the candidate rather than the medical school. Experienced head teachers will say that they expect medical schools to 'read between the lines', so that it is not what is said that matters, but what is left unsaid or understated. Such an approach inevitably means reliability is low, validity very dubious and acceptability ambiguous. They are expensive in terms of referees' time but not the medical school's.

Interviewing

Only about two-thirds of UK medical schools hold interviews, suggesting genuine uncertainty about their usefulness. They can, however, be more reliable than suspected. Marchese & Muchinsky (1993) report that reliability and validity are mostly dependent on training of interviewers and on a clear structure. Behavioural interviewing, where the emphasis is upon how the candidate has behaved in concrete situations in the past, is usually more effective than interviews asking about hypothetical situations in the remote future. Although expensive in terms of staff time, interviews are highly acceptable to the general public who are not happy with doctors being selected purely on academic grounds. However, they are often criticised after the event by candidates, parents and teachers.

Psychometric testing

Typically this involves questionnaires for assessing motivation and personality, timed assessments of intellectual ability or psychomotor tests of manual dexterity. The validity of these tests has often been formally assessed with regard to jobs in general and undoubtedly they are very reliable if well developed. However, they are time-consuming to administer and may be unpopular with candidates, who may feel that there are 'trick' questions and that the characteristics being assessed are not necessarily relevant to a career in medicine.

"There is a most odd tendency on the part of the British selectors to accept the headmaster's report as 'extraordinarily accurate', except in some particular instances, which the selectors seem to assume they can always recognise. This is part of a general delusion of selectors; that they are able to use imperfect materials such as other people's opinions (or, in the case of some headmaster's reports, other people's opinions of other people's opinion) but somehow, miraculously, in their hands, these base metals are transmuted in the finest gold"

Simpson 1972

> *"Prolonged observation of candidates in different situations by trained selectors makes the final . . . decision relatively easy. This contrasts with the brief interviews done by . . . medical schools where dubious decisions are often based on inadequate evidence. The experience of assessment centres is that early opinions may be suspect . . . The time has come to establish on an experimental basis a Medical Selection Board along the lines of the assessment centres of the Army, Civil Service and British Airways"*

Roberts & Porter 1989

> *"It is impossible to separate selection from training . . . In this country the only case I know of a thoroughly validated selection procedure from first to last was one in which selection and training were treated as a single problem"*

Sir Frederick Bartlett 1946

Assessment centres

Candidates are brought together in groups of 4–12, over a period of 1–3 days, and are asked to carry out a series of novel exercises, often involving group work (Roberts & Porter 1989). This is the core approach of the army, civil service and major companies. Assessment centres are particularly appropriate if the emphasis is upon assessing ability under competitive time stress or upon collaborating in group activities. Their reliability is good since assessors are highly trained but they are very time-consuming for staff and applicants and also expensive.

The cost(s) of selection

The direct costs of selection for a medical school are difficult to assess, but are probably between about £500 and £1000 per entrant, mostly accounted for by staff time. The implicit criterion of success is that graduates will practise high-quality medicine in the National Health Service from graduation until retirement, perhaps 40 years later. This contrasts with the £40 000 or so spent by British companies whose criterion of success is that the graduate stays with the company for five years.

There are two reasons why so little is spent on medical student selection. At present student selection is an 'open loop system', without feedback. A bad doctor may cost society very large amounts of money, but none of that cost comes back to the medical school. Selection costs are therefore seen as of little benefit to an institution and the temptation is to minimise them. If life-long medical practice were a closed-loop system, with graduates incurring costs and providing rewards to their medical school throughout their career, then selection and undergraduate training would be at the core of a edical school's activities, instead of being marginalised.

Routine monitoring of selection

Because selection is so vulnerable to criticism and possibly even to legal challenge, it is essential not only that clear policies are in place, but that routine data are collected for the monitoring of the process. Monitoring should look at the overall pattern of selection, assessing whether particular groups of applicants (women, ethnic minorities, students with disabilities etc.) are being systematically advantaged or disadvantaged. A simple head count is not sufficient for this purpose, since groups may also differ in a range of relevant background factors; multivariate analysis is the appropriate procedure, both for identifying possible disadvantage and understanding its locus (McManus 1998).

Studying selection and learning from research

Medicine can be notoriously insular. Research and experience outside of medicine are often ignored, and there are medical schools which will not even consider experience gained at other medical schools, never mind in industry, commerce and the public sectors in general. Personnel selection has been much studied and there is a vast literature. A good place to start is the regular series of articles in the *Annual Review of Psychology*, which are frequently updated (Borman Hanson & Hedge 1997).

Evidence-based medicine and the scientific study of selection

Evidence-based medicine is the current dogma in all areas of medicine. Student selection and medical education should be no different. The limitations should be recognised. If randomised controlled trials are taken as the only criterion of evidence then the vast majority of medical education would not be valid – with the inevitable result that opinion, prejudice and anecdote end up as the bases for action. Observational studies and the powerful methods of epidemiology are also useful, particularly when embedded in robust theories based in psychology, sociology and other basic sciences. A frequently encountered error when discussing, say, a prospective study of selection is to use both of the following arguments simultaneously:

- 'These students have only been followed up for 5 years, but our selection process was assessing who would become good practising doctors in the future. These results do not look far enough into the future.'
- 'This study was carried out over 5 years ago, and since then we have changed our selection process and our undergraduate curriculum, and the doctors will be working in a medical system that has also changed. These results are only of historical interest.'

When put like this the sophistry is immediately apparent – prospective, longitudinal studies for N years must, of necessity, have been started more than N years ago. Of course, the same arguments are not used in medical practice – chemotherapeutic regimes looking at 5 year survival must be subject to the same problems, but these trials are still done.

A further problem with studying selection is that it is very vulnerable, as are the egos of the individuals carrying it out. No one likes to think that their actions have been wasted or that their best-considered schemes are worthless. Neither does any institution like to see results published suggesting that it has not been doing a perfect job, particularly when its rivals' results are not publicly displayed. A common reflex response is to demand an unreasonably high criterion of evidence, which is a paragon of perfection. The scientific studying of selection is no different from any other science. One is not searching for proof of absolute truth, but identifying working, explanatory, hypotheses compatible with evidence, which have acceptable methodology, take known problems into account, and are therefore robust against straightforward refutation and make useful predictions. That is then a basis for practical action and further research.

Summary

Selection is an important yet usually under-resourced aspect of medical school activity.

Applicants may select medical schools because of their particular courses or their invitation to attend an interview. Medical schools may select applicants by their intelligence, their learning style and motivation, their ability to communicate and by evidence that they are conscientious.

A variety of methods of selection may be used by schools ranging from a purely administrative review of application form details, through assessment of personal biodata, to psychometric testing of candidates.

Whatever process is used it is likely to be costly and should be routinely monitored, evaluated and compared with examples of best evidence-based practice.

References and further reading

Bartlett F C 1946 Selection of medical students. British Medical Journal iii: 665–666

Biggs J B 1987 Study process questionnaire: manual. Australian Council for Educational Research, Melbourne

Borman W C, Hanson M A, Hedge J W 1997 Personnel selection. Annual Review of Psychology 48:299–337

Cook M 1990 Personnel selection and productivity: John Wiley, Chichester

Downie R S, Charlton B 1992 The making of a doctor: medical education in theory and practice. Oxford University Press, Oxford

Johnson M L 1971 Non-academic factors in medical school selection: a report on rejected applicants. British Journal of Medical Education 5:264–268

Marchese M C, Muchinsky P M 1993 The validity of the employment interview: a meta-analysis. International Journal of Selection and Assessment 1:18–26

Matthews G, Deary I J 1998 Personality traits. Cambridge University Press, Cambridge

McManus I C 1998 Factors affecting likelihood of applicants being offered a place in medical schools in the United Kingdom in 1996 and 1997: retrospective study. British Medical Journal 317: 1111–1116

McManus I C, Kidd J M, Aldous I R 1997 Self-perception of communicative ability: evaluation of a questionnaire completed by medical students and general practitioners. British Journal of Health Psychology 2:301–315

McManus I C, Richards P, Winder B C, Sproston K A 1999 Do UK medical school applicants prefer interviewing to non-interviewing schools? Advances in Health Sciences Education 4:155–165

McManus I C, Vincent C A 1993 Selecting and educating safer doctors. In: Vincent C A, Ennis M, Audley R J (eds) Medical accidents. Oxford University Press, Oxford, pp. 80–105

Newble D I, Entwistle N J 1986 Learning styles and approaches: implications for medical education. Medical Education 20:162–175

Powis D 1998 How to do it: select medical students. British Medical Journal 317: 1149–1150

Roberts G D, Porter A M W 1989 Medical student selection – time for change: discussion paper. Journal of the Royal Society of Medicine 82:288–291

Schmidt F L, Hunter J E 1998 The validity and utility of selection methods in personnel psychology: practical and theoretical implications of 85 years of research findings. Psychological Bulletin 124:262–274

Simpson M A 1972 Medical education: a critical approach. Butterworths, London

Chapter 36
Student support

J. A. Dent   S. Rennie

Introduction

Why is student support necessary?

Medical students are exposed to a variety of pressures, many of which may cause stress. These 'stresses', examinations, competition, information overload, time management, financial difficulties, relationship problems and career decisions, are similar to the pressures encountered by all students. In addition, it is recognised that medical students face other issues including relating to professionals in their workplace, dealing with death and dying, facing uncertainty, making mistakes and lack of time for recreation, relationships and family.

Medical students spend most of their time studying away from the university campus and are periodically at peripheral hospitals or in general practice placements. This, combined with unsociable hours of study, means that they are often away from their familiar social contacts and the support services provided by the university. In addition university services may not be able to provide help for problems specific to medical students such as careers advice on medical specialties.

Problems experienced by medical students commonly fall into five categories: academic, careers, professional, personal and administrative:

- Academic support may include identifying and helping students in academic difficulty, providing feedback and advice after examinations, study skills advice or guidance on the selection of elective components of the course including special study modules, projects and elective periods of study.

"Medical students enrolled today have greater expectations for student personal services than previously and a high attrition rate in medical education is not tolerated"

Heins et al 1980

- Careers counselling may include advice about the early years of postgraduate training as well as future career paths. It may involve help in preparing a curriculum vitae, writing references for the students and giving advice about interview technique.
- Professional counselling may be required to help students develop attitudes and behaviour appropriate for a doctor or to consider professional conduct and ethical issues. Patients expect to be treated politely and considerately and expect their doctor to be honest and trustworthy. It is important for students to develop a professional approach to patients early in their undergraduate career. Some students require support from a tutor in these areas as they develop a capacity for self-audit and an awareness of personal limitations.
- Personal problems experienced by students include adjustment to medical school, relationship concerns, financial difficulties and accommodation worries.
- Administrative problems deal mainly with the 'how', 'where', 'who', 'what' and 'when' questions that students have about the organisation of the course and university administration. These questions may seem trivial but can often cause students unnecessary concern and stress.

"Physicians must view the mentor/student relationship as a valuable opportunity to nurture the total growth of a young physician rather than merely to focus on the student's academic or personal problems"

Flach et al 1982

However, it is important not to view a student support system as a scheme primarily for students in trouble. Stress is a central component of a doctor's job and learning to cope with it is an important part of the training of a doctor. The ways in which medical students cope often provide a blueprint for how they deal with future professional and personal stress.

The aim of a student support system should therefore be to facilitate medical students' development, to ensure that their education is a positive experience and to create relationships which may be beneficial in the future. The support system can help the student adjust to medical school, learn stress management strategies and develop competencies for future use as a doctor. In addition, the scheme can provide a forum for feedback, advice and enhanced communications between faculty and students.

How can students be supported?

Students can be supported in a number of different ways: through tutor schemes and specialist tutors, a student advisory office, university and external support services, peer support systems and via e-mail or the Internet. These strategies may be used by faculties individually or in combination to provide a support system tailored to the needs of the students and the resources of the faculty.

Tutor schemes

These involve the allocation of staff from within the faculty to act as tutors to students in either a one-to-one or a group basis. Groups may be horizontal, with students drawn entirely from one year, or vertical, with a mix of students from all years. Tutors may meet with students individually to discuss specific problems. On occasion students may develop a relationship with another staff member who may become an 'unofficial tutor'.

There are advantages to a group system. In this age of increasing numbers of medical students, it reduces the number of tutors needed to provide a support scheme. It also enables peer support within the group. Peer support within horizontal systems often comes from identifying common problems and concerns, whereas a vertical system enables senior students to give empathy and advice to more junior students.

The tutor generally follows the students through the course ensuring the continuity which can lead to the development of a solid relationship with them. This relationship can be strengthened by engaging in social as well as educational activities. A tutor can help students with problems which may be academic, career-related, professional, personal or administrative either by providing that help individually or by referring them on to other resources (see Fig. 36.1). A tutor may also be required to act as an advocate for students in particular difficulties by making representations to appropriate faculty or senate committees.

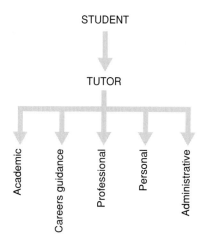

Fig. 36.1   Referral pathways for particular questions

Student advisory office

A student advisory office staffed by a small number of full-time advisers with an extensive knowledge of the medical course and its administration may be used as an initial contact point for students with queries or problems. These advisers can act as a filter for medical students dealing with their academic, career, professional, personal and administrative concerns or directing them to the most appropriate person within the faculty or the university services or in outside agencies. An advantage of this system is that advisers for students are readily available and accessible. This office may also be responsible for coordinating the tutor scheme and providing staff support and training.

The advisers may include non-medical staff members who are perceived as having the advantage of being separate from the staff members students may subsequently see, either during assessment or in their future career. One such member is a study skills tutor who works with students on an individual or group basis to help with the development of study methods, time management skills and revision and examination techniques. It is also useful to have a list of specialty advisers who are willing to speak to students about careers in their field of medicine.

University and external support services

Most universities have a variety of student welfare services including financial advisers, accommodation offices, disability support, legal advice, a health service, a chaplaincy and a counselling service. The finance officer is able to help students budget, manage debt and find grants. Accommodation offices provide lists of landlords and of accommodation to let. The university counselling service provides independent trained counsellors who are able to assist students with emotional and practical problems.

There is also a wide range of external advice agencies available such as the Citizens' Advice Bureau and the Samaritans. Students may access these services directly or be referred by their tutor. It may be useful in some cases for the tutor to act as an advocate for a student approaching any of these services.

Peer support systems

'Senior–junior', 'Big sibs' or 'Parenting' schemes provide great benefits to junior students if they are organised effectively. They involve the pairing of first-year students with a second- or third-year student, either on a one-to-one basis or in groups. These schemes have mixed success and usually work better when the senior students are volunteers. Senior students are often a good source of advice to junior students as they have personal experience of many of the problems students may face. Junior doctors may also provide excellent advice to medical students about the medical course, electives and securing jobs. Most universities have a wide range of student interest or 'affinity' groups (sports, music, social activities and minority groups) which can all contribute to student support.

Medical student councils or associations should be encouraged and supported by faculty. They can provide a focus for student support through academic, recreational and social events. They often produce newsletters and information leaflets which deal with concerns and enhance communication. A 'medical student survival guide' can provide information, advice and useful tips on a whole range of issues, such as which books to buy, how to study for examinations, where to look for grants and information specific to the medical school. A student guide is especially useful in helping first-year students orientate themselves and in providing answers to many of their questions.

E-mail and the Internet

Computers have rapidly become an essential part of medicine and most medical students are now conversant with e-mail and the Internet. E-mail provides an ideal interface for dealing with administrative queries and concerns. An e-mail address to which concerns can be directed should be given to students and administered directly by faculty's administrative staff. Most medical schools have websites which can also be utilised to provide 'bulletin boards' or 'talkshops' where problems and concerns can be aired and advice given by other students or staff.

"The value of peer-group relationships in providing support and growth during the educational process should not be underestimated"

Adsett 1968

A 'tutor support pack' can be made providing information on:

- how to be a tutor
- sources of specialist support
- staff development opportunities.

"the best advisers are individuals who are warm, empathetic, and spontaneous, who have constructive, sound judgement, and who get satisfaction out of watching medical students grow into mature adults as well as competent physicians"

Eckenfels, Blacklow and Gotterer 1984

Tutors are not required to:

- have a specialist knowledge of the content of each part of the course
- have first-hand experience of the training requirements of all specialties
- be a health, financial or marital counsellor
- have a degree in psychotherapy
- understand the administrative details of the medical school.

How to organise a tutor scheme

How to be an effective tutor?

The most effective tutors are volunteers who are committed, enthusiastic, self-motivated and accessible to students. They must be sensitive to the stresses and needs of medical students and have a genuine desire to help them grow into well-rounded doctors. Tutors, if they are to be successful, must from the outset be perceived as credible by the student body. Good tutors must be effective listeners as often this is all that the student requires. It is expected of course that a tutor will be trustworthy and will handle any confidential information appropriately. Tutors must be aware that students may view them as role models, confidants, friends and advocates.

What does a tutor need?

Basics requirements

Tutors need to understand the faculty's chosen student support scheme and know where they fit into it. It is important that they understand that their role is initially to provide a point of contact and support for all students' not just those with problems, and subsequently to be able to direct them to any of the five specialist areas of support already described:

- Academic. Tutors may be able to help with questions about study technique or with questions of a general nature about course content. They should have a working knowledge of the structure and content of the curriculum and be familiar with its objectives and with the range of options available for elective components of the course.
- Career. Tutors should have some knowledge of the range of junior training posts available in the area.
- Professional. Tutors should be able to give advice and guidance about standards of professional behaviour and be aware that they are often seen as role models.
- Personal. Active listening and the ability to empathise is probably all that is required for the majority of personal problems.

- Administrative. Tutors should know the basics of the organisation of the curriculum and the names of key people such as medical school office bearers, curriculum administrators and course secretaries.

Additional resources

Tutors need to have access to information which will help them direct students to sources of specialist information (see Fig. 36.2).

- Academic. Tutors require lists of names of the systems teachers and other content experts for the course and of block or phase coordinators.
- Career. Specific questions regarding entry requirements to training programmes are best referred to specialty career advisors. Questions about junior postgraduate training posts and how to apply for them should be referred to the postgraduate dean's office.
- Professional. Persisting problems with a student's professional behaviour, e.g. if there is a problem of plagiarism, are best referred to the dean or faculty secretary for appropriate action.
- Personal. Accommodation, financial or health problems should be referred to the appropriate university support services. More serious personal or emotional problems probably require the help of the professional counselling services which may be available in the university.
- Administrative. Specific details pertaining to the administration of the course are best referred to the medical school office secretaries and phase coordinators.

Student information

Tutors need to know the names of the students allocated to them and the best method to get in touch with them quickly. Information about their students should be provided for the tutors but previous counselling information from meetings with other members of staff should only be passed between tutors with the student's consent. A note of their academic progress to date is valuable and competency profiles should be made

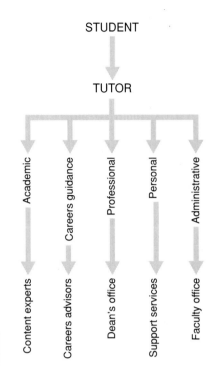

Fig. 36.2 Referral pathways for particular questions

A 'getting started pack' can be circulated to tutors and should include:

- suggestions on possible times and non-threatening venues for the first meeting
- names and e-mail address of group members
- list of key people in the medical school
- outline of other support services
- list of specialty advisers
- how to contact the scheme coordinator
- a model invitation to send out prior to the first meeting
- instructions for the content and frequency of meetings.

available for post-assessment discussion and feedback. Knowledge of the student's performance may be of help if the tutor is called on for any advocacy role. However, it must be emphasised that all such information must be handled according to the university's policy on confidentiality.

What does the scheme need?

Recognition
To be a success the scheme must be valued, tutors must be appreciated, their efforts must be recognised and events aimed to raise the profile of the scheme must be appropriately promoted and supported by the dean and faculty.

Similarly, it is important that the student body understand and participate appropriately in the scheme if they are to benefit by it. Student involvement with the scheme can be enhanced by inviting them, or a representative group, to meetings with faculty members for discussion on the development of the scheme or for feedback.

Flexibility
Not all students require the same extent of contact with their tutors and most are content to know that they have one available if necessary. The scheme should recognise that, whatever the system, there are three levels of student/tutor interaction which will develop (see Fig. 36.3):

- Close relationship. One-third of students establish a personal relationship with their tutor; this follows meetings to discuss personal or academic problems or simply because they naturally get on well together.
- Contractual relationship. About half of the students only see their tutor as requested and would rarely initiate contact.
- Constrained relationship. A small peripheral group choose not to participate and are only seen when important information is being disseminated or when they perceive that it is to their advantage to be present. This last group probably represents a variety of

"Despite the heavy load of responsibilities they carry, faculty must show interest in the students and their activities to the degree that they do not let other responsibilities always crowd out their attending student functions or having informal chats with students"

Adsett 1968

"serving as a mentor is included as one of the recognized criteria for faculty promotions"

Flach et al 1982

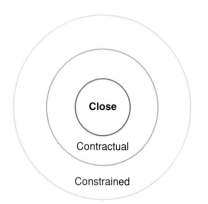

Fig. 36.3 Student/tutor relationships

personalities including those who are very self-sufficient or independent students, those who are reserved or intimidated and those who have chosen not to participate in any aspect of medical school life. It is important for tutors to seek to reduce the size of this group and to recognise and address the problems and needs which they present. However, some students in this group may have developed relationships with other faculty members who act as unofficial tutors.

Not all tutors are able to relate with equal effectiveness to students and a flexible rather than a rigidly applied scheme is more likely to be successful. Individual tutors can then adapt the scheme to their own style while still following the main principles of providing support as required. Some tutors use academic exercises, such as discussion of a learning styles questionnaire, to facilitate their initial interaction with the group. Others are comfortable with an informal meeting in a coffee-shop venue. Whatever ploys are adopted the scheme should aim to be social as well as educational so that students are encouraged to move from the outer towards the inner circles of interaction.

Administration

An enthusiastic coordinator should be appointed who will identify the most appropriate scheme for the medical school, invite suitable members of staff to become tutors and gain the support and recognition of the faculty so that the initiating momentum of the scheme is maintained. The coordinator will have to act as a resource back-up for tutors and be able to supply additional information to them as required. For this to be possible (or tolerable!) appropriate secretarial assistance is necessary to provide a filter for enquiries from tutors and students. Secretarial assistance is also required for compiling the 'tutor support pack'. An information pack for students is also necessary to explain the purpose and benefits of the scheme and what can be expected from it. Staff development programmes are also required. These are best structured as informal meetings to provide feedback, discussion and training opportunities which

The university year can begin with a social evening for all tutors and peer supporters to meet their new students.

"Graduating seniors have expressed regret that they did not put more effort into the mentor relationship"

Flach et al 1982

"Meet the person who will get you your first PRHO job"

From a tutor's invitation to a second-year student group

are especially important for first-time tutors. A newsletter can be used to follow up these sessions, expand on issues raised in discussion and remind tutors of impending events which may have a bearing on student well-being such as forthcoming examinations. Finally information for both students and tutors should be available in the library and on the university website.

Summary

Student support is required in relation to five areas of potential stress: academic problems, careers advice, personal worries, professional issues and administrative questions. Support can be provided in a variety of ways by tutor schemes, student advisory officers, university and external support services, peer support groups or via the Internet. Successful tutors are required to be good listeners and set a good example as role models. They should be able to provide first-line help in each of the areas of student concern but need additional resources which will help them direct students as required to further sources of expert help.

For their part, students should participate appropriately in the scheme and realise that it is not just for students in trouble but may help all students to develop stress management strategies that will be useful in their later career. The scheme must be appropriately resourced, administered and recognised as important by faculty. Each individual faculty can make a selection of an appropriate mixture of several of the methods described and the final scheme should be administered with some flexibility so that all students and tutors involved can participate in it to the extent they are comfortable.

References and further reading

Adsett C A 1968. Psychological health of medical students in relation to the medical education process. Journal of Medical Education 43:728–734

Coombs R H, Virshup B B 1994. Enhancing the psychological health of medical students: the student well-being committee. Medical Education 28:47–54

Cotterel D J, McCrorie P, Perrin F 1994 The personal tutor system: an evaluation. Medical Education 28:544–549

Eckenfels E J, Blacklow R S, Gotterer G S 1984. Medical student counseling: the Rush medical college adviser program. Journal of Medical Education 59:573–581

Flach D H, Smith M F, Smith W G, Glasser M L 1982. Faculty mentors for medical students. Journal of Medical Education 57:514–520

Heins M, Clifton R, Simmons J, Thomas J, Wagner G, Zerega D 1980. Expansion of services for medical students. Journal of Medical Education 55:428–433

Michie S, Sandhu S 1994 Stress management for clinical medical students. Medical Education 28:528–533

Plaut S M, Walker-Bastnick L, Helman L, Ginsberg R, Rapoport R G, Plaut J M, Cannon M J 1980. Improving staff–student relations: effects of a humanistic medicine programme. Medical Teacher 2: 32–39

Rathburn J 1995. Helping medical students develop lifelong strategies to cope with stress. Academic Medicine 70:955–956

Weston J A, Paterson C A 1980. A medical student support system at the University of Colorado school of medicine. Journal of Medical Education 55:624–626

Chapter 37
Study skills

R. C. Bandaranayake

Introduction

Learning for life

In most areas of science knowledge grows exponentially, and medicine is no exception. With increasing knowledge it is imperative for the medical students to develop sound learning habits, which will stand them in good stead throughout their professional life. Such habits include both the selection of what is learnt as well as how it is learnt. The latter is one factor which determines whether what is learnt will be remembered long enough to become part of the student's repertoire of knowledge (long-term memory) or will be discarded as soon as it ceases to be of immediate use (short-term memory).

Growth of knowledge

Knowledge in every discipline has grown to such an extent that subdisciplines have grown out of erstwhile disciplines and departments have split into subdepartments. The daunting task facing today's medical student is often compounded by the discipline specialist, who has expectations of the student far beyond that required for the basic doctor.

In facing this challenge the average student resorts to the most expedient strategy of studying to satisfy immediate concerns of assessment. After the examination much of what is learnt is forgotten, and only that which is used in the period immediately following is remembered. Students and clinical teachers frequently complain of the futility of forgotten

"Scientific knowledge grows exponentially, with a doubling time of fifteen years"

Unattributed

"Departmental allegiance often takes precedence over institutional allegiance, as academicians train the medical student to be a clone of their own speciality or sub-speciality"

Bandaranayake 1999

Constantly encourage students to recall the basic science concepts underlying the clinical knowledge and skills they encounter.

preclinical anatomy and biochemistry. Preclinical teachers argue that such learning is more easily recalled if required during the postgraduate phase.

Can students study these subjects in a way which enables the retention of learning essential for professional practice, so that re-learning does not become a major endeavour but is seen as part of the continuum of learning?

The continuum of learning

Learning is continuous with new learning built on what has already been learned. Medical education is a continuum, which starts at entry to medical school and ends with cessation of professional practice. Only a relatively small, though important, part of this continuum takes place in the undergraduate medical school. However, both the content of what is learnt and the process of learning make a significant impact on the remaining phases of the continuum.

Most medical students have not decided, during their undergraduate training, which specialty they will follow, partly because they have not yet experienced those specialties. Some medical schools offer students the opportunity to experience the specialties initially, before focusing on their chosen one, through a system of electives comprising a large part of the curriculum. This practice suffers from the disadvantage of specialisation without adequate exposure to the basic medicine which is required even of a specialist. Thus selection of what is to be learnt to be a sound specialist in any field becomes critical.

Component study skills

Many important process skills must be developed in the medical student:

- self-directed learning
- learning with understanding (deep learning), leading to long-term retention, rather than through rote (surface) learning, which is likely to result in short-term retention

- seeking and retrieving information from an increasing variety of sources
- critically reviewing what is read, rather than blindly accepting the written word
- integrating new learning with existing knowledge by seeking links between them, and dealing with dissonance
- assessing oneself on learning that has occurred to ensure that it can be remembered and applied to the situations likely to be encountered in professional practice.

Study plan

The medical student, constantly faced with new areas for learning across a spectrum of subjects, must develop a study plan for each significant period of time, such as a week. Often subjects are not organised in a way that enables the student to see the links between them. In some curricula integration among subjects is achieved through themes, such as organ systems or clinical problems. Yet the student must learn to establish priorities for study, based not on expediency but on **importance, difficulty** and **timeliness**.

Importance must be judged in terms of:

- usefulness for professional practice
- the degree of understanding required for further learning
- the place of new learning in the unfolding of a continuing story.

Difficulty depends on:

- the existence of prerequisite learning
- the predilection of the individual for the subject
- the level of abstraction of the subject
- the degree and nature of the initial exposure to the subject.

Each student has to learn to identify areas of individual difficulty and plan study in such a way as to devote more time to such areas.

"Systematic methods of learning may require more effort and patience in the beginning, but soon they become habitual and effective"

Smith, Shores & Brittain 1951

Timeliness relates to a number of factors, which include:

- readiness for the next phase of study, i.e. what is about to be learnt is considered prerequisite to what is to follow
- synchronisation among different subject areas related to a common integrating theme
- assessment points during the course of study which drive the student to concentrate on certain areas.

Readiness for learning depends on intrinsic motivation, an inner urge to learn, as well as the acquisition of prerequisite learning on which new learning is built. This includes the basic skills of language and communication and the ability of the learner to identify discrepancies between what he or she knows and does not know.

In developing a study plan, the student must:

- identify the focus of study
- determine the depth to which study of a particular topic is to be undertaken
- understand the inter-relationships of topics by designing a logical sequence of topics for study.

Focus of study is determined by learning objectives. However, a student confronted with a daunting array of objectives must determine priorities among them, based on both their relative importance for progressive learning, for future application and perceived gaps in knowledge which hinder further learning.

Depth of study is that which is required for understanding and depends on the complexity of the subject matter. As this cannot often be judged prior to actually undertaking study, the student must build into the plan study time in proportion to the relative difficulty of each subject area as experienced previously. The temptation to memorise without understanding should be resisted.

"the most significant and common factors hindering academic growth result from the lack of adequate secondary school preparation in the basic skills of language"

Wilcox 1958

Avoid requiring students to provide lists from memory, such as investigations, without providing the reason for each item in the list.

Encourage the student to link the subject you teach with related learning outside your specialty.

"*Learning may be enhanced if a variety of presentation methods is used with students. . . . Learning occurs when students use a combination of senses*"

Lock 1981

Provide a variety of learning experiences for your students when you help them learn a given topic.

Learning occurs as new material is related to previously learned material. If the steps are properly sequenced and studies undertaken accordingly, both horizontal and vertical integration will be facilitated. In other words, the learner will be able to see the links between progressive learning as well as among parallel learning in related areas. Often, lack of synchronisation across disciplines hinders horizontal integration between them. The student must learn to develop a study plan which brings these relationships to the fore, even if it may not correspond to the school's formal timetable.

Resources for study

For the individual student multiple stimuli aid learning as long as there is no dissonance among them. For example, when concepts are presented as descriptive text, graphs and three-dimensional models, students are better able to grasp them. Learning which is reinforced by multiple stimuli is likely to be retained longer.

At the same time, individual students may learn best in different ways. For example, in anatomy through:

- dissection
- prosected specimens
- projected images
- two-dimensional pictures
- printed text.

Teachers should help students identify the method(s) of study by which they learn best. Methods are determined by:

- type of learning objective
- individual preferences and style
- practicalities of a given situation
- priorities in the purpose of learning
- time available for learning.

A skill of paramount importance to the medical student during a lifetime of continuing education is the ability to seek, retrieve and store information. Students must learn to undertake this task efficiently early in their medical education. Many, not having acquired these skills during secondary education, need training in them. While orientation courses at entry to medical school include visits to libraries, relatively few include training in these skills. Locating information from different sources includes the skills of using library filing systems, referring to indices, scanning reading material to determine relevance and importance, and referencing for subsequent easy retrieval (Saunders, Northup & Mennin 1984). The tendency to accumulate photocopied material for later use without adequate discrimination should be avoided. Immediate study of the material, highlighting important points and noting them on index cards, would save hours of wading through piles of accumulated material subsequently.

Learning style

A considerable body of literature now exists in the field of medical education on the approaches which students adopt to learning. It was thought earlier that students had different learning styles, and attempts were made to classify students accordingly, by such instruments as Kolb's (1976) learning inventory. It is now thought that a learning approach does not describe a particular attribute of the student, but a relationship between the learner and the learning task (Ramsden 1987). In other words, a given student may adopt a particular learning approach for one learning task and a different approach for another.

Learning approaches include:

- information processing, such as organising and elaborating information
- strategies for learning, such as memorising and note-taking
- support strategies, such as organising study time (Wilcox 1958).

Three approaches, related to the student's motivation and purpose for study, have been described (Entwistle 1988):

"in many of the problem-based medical schools the ability of the student to identify and utilize appropriate learning resources is an established component of student assessment"

Saunders, Northup & Mennin 1984

Give your students assignments which require them to study beyond their textbooks and class notes.

- surface learning, where the learner undertakes rote learning with little understanding, and relies on memory for reproducing that which is learnt
- deep learning, where the learner undertakes an active search for meaning in trying to understand what is learnt
- strategic learning, where the learner is motivated by achievement of a goal and adopts a strategy to achieve it.

Study skill courses should focus on developing students' awareness of these approaches so that they could select that which is most suited to a given learning task.

Superficial reading of text does not guarantee that what is read, and even understood, will be retained in the long-term memory. Students must develop the practice of reflecting on the subject matter, connecting it with what they already know and summarising new learning in their own words.

Few would disagree that the attributes and study skills we would desire in a medical student are those embedded in the deep approach to learning. However, many curricula are planned and implemented in ways that promote surface or strategic approaches (Stiernborg & Bandaranayake 1996). The recent surge of curricula adopting problem-based learning to varying extents favours the deep approach (Newble & Clarke 1987). There is no reason, however, for not inculcating such an approach even in the more conventional curricula.

While the most *efficient* reader may be the 'one who can gather the most amount of information from the printed page in the least amount of time' (Wilcox 1958), he or she may not be the most *effective* learner, as much of that information may last only a short span of time. The reflective process involved in the deep approach to learning may, ostensibly, be more time-consuming. However, longer retention of learning makes this approach more effective in the long term. One reason why students complain of the tedious nature of basic

"The (anatomy) student (who learns) to reason anatomically . . . will find the acquisition of new and related facts an easier task"

Grant 1937

In clinical teaching challenge students with problem-solving exercises based not only on what they already know, but also on what they should but do not know.

science courses may be the lack of time and opportunity for reflection.

The key to the development of any skill is practice until perfection is achieved. This applies to both cognitive and psychomotor skills. Students accustomed to surface learning may have initial difficulty adopting a deep approach. Effective ways of reflecting on newly learned material are writing essays, discussion with peers, teaching others and entertaining questions.

Teachers have an important role to play in this process, as they must devise assignments which compel students to reflect on their learning. Such reflection is encouraged by requiring students to apply their new learning to problems and situations which they have not encountered hitherto. Teachers must also help students relate such learning to their personal goals, to enhance motivation.

Practice of psychomotor skills is a three-stage process of:

1. observation of a demonstration
2. practice under supervision
3. independent practice until perfect.

In the clinical situation the last step depends on the student's initiative and industry. Recent development of clinical skills laboratories has contributed to expanding opportunities available to students to hone their clinical skills.

Review of learning

Review and application of new learning must take place periodically if it is to be built into the student's cognitive framework. Memory is enhanced not only by actively seeking links between new learning and previous learning and experience, but also by deriving logical associations among areas of new learning. For example, the student who is learning about renal function for the first time should seek relationships, on the one hand, with the circulatory system (which may have been learnt earlier) and, on the other, with the microscopic structure of the nephron (which may be introduced at the same

"The best way to learn to appreciate and understand scientific method is to practice until it becomes habitual"

Smith, Shores & Brittain 1951

When you have demonstrated a clinical skill to your students, let each in turn practise it under your supervision and then encourage them to practise it by themselves.

"Of two men with the same outward experiences and the same amount of mere native tenacity, the one who thinks over his experiences most, and weaves them into systematic relations with each other, will be the one with the best memory"

W James in Smith, Shores & Brittain 1951

time). This helps in acquisition of the new learning as well as review of the old.

In reviewing learning, the student is often confronted with the problem of deciding what topics are important for review. Importance is a matter of perception: to the practitioner, that which is applicable to practice; to the teacher, that which is essential for understanding the subject; to the student, that which is likely to be examined.

In a course which purports to prepare future professionals, rationality dictates that importance be related to practice. However, preparation for practice without understanding the basis of that practice merely results in a technician rather than a professional. Hence emphasis should be placed on understanding the basic sciences rather than memorising that which is applicable.

Many problem-centred curricula adopt the concept of the spiral problem. The same problem is introduced at increasingly complex levels during successive phases of the curriculum. This helps the student identify content which is considered important for review. When the same content is required for different problems, opportunities are provided for students to review and practise its application in different situations.

A useful technique for review is to organise information that has been learnt into chunks, around certain principles, generalisations or cues. These form pegs on which more detailed information may be hung. Such organisation aids easy retrieval of the information, as the pegs are more easily recalled. Thus the student learning about the joints of the body may remember a few principles which govern classification of joints in relation to movement. Even if the details pertaining to a particular joint may be forgotten, recalling the principles would facilitate their retrieval.

Assessment of learning

Assessing oneself is perhaps the most difficult, yet most important, skill that must be undertaken for effective study. Active participation in the process of learning requires insight into one's strengths and weaknesses through self-analysis. Development takes place through capitalising on strengths and eliminating weaknesses. To identify deficiencies one must not only be a good judge of oneself, but also be aware that a deficiency exists. Students who are coached by a teacher have these deficiencies pointed out to them; those studying in groups are often helped thus by their peers; the individual learner, however, has to depend on certain cues, such as an inability to understand a difficult topic, to identify deficiencies in prior learning. A sound practice is to test oneself on what one has just read using pre-designed questions or exercises. Frequent reviews help students follow their progress.

Formative assessment is now a regular feature of many medical curricula. Unfortunately, it is often misused in that feedback from such assessment is not provided to students in a way which helps them identify deficiencies. In many instances, formative assessment consists of a series of summative exercises, which contribute to a final grade on which pass–fail decisions are based. While such a practice has the advantage of increased sampling of topics tested, it fails to serve a formative purpose. The problem is compounded by students attempting to hide rather than display their weaknesses, as they are aware of the important decisions that are based on the results.

If student assessment is to play a role in helping students learn, class tests conducted before and during a unit should provide feedback detailed enough to point out areas or skills where deficiencies in learning exist.

It is well known that assessment is the strongest motivator of student learning. While this is unfortunate, teachers should capitalise on this fact and set tests which call upon the students' higher cognitive skills, rather than on the ability to reproduce what is learnt. Assessment should encourage students to search for application of what they learn both in their personal lives and in the context of their future practice, and test their ability to discriminate between fact and opinion, between assumption and established truth. The critical appraisal of ideas should be an essential ingredient of

"Boiling down ideas to a few words is a practical test of your understanding of the material"

Crawford in Smith,
Shores & Brittain 1951

When you teach, question your students regularly, but react to their responses in such a way that they feel comfortable to display, rather than hide, deficiencies. Only then will they be able to take remedial action.

the total assessment package, as should the ability to gather information pertaining to a given problem.

Unfortunately most tests in medical education call upon the lower cognitive skills of recall and recognition. We fail to harness the greatest motivator of student learning to bring about desirable learning habits in our medical students. Most study skill courses aim at helping students pass these types of examinations rather than pursue learning which would arm them with the skills and attributes for a lifetime of continuing education.

Summary

In facing the challenges created by the explosion of medical knowledge, students resort to the expedient strategy of acquiring knowledge to satisfy immediate concerns of assessment, with much of it forgotten thereafter. This chapter provides suggestions for teachers to help students learn with understanding that which is essential for professional practice, while minimising the amount forgotten. The component study skills which are emphasised in this chapter are those of self-directed learning, learning with understanding and reflection, seeking and retrieving information, critical review, integration of new learning with old and the use of feedback.

A weekly plan of study designed by the student should be based on priorities determined by the importance of the topic for both understanding and application, its relative difficulty and its timeliness. The student should be helped to make decisions with regard to the focus of study as determined by objectives, its depth for understanding and its sequence. While teachers should ensure that students are exposed to a variety of sources for studying a given topic, the individual nature of learning determines which of these is optimal for a given student. Study skill courses should utilise recent findings on the relationship between the learner and the learning task to inform students of the different approaches to learning, and help each of them select that which is best suited for a given task.

Opportunities for repeated independent practice of both cognitive and psychomotor skills should be provided, the former through assignments, which call upon the student to apply learning to unfamiliar situations, and the latter through such facilities as skill laboratories. Review of learning should emphasise links between concurrently and progressively learnt topics, thereby promoting horizontal and vertical integration. Formative assessment by teachers, peers and self should be geared to providing feedback on individual strengths and weaknesses. The powerful effect summative assessment has on driving student learning should be capitalised on to promote desirable learning habits by testing higher cognitive skills in examinations.

References and further reading

Bandaranayake R C 1999 Basic sciences in the undergraduate medical curriculum: relevance and motivation. In: Medical Education in GCC Countries, First GCC Conference of Faculties of Medicine, Kuwait University

Entwistle N J 1988 Motivational factors in students' approaches to learning. In: Schmeck R R (ed.) Learning Strategies and Learning Styles, Plenum, New York

Grant J C B 1937 Grant's method of anatomy. Williams & Wilkins, Baltimore

Kolb D 1976 Learning style inventory. Technical Manual. McBer, Boston

Lock C 1981 Study skills. Kappa Delta Pi Northeastern University Publishing Group

Newble D, Clarke R 1987 Approaches to learning in a traditional and an innovative medical school In: Richardson J T E, Eysenck M W, Piper D W (eds) Student Learning: Research in Education and Cognitive Psychology. Society for Research into Higher Education and Open University, Milton Keynes

Ramsden P 1987 Improving teaching and learning in higher education: the case for a relational perspective Studies in Higher Education 12:275–286

Saunders K, Northup D E, Mennin S P 1984 The library in a problem-based curriculum. In: Kaufman A (ed.) Implementing Problem-Based Medical Education. Springer, New York

Smith S, Shores L, Brittain R 1951 An outline of best methods of study, 2nd edn. Barnes & Noble, New York

Stiernborg M, Bandaranayake R C 1996 Medical students' approaches to studying. Medical Teacher 18:229–236

Wilcox G W 1958 Basic study skills. Allyn & Bacon, Boston

Chapter 38

Staff development

J. R. Crosby

Introduction

What is staff development?

Staff development can be defined as the process designed to prepare members of staff for various academic roles and to enhance their productivity and vitality in these roles (Bland et al 1990). An academic role may include research, teaching, administration or management components. For the purpose of this chapter the academic role considered is that of a teacher.

Traditional teaching methods adopted in medical schools were didactic for preclinical material and opportunistic and unstructured for clinical work.

Recent changes in medical education (see Chapter 1) include a shift towards students taking responsibility for their own learning. In order to meet these challenges the role of the teacher has changed.

Twelve diverse roles of the teacher have been proposed (Harden and Crosby 2000). These roles include not only the familiar face-to-face components and organisational issues but also the development of resource material and facilitation required for active, student-centred modes of learning.

Consequently, members of staff may be asked to assume duties for which they have received no formal training (Wilkerson & Irby 1998). Staff development programmes are therefore required to include the whole gamut of learning opportunities available to staff ranging from conferences on education to informal discussions on the development of materials to support a course. However, for staff development to be meaningful it requires more than simple attendance;

"programmes designed to prepare faculty for various academic roles and to sustain their productivity and vitality"

Bland et al 1990

"Twelve roles of the teacher:
1 *Lecturer*
2 *Teacher – clinical*
3 *Role model – clinical*
4 *Role model – teaching*
5 *Tutor/mentor*
6 *Learning facilitator*
7 *Examiner*
8 *Evaluator*
9 *Planner*
10 *Organiser*
11 *Developing study guides*
12 *Developing learning resource material"*

Harden 1997

a degree of reflection and development is also needed to ensure continuity for personal development.

Why is it important?

The most persuasive reason for staff development is that it may ensure better educational programmes for students. The educational programme will influence student learning with an improved likelihood of the development of a competent medical practitioner.

It is interesting to compare the training of a doctor with that of a lecturer in higher education.

To become a doctor a 5-year undergraduate course is followed by a period of on-the-job training before qualifying. Once the basic 'nuts and bolts' have been attained there is an on-going period of postgraduate education and continuing medical education. This is necessary to ensure that an acceptable standard of patient care is maintained over the years. No doctor would believe that the knowledge and skills obtained at graduation would be sufficient for 50 years of practice.

When required to add teaching to their responsibilities, however, doctors will invariably have no formal qualifications in teaching when appointed. From this shaky start the requirement to obtain training in education is frequently not endorsed and any bad practices developed will be perpetuated. In the medical scenario this is equitable with a non-qualified person offering patient care with no on-going training to improve their performance.

The concern of training university staff in higher education formed part of the Dearing report into higher education (Dearing 1997). This places professionalism in teacher education in higher education at the top of the agenda and includes the following principle as a term of reference: 'higher education should be able to recruit, retain and motivate staff of the appropriate calibre.' The key recommendation is that all new members of university staff at lecturer level should hold a certificate or equivalent award in higher education.

"A society cultivates whatever is honoured there"

Plato c.427–c.347 BC

"For an institute to receive accreditation from the ILT for its training courses . . . a person will carry out a one day visit"

Utley 1998

Consider multiprofessional or uniprofessional sessions with groups other than medically trained individuals.

Be sure you know why a member of staff has a problem with staff development.

A further recommendation was that higher education institutions in the UK establish or seek access to programmes accredited by the proposed Institute for Learning and Teaching (ILT) that supports teaching excellence. Membership of the ILT may become mandatory for university staff with appropriate teaching awards being a criterion for membership.

Who is it for?

An undergraduate medical course is different from other undergraduate courses in that staff employed by the National Health Service rather than the university conduct the majority of the teaching. The rewards for teaching on the undergraduate course are frequently intangible for this cohort of teachers.

Staff development should not only include both these groups of staff but also encompass all the roles of the teacher. Sometimes the teacher's roles in the planning and management of a curriculum may be overlooked to concentrate on instructional elements (how to deliver better lectures, for example). A teacher's performance is usually based on face-to-face contact rather than on the logistics or educational strategies adopted.

Objections to staff development

Commonly heard objections

Staff development is sometimes considered a necessary evil. Everyone knows it should happen but is reluctant to take part. A variety of objections or barriers to involvement in staff development are frequently heard.

'I know it all'

This dangerous way of thinking is characterised by staff who have been influenced in their teaching strategy by the way they were taught and have followed the same strategies since then. Despite the fact that these strategies may be good, bad or indifferent these teachers do not believe that they need to change.

'I haven't enough time'

These teachers contribute minimally to the teaching programme but may have a genuine desire to improve their teaching were it not for other demands on their time.

'I am not interested'

These people are not motivated to contribute to the teaching programme because, although they are members or honorary members of staff, they have greater interests in research or clinical practice.

'It is all common sense'

Some people assume this arrogant stance which is a limitation rather than an advantage in that they may not progress beyond their own interface with education. Progressing in an educational environment can be helpful in formulating educational ideas, and some people naturally thrive and grow in that environment.

'I do not agree with the changes'

Change is often a painful process. Some staff may express reasonable or unreasonable concerns about the changes.

Answering these objections

It is often possible to refute these objections and thereby reduce some of the barriers to staff development.

'I know it all'

Staff development may act effectively by reinforcing the good practice of a competent teacher and for some it may also highlight practice that could be improved. The belief that you can learn just from experience may lead some teachers to think they have little to learn about teaching (Grossman 1990). With these individuals it may be worth while probing their understanding of educational parameters to ascertain the depth of their understanding. It may be necessary to expose constructively their lack of appreciation of educational issues. Lack of involvement in staff development is indicative of an attitude towards

Listen – do not condemn those views which are different to your own.

Make sure the dean is, and is seen to be, supportive of staff development.

Consider the reward systems that operate for teaching. Are the rewards enough to motivate?

"The primary source of knowledge about teaching came from observing teachers when they were learners"

Irby 1996

Attempt to convert the antagonists to protagonists.

personal development which may also be evident in other areas.

'I haven't enough time'

Ascertain that time is the real reason for lack of commitment to staff development and not a lack of motivation. A real lack of time is more a management issue than a problem with the individual and requires a policy decision to be taken by the medical school on the relative importance of teaching compared to activities competing for a teacher's time. It may involve asking some members of staff to do less in other areas.

'I am not interested'

Staff development is comparable to any personal development issue. If someone does not want to do it time must be spent determining why there is this lack of motivation. Once a root cause is identified two options exist – remove the staff member from the teaching programme or attempt to remotivate. The latter is preferable and it may require a person in a position of responsibility to highlight the importance of teaching.

'It is all common sense'

To a certain degree learning is common sense. However, as a teacher, fundamental mistakes may be made in facilitating learning. Individuals may be exposed to bad habits which become reinforced. Staff should be disabused of the notion that education is common sense.

'I do not agree with the changes'

Staff who do not agree with curriculum changes must be heard. Education and learning are epitomised by freedom of speech, a democratic approach, the ability to critique material presented and to share differences of opinions. It may be the antagonists of a curriculum who will act to refine and develop it. Whilst the antagonists should be heard a riposte must be forthcoming. If a riposte is not evident, consideration must be taken of the comments. Staff who do not agree with the changes may be very good teachers who are familiar with the curriculum. Their lack of support for the changes may have no detrimental effect on their ability to facilitate learning. However, action is necessary if anyone inadvertently or deliberately undermines the curriculum to those students currently engaged in it.

The relationship between staff development and quality

Quality issues

Staff are, arguably, the most important resource of a medical school. It is the quality of staff which is the most important determinant of success. It is not enough simply to recruit good-quality staff; it is necessary to ensure that they remain motivated and trained.

Traditionally staff have been left to follow a laissez-faire approach to their development, being left to their own devices without much support. The challenge is to deepen the educational experience with the innovative approaches necessary to develop new skills.

New staff need support, perhaps by setting up a mentor system which will provide them with a personal guide as to how things get done and how best to develop their career opportunities.

Finally a systematic practice of reviewing staff performance is required.

Managing quality

The philosophy of quality in staff development requires a responsiveness between management and staff, and between staff and students. Quality has to be established by first determining the standard expected. The standards considered may be framed using the 12 roles of the teacher (Harden and Crosby 2000). Criteria for each role can then be formulated, for example:

Role: small group facilitator
Criteria:

- Personal introductions were made.
- The objectives were clear.
- The task was explained.

- The number of students allocated to the task was appropriate.
- Adequate time was allocated to complete the task.
- All students participated.
- Adequate facilitation was given by the tutor.
- Group difficulties were dealt with.
- Individual difficulties were dealt with.
- There was a good overall rapport.
- The tutor stimulated the students.
- The students appeared interested.

It is advantageous to use a variety of methods to evaluate the quality of teaching (see Fig. 38.1):

1 Student feedback. A variety of methods can be adopted to determine the student view of an educational session. These may include quantitative questions or a more qualitative approach.
2 Self-assessment. Self-assessment frequently is a minimised form of evaluation. In teaching, self-assessment is a powerful way of gauging performance.
3 Peer support. Peer review of sessions is the method whereby the university can regularly review its teachers. Checklists are provided to offer support for the reviewer in giving feedback. Confidentiality is a key aspect of the peer support system in the UK and relies on a degree of professionalism on the part of both the reviewer and reviewee.
4 Funding bodies. Universities are to be more accountable and funding bodies are becoming an aspect of university life. Effective accounting procedures have therefore become a requirement.

Introducing staff development programmes

Although wonderful staff development programmes can be evolved, without attendance or engagement they will be meaningless. Any staff development programme therefore should be pragmatic and reflective of what can be achieved. Several key steps can be considered.

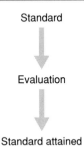

Determining Quality

Standard

Evaluation

Standard attained

Fig. 38.1   Determining quality

Determining needs – the evolving scenario
Staff development sessions can be set up without much thought and may include sessions on 'Effective lecturing' or , 'Small group teaching'. On the surface these may seem suitable but are they pertinent to staff requirements? As with curriculum development, staff development is a dynamic and evolving process. Various approaches can be adopted to determine needs (Dunn, Hamilton & Harden 1985). The following are some approaches which may be considered.

Task analysis
Consider any new approaches that are to be introduced into the teaching programme. Determine the tasks the teacher must perform. Sessions can then be arranged before implementation of the educational initiative. However, experience has shown that individuals do not necessarily perceive needs until a personal need (deficit) has been identified. Carroll (1993) suggests a 'need to know' culture requires to be created to increase receptiveness to learning. Unfortunately this may come from lack of communication and forward planning rather than any forward insight. This 'need to know' culture requires staff development sessions to be run during and after initial implementation.

Critical incidents
Ask staff to identify critical incidents that have arisen. In task analysis, an assumption may be made that staff do not have the necessary skills. This assumption may be correct but involving staff will raise the profile of staff development as well as basing staff development on an individual perception of needs. Sometimes the best people to identify a need are the teachers themselves so programmes must be devised which respond to this.

Study of error in practice
Ask staff or students. Often students, the recipients of teaching, are best able to identify areas of weakness. Many curriculum committees have student members. Staff development should be no exception.

Include staff development as one of your course reporting elements – see Chapter 39.

"Four levels of development:

- *instructional*
- *professional*
- *leadership*
- *organisation"*

Irby 1996

Consider how your school is performing at the four different levels of need.

Additional needs

- Implementation of the curriculum. This is intended to increase or update expertise in subject areas depending on the requirements of the curriculum and to gain cooperation for essential programme elements or to model a successful implementation.
- Instructional improvement. This is to enable staff to practise technical skills or gain experience in a repertoire of instructional strategies, to build competence and strengths in weaker areas or develop collaborative structures and supportive relationships.
- Professional development. This focuses on how to establish norms of continuous adult learning, experimentation and an openness for new ideas or feedback, and how to develop skills; for improvements by reflective self-analysis, self-assessment or goal-setting.
- Organisational issues. This may include improvement in integration and commitment to curricula goals at all levels, the quality of interactions and relationships within the professional working climate and the elimination of dysfunctional structures and practices.

Negotiation – getting agreement

Teachers may feel disenfranchised with recent curriculum development if many changes have taken place quickly or without proper negotiation and dissemination of material. Some types of staff development may not be successful without negotiation. Peer support, for example, may be considered threatening if the process and the rationale for its introduction are not explained.

Endorsement – getting support

Endorsement of the staff development programme by faculty is essential and the dean must play an obvious and positive role in the programme. Concrete rewards such as credits for attendance should be seen to be awarded and be valuable for promotion.

Development
Development should consider both content and delivery. The development of a staff development programme may benefit from the involvement of key members of staff.

Publicity
This requires an administrative framework for all staff to be regularly informed of any developments.

Implementation
Implementation of a staff development programme may include the delivery of sessions, circulation of reading material, one-to-one meetings or organisation of peer review.

Evaluation
The effectiveness of the programme should be evaluated not so much by attendance at sessions or the gaining of certificates as by staff perceptions and a perceived change in behaviour.

Staff perceptions
A recorded perception by staff of the value of the programme is made. An individual is asked to judge the value of the programme by rating, usually using a Likert scale (p. 83), various aspects of the programme. Free text comments are also often adopted: 'how will you change your behaviour in future?' etc. These forms of evaluation are easy to administer and analyse. The value of the analysis may indicate the success of implementation of the programme but not necessarily of a change in the person's future behaviour.

A perceived change in behaviour
A more valid measure of the success of a staff development programme is a behavioural change in the member of staff. It is feasible that some members of staff are adopting good educational practice. In these cases the staff development may serve to reinforce this good practice rather than elicit any change in behaviour. A

change in behaviour is desirable for many staff and may be measured in two ways:

- Observational techniques. Members of staff may be reviewed before and after a staff development programme. Their performance may be judged. A peer member of staff or a recipient of the teaching may conduct this review.
- A change in the quality of learning demonstrated by students. Ideally the end product of the teaching should be assessed. Unfortunately there are many variables which may affect this parameter: for example, change in curriculum content, change in assessment techniques or change in student profile. As a consequence this is perhaps a rather unreliable method.

Summary

Traditionally teaching methods adopted in medical schools were didactic for preclinical material and opportunistic and unstructured for clinical work. However, in recent years the role of the teacher has expanded and with this expansion an increased requirement for staff development has emerged. In addition educational establishments are being made more accountable for the standard of education delivered. However, this increase in requirement may not be matched with an increase in demand for or involvement in staff development programmes.

Staff development not only means attendance at formal sessions but can include a whole range of learning opportunities. A variety of approaches should be adopted in order to maximise the opportunity for all staff to become involved.

In devising staff development programmes the following should be considered:

- needs
- negotiation
- endorsement
- development
- publicising

- implementation
- evaluation.

References and further reading

Bland C J, Schmitz C C, Stritter F T, Henry R C, Aluise J J 1990 Successful faculty in academic medicine: essential skills and how to acquire them. Springer, New York

Carroll R G 1993 Implications of adult education: themes for medical school faculty development programmes. Medical Teacher 15:163

Dearing R 1997 National report – Staff in higher education. http://www.leeds.ac.uk/educol/ncithe

Dunn W R, Hamilton D D, Harden R M 1985 Techniques of identifying competencies needed for a doctor. Medical Teacher 7:15–25

General Medical Council 1993 Tomorrow's doctors GMC, London

Grossman P L 1990 The maturing of a teacher: teacher knowledge and teacher education. Teachers College, New York

Harden R M, Crosby J R 2000 The good teacher is more than a lecturer – the twelve roles of the teacher. Medical Teacher 22:334–347

Irby D M 1996 Models of faculty development for problem-based learning. Advances in Health Sciences Education 1:69–81

Nieman L Z, Donoghue G D, Ross L L, Morahan P S 1997 Implementing a comprehensive approach to managing faculty roles, rewards and developments in a year of change. Academic Medicine June 72(6):496–504

Utley A 1998 Cash carrot to enforce training. Times Higher Education Supplement 11 September:1

Wilkerson L, Irby D M 1998 Strategies for improving teaching practices: a comprehensive approach to faculty development. Academic Medicine April 73(4):387–396

Chapter 39
Academic standards – course monitoring and evaluation

A. T. Davidson   D. C. Old

What can we learn from this cycle of teaching?

"quality assurance and quality enhancement go hand-in-hand"

Higher Education Quality Council
1996

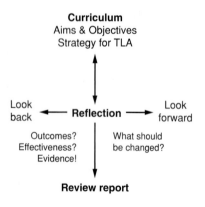

Curriculum
Aims & Objectives
Strategy for TLA

Look back ← **Reflection** → Look forward

Outcomes?   What should
Effectiveness?   be changed?
Evidence!

Review report

TLA - Teaching, learning and assessment

Fig. 39.1   A model of the review process

Introduction

Review is part of learning
Reflection is an essential phase of effective student learning. Evaluation and review by teachers can be viewed as a form of learning in itself:

- learning about the outcomes of curriculum delivery.
- learning about the effectiveness of curriculum delivery.

This learning can then be applied through:

- actions to enhance future delivery of the curriculum
- professional development by the teachers.

Public sector organisations world-wide are facing increasing demands for accountability, and medical teachers will typically be involved in a variety of accountability or audit processes associated with their clinical, research, teaching and professional roles. Effective review of teaching keeps the focus on learning, and in particular on action for enhancement; it does not adopt a bureaucratic, procedural approach, which sees the production of a review report as the endpoint.

Review of teaching should ask a set of questions (see Fig. 39.1):

- What are the outcomes of the teaching in terms of student achievement and attainment?
- How effective was teaching?

- What were the successes? How could they be extended?
- What were the problems or limitations? How could they be addressed?
- What action should be taken? What changes should be implemented?
- What is needed (resources, further learning or development) to help effect these changes?

Systematic review

Review should therefore be seen as an integral part of the 'normal' teaching cycle. A systematic and rigorous approach need not lead to a bureaucratic approach and if properly implemented, will be:

- Helpful. A structured approach to review will help enhancement of the teaching and learning process.
- Useful. Review processes can inform staff with management responsibilities – 'what is going on?', 'to what extent are we fulfilling our responsibilities?', 'what should we be changing?'
- Efficient. Internal review processes can routinely collect a range of information and can stimulate reflection and early action.

Effective internal review processes within universities are also now expected by external bodies such as funding organisations and professional and statutory bodies (PSBs). Indeed the reports from internal review processes are generally a prescribed submission in external reviews and such reports are frequently judged as a primary indicator of a faculty's capability to be self-aware, reflective and committed to quality.

"it is widely recognised that credible self-regulation in a higher education system must be underpinned by robust and effective mechanisms for evaluating the quality and standards of provision"

Jackson 1997

Requirements for effective review

What is needed to enable effective review and evaluation?

Clear communication of the curriculum

Since evaluation is carried out with reference to the aims, objectives and strategies of the curriculum, it is essential that these are clearly and comprehensively stated for

"In the design of programmes of study, there should be explicit and reasoned coherence between the aims and intended learning objectives/outcomes, the modes and criteria of assessment, the strategies for teaching, and the resources for learning"

Higher Education Quality Council 1996

both teachers and students. The following should be made explicit:

- aims and objectives – student outcomes
- strategies for teaching, learning and assessment – approaches to, and procedures for, the delivery of the curriculum.

This information should be defined at levels of detail appropriate to each individual level. This may be at a relatively broad brush level for the complete degree programme with more detail at the level of the individual unit or module. Besides being an essential reference point for monitoring, clear statements of aims and objectives greatly aid student learning, and are also key reference documents for any external review and accreditation by funding bodies or PSBs.

Organisation

A typical medical school is a complex organisation; the collective set of teachers is likely to be associated with several employer organisations, over a number of dispersed sites. Effective communication between the teachers is essential, including:

- definitions of roles and responsibilities, at the levels of both executive management and the individual teachers; this should include identification of responsibilities for evaluation and review
- curriculum activities, timetable
- information on students
- information on student performance, including assessment results
- on-going developments and changes.

Culture

Effective review requires a culture which values and encourages:

- commitment to student learning
- self-awareness, reflection and professional learning
- constructive criticism.

The culture must also:

- be realistic and evidence-based, not based on assertion or opinions
- view monitoring and review from a learning perspective, as a means of enhancement and demonstration of commitment and concern, not a bureaucratic 'chore'.

Resources

Review processes themselves require resources, principally in terms of teaching staff time and administrative support. Medical teachers are inevitably extremely busy people. Their participation in review processes should be made as straightforward and efficient as possible.

Rigour

Effective internal review should incorporate an element of internal scrutiny and questioning, including internal audit committees or external participation. Besides helping prevent complacency, such an impartial perspective can itself aid learning, both via directed questioning and fresh insights to discussion.

Levels, dimensions and cycles of review

Levels in the curriculum

A typical medical curriculum, and its location in the wider environment, can be modelled as a series of levels, located both within and outside the medical school, and each with its own group of staff and specific concerns (see Fig. 39.2):

- external to the university
  — PSBs
  — funding bodies
- the university – at the institutional level
- the medical school – at the overall faculty/school level
- the medical curriculum:
  — at programme level – i.e. the complete programme of studies leading to degree award
  — major blocks or phases within the programme
  — discrete units or modules within the blocks.

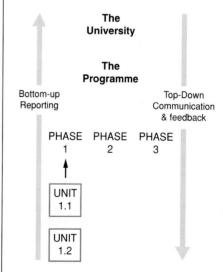

Fig. 39.2 Levels within the curriculum

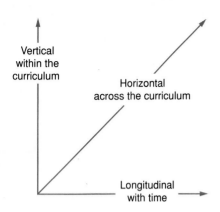

Fig. 39.3   Dimensions of review

Dimensions

Dimensions of evaluation, communication and reporting can be considered along three axes (see Fig. 39.3):

- vertical: upwards and downwards between levels within the curriculum and outside the curriculum, e.g. to the university and relevant external bodies – typically funding bodies and PSBs
- horizontal: across the curriculum, between units offered at the same level of study, such as between different subjects
- longitudinal: across different periods of time, looking back on trends over recent years, also looking forwards to future contexts and developments.

Frequency

Frequency of reviews in the longitudinal dimension can be considered in two basic intervals:

- Routine – each cycle of delivery (typically annually); review the previous cycle; plan minor changes, generally for the next cycle.
- Periodic – typically at 5 yearly intervals. Stand back and take an overview of the complete curriculum; plan significant, longer-term changes.

Routine (annual) review

Routine review describes review carried out at the end of each cycle of implementation (typically annually).

Focus and reference

The focus is normally on:

- review of implementation this cycle
- identification of actions for the next cycle.

Routine review should be undertaken with reference to explicit statements of the curriculum:

- aims and objectives
- strategies for teaching, learning and assessment.

Routine review:
How did it go this time?
What can we learn from this?
What should we do next time?

"The audit teams unanimously commended annual reviews conducted by programme teams in between larger periodic audits. . . . The best annual reviews combined elements of qualitative assessment of the year with interpretation of statistics"

Higher Education Quality
Council 1994

Questions

Outcomes
- What were the outcomes – in terms of student achievement and attainment this year?
- To what extent were the stated aims and objectives achieved?

Effectiveness
- How effective were teaching, learning and assessment this year?

Strengths/weaknesses
- What were the successes/strengths this year? What potential is there for extending these?
- To what extent were those strengths identified last year (or in previous years) maximised?
- What were the problems/weaknesses this year? How might they be addressed?
- To what extent were those problems identified last year (or in previous years) addressed?

Actions
- What changes should be implemented? When? By whom?

Needs
- What additional resources or information are required?

Levels of review
The same basic questions are applicable to all levels within the curriculum, but with extent of focus and detail appropriate to the level of the curriculum under scrutiny.

Periodic review

Periodic review describes a fundamental review carried out at discrete intervals. These are typically of the order of 5 years.

"Programmes should be regularly monitored and reviewed, with any necessary modifications being incorporated"

Higher Education Quality Council 1996

Focus and objective

The focus is normally on the curriculum as a whole, involving:

- reflection on the past period (since the last periodic review)
- a look forward to the future period
- the objective of planning the optimum curriculum and strategies for teaching, learning and assessment for the future period (to the next review).

Look back

- What have been the outcomes?
- What changes or developments have taken place?
- What are the key strengths/successes?
- What are the key weaknesses/problems?
- What are the key messages from routine reviews?

Look forward

- What changes are envisaged for the future period which might affect:
  - discipline
  - learning environment and resources
  - staff
  - students
  - employment etc.
- What curriculum should be delivered in the future?

The review process

This can be a lengthy process and can usefully be split into discrete phases, tasks and groupings etc.:

- An external perspective can be beneficial, such as participation from other faculties and from other medical schools. Besides providing fresh insights, this can provide an element of challenge and rigour.
- The process needs to be effectively documented – both for communication and audit purposes. The emphasis in documentation should be on reflection and conclusions, rather than describing the review process and data inputs.
- Group discussion or 'away-days' can be effective.

"Internal processes for the approval and review of programmes should involve an element of scrutiny external to the institution, and where they exist, the programme partners"

Higher Education Quality Council 1996

The review report
- Content:
  - a summary of the conclusions from the evaluation and reflection – with references to the evidence considered.
  - explicit statements of the curriculum and strategies for teaching, learning and assessment for the future period
  - an implementation plan for any proposed major changes
- Style:
  - a good review report will be a 'useful' document, it will clearly point to the future, and will be a helpful reference to staff in the future
- Significance:
  - periodic review reports are frequently key references for external reviews such as PSBs.

Inputs to review

Review is basically about asking questions; the answers to these questions can be obtained from a range of inputs.

Statistics and performance data
Student performance in assessments etc. may be useful.

Surveys
Use surveys of views and opinions by paper or PC questionnaires, or obtained by discussion or interview:
- student feedback on effectiveness of teaching
- graduate and employer feedback on appropriateness of the curriculum.

Consultative groups
- Student – liaison or consultative committees
- Employer and professional – liaison or consultative committees.

Staff observations and reflection
- Feedback from staff via peer review and team discussion of teaching

"(External) academic reviewers will form their judgements through observation of the institution's own programme validation and review events"

Quality Assurance Agency for
Higher Education 1998

- Personal reflection – observations at the time, such as a teaching log, noting 'how it went', 'the next time I teach this I will...'
- Reflection on good practice observed elsewhere – e.g. by staff who have undertaken visits or who have acted as external examiners or reviewers.

External reviews
These may include reviews by funding bodies or PSBs.

Reports, textbooks, journal articles
Review documents/literature on good practice in teaching from PSBs, employer organisations or journals. This could include any published reviews of other medical schools which have been acclaimed – what can we learn from them? Increasingly external reviews are being made readily accessible via websites.

External consultants
External experts may be used as consultants.

Specific considerations in review of medical teaching

The comments noted above are generally applicable to review of any university subject. What specific characteristics of medical education can influence approaches to review?

The range of staff associated with the curriculum
The total complement of teachers associated with a medical curriculum typically:
- includes a large number of individuals
- may change frequently as many staff will be 'rotating through' in clinical training posts
- includes a wide range of professional and specialist disciplines
- is employed by several organisations
- is located across a number of dispersed sites, including university and a range of hospital or primary care settings.

Forms and situations of teaching

Medical education typically has a great variety of types and settings of teaching from formal lecture through ward-based clinical teaching to private study.

Multiple demands on medical teachers

The typical medical teacher may be expected to be active and effective in a range of roles:

- clinical work
- research
- teaching
- professional activities etc.

Each of these has its own set of performance and review requirements.

The answers

The factors noted above add up to a diverse and complex situation and inevitably review in such an environment will be demanding and complex. There are no 'magic' answers. It is perhaps stating the obvious to stress the importance of:

- clarity and simplicity of procedures
- clarity of organisation and management – including, crucially, definitions of responsibilities for review
- provision of resources to support review
- 'filtering' and 'streamlining' of information and reporting – focus on priorities and 'need to know' information.

Indeed effective internal review procedures should be seen as a key 'tool' to help manage the complexity, not as an 'add-on' bureaucratic chore.

In many ways, review is similar to research, and involves similar skills and attitudes:

- Staff are collecting data (on the outcomes and effectiveness of their teaching).
- They are analysing this data.
- They are drawing conclusions (which should be orientated towards actions for enhancement).

Good review

Good internal review:
- is reflective and is orientated towards actions which will lead to enhancement
- is honest and evidence-based:
  - it is not used as a vehicle for personal assertions or complaints or as a lever for resources or power
- is inclusive:
  - all participants should have the opportunity, and be encouraged, to contribute
- is seen as important and useful:
  - deans, teaching deans and other senior staff must promote and encourage effective review – as a tool for enhancement, not as bureaucracy
- is efficient:
  - it is focused on the appropriate level
  - it is concise and clearly organised
  - it relates to any relevant external review requirements or frameworks – 'do it once only'
- 'closes the loop'
  - it provides feedback and responses to all participants
- it is clearly documented and archived
  - this facilitates internal communication and learning
  - it also supports audit – both internal and external
- it is itself reflective
  - the effectiveness and efficiency of both the design and implementation of the review processes are evaluated.

Summary

Review and evaluation can be perceived as a bureaucratic exercise, focused on reporting past events. Alternatively, they can be seen as key tools to help enhance standards and quality. The challenge to teachers is to design and use the internal review process to achieve the latter and simultaneously satisfy external demands for accountability.

References and further reading

Higher Education Quality Council (HEQC) 1994 Learning from audit. HEQC, London

Higher Education Quality Council (HEQC) 1996 Guidelines on quality assurance 1996. HEQC, London

Jackson N 1997 'The role of evaluation in self-regulating higher education institutions'. In: HEQC Managing Quality and Standards in UK Higher Education. HEQC, London

Power M 1994 The audit explosion. Demos, London

Quality Assurance Agency for Higher Education 1998 Higher quality. IAA, Gloucester

Websites

Higher Education Funding Council for England (HEFCE)
http: hefce.ac.uk
Scottish Higher Education Funding Council (SHEFC) *Results XX*
http:shefc.ac.uk

Appendix

Some useful Websites for teaching

Educational Websites
- Omni http://omni.ac.uk/
  The organising medical networked information project is a UK initiative which acts as a gateway to sources of biomedical information.
- Bristol Biomedical Image archive http://www.ets.bris.ac.uk/brisbio.htm 20 000 images for teaching.
- The virtual heart http://sln.fi.edu/biosci/heart.html Descriptions of cardiac function and pathology with audio and visual clips.
- GHIFT, Gateway to health informatics. http://www.chime.ucl.ac.uk/ghift/ Database of information and resources to support education and training in informatics in the UK.
- Guide to Medical informatics, the internet and telemedicine, http://www.coiera.com/
- The Risk Files (http://www.cybermedic.org/) is a free publication dedicated to informing health-care professionals about the internet and related issues. It is compiled and issued monthly by Ahmad Risk and delivered by email.
- http://cebm.jr2.ox.ac.uk
  The centre for evidence-based medicine website.

Free Access to Medline
- Pubmed http://www.ncbi.nlm.nih.gov/PubMed/
  The National Library of Medicine's search service of 9000 journals since 1967 based in Bethesda, USA. Very fast.
- BioMedNet's Evaluated Medline – http://biomednet.com/gateways/db/medline

INDEX